REVOLUTIONARY

CONCEPTIONS

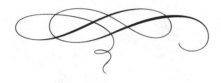

Published for the

OMOHUNDRO INSTITUTE

OF EARLY AMERICAN HISTORY

AND CULTURE,

Williamsburg, Virginia,   *by the*

UNIVERSITY OF

NORTH CAROLINA PRESS,

Chapel Hill

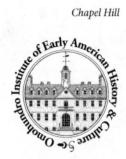

— SUSAN E. KLEPP —

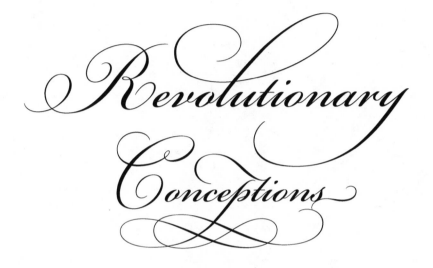

Revolutionary Conceptions

WOMEN, FERTILITY,

AND

FAMILY LIMITATION IN AMERICA,

1760-1820

THE OMOHUNDRO INSTITUTE OF EARLY AMERICAN HISTORY AND CULTURE

is sponsored jointly by the College of William and Mary

and the Colonial Williamsburg Foundation. On November 15, 1996,

the Institute adopted the present name

in honor of a bequest from Malvern H. Omohundro, Jr.

Designed by Courtney Leigh Baker and set in Minion Pro and Bickham Script Pro
by Tseng Information Systems, Inc. Manufactured in the United States of America

Library of Congress Cataloging-in-Publication Data
Klepp, Susan E.
Revolutionary conceptions : women, fertility, and family
limitation in America, 1760–1820 / Susan E. Klepp.
p. cm.
"Published for the Omohundro Institute of
Early American History and Culture, Williamsburg, Virginia."
Includes bibliographical references and index.
ISBN 978-0-8078-3322-3 (cloth : alk. paper) — ISBN 978-0-8078-5992-6 (pbk. : alk. paper)
1. Birth control—United States—History—18th century. 2. Women—United States—
Social conditions—18th century. 3. United States—Social conditions—To 1865. I. Title.
HQ766.5.U5K54 2009
304.6′66082097309033—dc22
2009024332

Parts of this book draw on my previously published work, "Revolutionary Bodies: Women
and the Fertility Transition in the Mid-Atlantic Region, 1760–1820," *Journal of American History*,
LXXXV (1998), 910–945; and "Lost, Hidden, Obstructed, and Repressed: Contraceptive and Abortive
Technology in the Early Delaware Valley," in Judith A. McGaw, ed., *Early American Technology:
Making and Doing Things from the Colonial Era to 1850* (Chapel Hill, N.C., 1994), 68–113.

The paper in this book meets the guidelines for permanence
and durability of the Committee on Production Guidelines for
Book Longevity of the Council on Library Resources.

The University of North Carolina Press has been
a member of the Green Press Initiative since 2003.

This volume received indirect support from an unrestricted
book publication grant awarded to the Institute by the L. J. Skaggs
and Mary C. Skaggs Foundation of Oakland, California.

cloth   13 12 11 10 09   1 2 3 4 5
paper   13 12 11 10 09   1 2 3 4 5

THIS BOOK WAS DIGITALLY PRINTED.

ACKNOWLEDGMENTS

This project has been gestating for a long time — too long. This is not because of a lack of helpful historian / midwives. Indeed, I have been exceptionally lucky in the assistance provided by friends and colleagues in finally birthing this book. Kathleen Brown and Toby Ditz read the entire manuscript as the outside readers for the Omohundro Institute of Early American History and Culture's Book Publications program. Their strong support and astute comments have been much appreciated and have helped make this a better book. The encouragement of Linda K. Kerber has likewise been important in pushing this project forward. Barbara Day-Hickman, Karin Wulf, Gloria L. Main, and Judith McGaw read and commented on various chapter drafts. A whole host of colleagues have listened to paper presentations (sometimes more than once), and their probing questions and careful comments have been extremely useful: Ava Baron, Leslie Patrick, Susan Branson, Billy G. Smith, Ann A. Verplanck, Simon Newman, Farley Grubb, Cornelia Dayton, Elaine F. Crane, David Waldstreicher, Roderick McDonald, and C. Dallett Hemphill are among many in the historical community who helped sharpen the argument. Others went out of their way to send citations, references, and documents: Konstantine Dierks, Ellen G. Miles, Ruth Wallis Hearndon, Dorothy Truman, Niki Eustace, Frank Fox, Gary Nash, Owen S. Ireland, and Susan Stabile are among those generous scholars. Emily Rush undertook some of the most tedious clerical tasks and provided her computer wizardry to many a frustrating problem. Fredrika Teute and Mendy Gladden were early supporters. The careful editing of Bridget Reddick and Virginia Montijo has sometimes succeeded in reining in my irregular prose. A study leave from Temple University provided valuable research time. The McNeil Center for Early American Studies has been an intellectual home for a long time; the Omohundro Institute for Early American History and Culture provided additional stimulus as have the staffs of the many archives in and around Philadelphia. A long time ago now Dorothy Swaine Thomas, Ann R. Miller, and Hope T. Eldridge — demographers all — provided inspiring examples of women as scholars, when there were none in any history department of my acquaintance.

My family has helped me through both by supporting my work and by taking me from it. To Phil, Ben, Karen, Emily, and new grandbaby Jackson this book is dedicated.

CONTENTS

ILLUSTRATIONS

— PLATES —

TABLES

REVOLUTIONARY

CONCEPTIONS

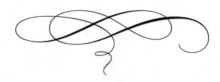

First to Fall

FERTILITY, AMERICAN WOMEN,

AND

REVOLUTION

A nineteenth-century historian entertained his readers with a comic interlude. His tale of bygone days told of the reunion of "Old Lydick," a humble Pennsylvania German veteran of the Revolutionary War, with George Washington, who had "once honoured [Lydick] with his favour." After mutual pleasantries, Lydick supposedly told the newly elected first president of the United States:

> It has been my happiness, once again, to meet and pay my duty to your Excellency. I have but one regret. You are childless! You leave your country no representative of your virtues! But *you* are not as old as Abraham [George Washington was in fact fifty-seven]; and *she* (gently touching the shoulder of Mrs. Washington) as old as Sarah [Martha Dandridge Custis Washington was fifty-eight]; and through the favour of the Almighty, I hope that a son may still be born to bless us.

Washington thanked him, and Lydick left, "praying, that fruitfulness might crown the last years of their existence with perfect felicity." It was not enough for Washington to be the figurative "father" of his country. According to this elderly baker and farmer, the president also needed to prove his virility by siring male offspring. Procreation towered above all other achievements.[1]

This story is undoubtedly fictitious, with its stock comic character of the simple, honest, but rustic and faintly ludicrous Pennsylvania Dutchman. Yet Lydick's character was meant to recall the old days, when fruitfulness was a civic virtue, not laughably uncouth, and when a man's standing as husband and father was measured by the number and rank of his sons as well as by the deference of his subordinates. It was a time, too, when a woman's first task in marriage was to follow biblical commandments to "increase and multiply" (as well as to be silent). By 1822, when this tale was published, Lydick's fecund and patriarchal sentiments, once so potent, were designed to evoke a wistful smile or hearty chuckle at old days, old ways. What had changed?[2]

In the actual, not fictive, late 1780s, Susanna Hopkins Mason took pen in hand to describe a very different ideal through the lens of her life on a Pennsylvania farm:

> Here frugal plenty on our board is seen,
> A house convenient, mostly, neat and clean;
> A few choice books, a few choice friends I boast,
> Which seem to vie which shall engage me most,
> Four darling objects of parental care,
> Blooming in youth, of either sex a pair, —
> My Egbert too, if I his worth might tell,
> In modest merit, few would him excel.

Mason's doggerel verse described a new mental and material world: a reasonably efficient and inviting domestic space, with books and with, no doubt, the teacups, teapots, teaspoons, sugar tongs, and tea tables that invited socializing with friends. The intellectual diversions of reading and sociability offered enticing options and shifted women's concerns, if not always their waking hours, from the daily drudgery of housework. Egalitarian ideals infused relationships: a loving husband and responsive father shared the joys of rearing carefully enumerated, beloved children, equally divided between

---

1. Alexander Garden, *Anecdotes of the Revolutionary War in America, with Sketches of Character of Persons the Most Distinguished, in the Southern States, for Civil and Military Services* (Charleston, S.C., 1822), 394–395.

2. There was a farmer and prosperous baker who was active in Pennsylvania politics and who had been associated with Washington. See [Benjamin Rush], "An Account of the Life and Character of Christopher Ludwick...," *Poulson's American Daily Advertiser* (Philadelphia), June 30, 1801. This much-republished brief biography does not include the reunion episode.

girls and boys. And in an age when most women, if they lived through their childbearing years, might still bear seven, eight, or nine children, Mason counted four offspring. All thrive because frugal restraint allowed plenty for everyone. Even though a son and daughter would unfortunately die during a later epidemic, Susanna Mason was done with childbearing. She was not alone.[3]

PROCREATION IS POWER. Childbearing helps define adulthood and shapes images of femininity and masculinity. Sons and daughters have been valued as cheap labor, as affectionate companions, as lovable responsibilities, as sources of pride and accomplishment, as offerings to the gods or the state, or as guarantors of a kind of immortality, among many other reasons for having offspring. But generation is of interest to more than just mothers and fathers. Kin, ethnic, religious, cultural, and national groups have a stake in either the survival or growth of specific populations. Fertility rates are a major factor in assessing the health of economies, in preserving languages, beliefs, and cultures, and in garnering strength in politics, diplomacy, and the military. Not surprisingly, moralists, theologians, and politicians attempt to enforce particular interpretations of marriage and parenthood that can promote the responsibilities of parents and children or parental contributions to specific interests and institutions.

Procreation is power, but who wields that power and for what ends? Women bear the brunt of procreation through gestation, labor, and birth. They typically breast-feed, nurse, cleanse, comfort, and train the young— sometimes willingly, sometimes not. There are many reasons to have children. There are also reasons for having few or none. Why did American colonists favor exceptionally large families for so long? Why were these same Americans or their descendants among the first in the world to reject high fertility and invent a new ideal of limited childbearing? Which Americans were willing to innovate, and what was the relationship of limited childbearing to the era of the American Revolution, circa 1763–1800?

BEFORE THE AMERICAN REVOLUTION, colonial women and men were exuberant about the "teeming," "flourishing," or "big" pregnant body. Large families were part of a bountiful natural order that celebrated abundance,

3. "A Just Representation of a Pennsylvania Farm; Addressed from a Friend in the Country, to Her Friend in the City" (late 1780s), in [Susanna Mason], *Selections from the Letters and Manuscripts of the Late Susanna Mason; with a Brief Memoir of Her Life, by Her Daughter* (Philadelphia, 1836), 143.

especially of sons. Women's essence was found in their productivity. Their duty was to marry and bear children. Men were simply human; women were "the Sex," and their physicality was their defining characteristic. Free women in the colonies bore nearly as many children as possible under the marriage and breast-feeding conventions of the time, typically marrying in their late teens or early twenties and nursing each child for a year or two before becoming pregnant again. If all was well, married women gave birth roughly every eighteen months or two years until menopause. Women were rewarded for their performance of their marital duty with praise and esteem. The resulting children were seen as a feminine contribution to the paternal lineage and as a form of wealth that benefited both parents. The dark side of celebratory abundance could be the callous treatment of supernumerary children, especially girls. Women's relationship to procreation was thought to be largely passive, and, although some wives might delay births during wars and other crises, most colonial women believed that fate determined the number of children they would bear.[4]

In many ways the colonial experience was unique, extreme, in the Western world. European women married later than most women in the colonies and gave birth, on average, in two- or three-year intervals through life if they married, although many more women in the Old World never wed. In North America, a youthful population, early and nearly universal marriage, and shorter intervals between births led to rapid growth—a colonial population of 251,000 in 1700 had increased to 2,464,000 in 1775, largely through natural increase rather than by either voluntary or forced immigration. The procreative prowess of colonial women was considered remarkable even at the time. But this state of affairs did not last. Before the end of the eighteenth century, many women came to advocate small families and limited childbearing.[5]

Why individuals and nations decide to switch from high fertility practices and goals to low, planned fertility has been a persistent question among scholars and of interest to social service agencies and governments. The timing of the switch from "natural" (and presumptively unmediated) childbearing to goal-oriented and limited family size has been investigated in study

4. Variations in the number of births during periods of war and peace are one of the many areas that needs more study. The best work on birth intervals can be found in Kristin Senecal, "Marriage and Fertility Patterns in Cumberland County, 1800–1859," *Pennsylvania History*, LXXI (2004), 191–211.

5. United States, Bureau of the Census, *Historical Statistics of the United States, Colonial Times to 1970, Bicentennial Edition* (Washington, D.C., 1976), Z1–Z19, 1168.

after study for localities across the globe. These analyses use different investigative assumptions and offer conflicting explanations for the change from high to low fertility, but most scholars have come to concur on timing. The crucial innovation in attitudes toward fertility—when family planning and curtailed childbearing replaced lifelong, abundant childbearing—began in Western Europe in the 1870s, in Eastern Europe, parts of Asia, and Latin America in the early twentieth century, and in much of Africa, South Asia, and other regions in the 1970s. Yet, in the United States and France, as research has shown, fertility levels began to decline in the second half of the eighteenth century, a century before the rest of the Western world and two centuries before much of the rest of the globe. Why were birthrates in these two countries the first to fall? Given the religious pronouncements in favor of abundant procreation, the economic perceptions of the wealth entailed in offspring, and the personal and social identities bound up with extensive parenthood, why did family limitation begin at all? And why were enslaved Americans on a different path, apparently raising fertility levels as the bonds of servitude hardened?[6]

Many of the ideas at stake in the decision to adopt family planning circulated widely in the eighteenth-century transatlantic world. Companionate marriages, sentimentalized childrearing, self-determination, consumerism, humanitarianism and anticruelty, physical comfort, radical egalitarianism—all these and more were known and discussed in Great Britain, on the Con-

---

6. The majority of scholars have come to agree that American fertility levels began to fall owing to family planning (although planning may only consist of delayed marriage) in the late eighteenth century. See Gloria L. Main, "Rocking the Cradle: Downsizing the New England Family," *Journal of Interdisciplinary History*, XXXVII (2006–2007), 35–58. See also Joan E. Cashin, "Households, Kinfolk, and Absent Teenagers: The Demographic Transition in the Old South," *Journal of Family History*, XXV (2000), 141–157. Recent syntheses of American demography include Herbert S. Klein, *A Population History of the United States* (Cambridge, Mass., 2004), 69, 79–87; Michael R. Haines and Richard H. Steckel, eds., *A Population History of North America* (Cambridge, Mass., 2000); and Michael Haines, "Fertility," in Joel Mokyr, ed., *Oxford Encyclopedia of Economic History* (New York, 2003), II, 284–291. Contrary views locate the fertility transition in the late nineteenth and early twentieth centuries, arguing that the earlier decline reflected only the passing of frontier conditions and the development of a European-style stasis in population in the early nineteenth century. See J. David Hacker, "Rethinking the 'Early' Decline of Marital Fertility in the United States," *Demography*, XL (2003), 605–620; Daniel Scott Smith, "A Malthusian-Frontier Interpretation of United States Demographic History before c. 1815," in Woodrow Borah, Jorge Hardoy, and Gilbert A. Stetler, eds., *Urbanization in the Americas: The Background in Comparative Perspective* (Ottawa, Ontario, 1980), 15–24. Both arguments accept declining numbers of children but raise the question of whether the decline was due to family planning or adjustment to something like European conditions. An exploration of the intentions of contemporaries will help settle these disputes.

tinent, in the colonies, and at ports of call around the Atlantic world. These concepts often remained distant abstractions, however, lost in the hubbub of daily routine, disassociated and countered by the tug of habit and counter-vailing ideas.

The American Revolution, like the later French Revolution, disrupted routine and challenged old assumptions. The existing critiques of politics, religion, economics, social hierarchies, and women's traditional roles were brought to the fore as Revolutionaries sometimes unwittingly undermined the status quo as they asserted universal rights of life, liberty, and happiness and invited debate, gossip, and reflection on foundational values. Ideas that had once been of moderate interest might now, in protests and a war based at least in part on competing ideologies, become matters of life and death.

From this turmoil, growing numbers of women came to advocate a dra-matic reformation in their definitions of femininity, including limitations on childbearing and wifely obligation. Women, like men, protested that they would not be enslaved and contrasted the bodily integrity and self-determination of free peoples with the chained flesh of the slave. Assertions of individual virtue and heartfelt sensibility could be claimed by women as well as men. Old assumptions of patriarchal authority and male preference were challenged. New ideals of mutuality between husband and wife, along with a growing recognition of the importance of daughters as well as sons, emerged from the seemingly self-evident truths embraced by the fractious coalition of harried taxpayers, expansionists, nationalists, free traders, slave-holders, freedmen, republicans, and democrats who fought for their own particular visions of liberty. It was in this revolutionary era, starting about 1763, that many American women rejected a lifetime of childbearing and began limiting births. In doing so, they were more than one hundred years in advance of every Western European nation but France and some two hun-dred years before the now nearly global shift to limited births. They spoke and wrote and introduced innovative ideas and behaviors to friends and family. Ideas of individuality, rationality, sensibility, planning for the future, and rights predated the Revolution, but the crises of the revolutionary era, 1763–1800, provided an urgency to the discussion and dissemination of new ideas, new behaviors.[7]

7. There is now a large literature on the multiple ways the American Revolution undermined traditional assertions of female inferiority and opened new possibilities for women. A few examples are Mary Beth Norton, *Liberty's Daughters: The Revolutionary Experience of American Women, 1750–1800* (Boston, 1980); Linda K. Kerber, *Women of the Republic: Intellect and Ideology in Revo-lutionary America* (Chapel Hill, N.C., 1980); Cathy N. Davidson, *Revolution and the Word: The*

Not all Americans, of course, shared in the revolutionary optimism of the last third of the eighteenth century. More than 90 percent of African Americans remained enslaved in the early Republic. The Constitution of 1787 only strengthened the power of slaveowners over their human property. To the enslaved, the Revolution must have meant little but disappointment. Birthrates among the enslaved were increasing, not declining. Although African Americans living in the northern states gradually gained their independence during and after the American Revolution and, from the limited evidence available, began limiting births just as their neighbors were doing, they were a small segment of the total population with African ancestry. For the vast majority of African Americans who lived in slave states, freedom came only in the mid-nineteenth century, and it was then, in another era of rights talk, grassroots organizing, and political access during the Civil War and its aftermath, that fertility rates began to decline.

Free women during and after the Revolution engaged in political debate, some helped enforce the nonimportation agreements, others picked up guns to protect property and family, while servants and slaves seized opportunities to run away, but very few imagined or urged equal political rights for females—even in New Jersey, where, from 1776 to 1807, wealthy single women could vote but could not hold office. Too many intervening inequalities needed attention. Women lagged in health, in schooling, in apprenticeships, in access to the courts, in civil rights, in propertyownership, in the availability of cash and credit, in choice of occupations, and in a host of other areas that would have required men to change fundamental legal assumptions and to share political power, wealth, and opportunity voluntarily. More feasible were reforms in marital obligations.

Using letters, poems, commonplace books, and novels, free women shaped public opinion by advocating significant changes in spousal relations. They emphasized balance, respect, and mutual consideration between wives and husbands. Women also sought a better life for their daughters. A crucial part of this reformation of marriage was the attempt, not always success-

---

Rise of the Novel in America (New York, 1986); Carol Berkin, Revolutionary Mothers: Women in the Struggle for America's Independence (New York, 2005); and Gary B. Nash, The Unknown American Revolution: The Unruly Birth of Democracy and the Struggle to Create America (New York, 2005). Only Norton briefly considers the effect of the Revolution on reproductive goals. Less-positive assessments of at least the civil, political, and economic positions of postrevolutionary women are Carroll Smith-Rosenberg, "Dis-Covering the Subject of the 'Great Constitutional Discussion,' 1786–1789," Journal of American History, LXXIX (1992), 841–873; Elaine Forman Crane, Ebb Tide in New England: Women, Seaports, and Social Change, 1630–1800 (Boston, 1998); and Rosemarie Zagarri, Revolutionary Backlash: Women and Politics in the Early American Republic (Philadelphia, 2007).

ful, to control childbearing by limiting the number of pregnancies. Fruitful abundance and lifelong childbearing were being replaced by a rationalized marshaling of resources through family planning. A passive attendance on divine favor was exchanged for loving and prudent management founded on ideals, typically grounded in deep religious faith, of selfless sacrifice for the rising generation. New visions of femininity and family, even though contested and often resisted, would be the engines that launched the shift from high fertility (those seven, eight, or more children over the course of a colonial woman's lifetime—if she lived to age fifty) to falling fertility measured by an average of seven children in 1800, five by 1850, three and a half by 1900, just over two by the late twentieth century, and still fewer for most women in the United States in the early years of the twenty-first century.[8]

Family limitation, or restricted fertility, was not new to Americans in the nineteenth century, when most European nations experienced declining fertility, nor in the early twentieth century, when virtually all of the rest of the Western world experienced the same transition in fertility. This book investigates the original intentions of that founding generation of American women (and some men) who rejected the abundant and redundant fertility of the colonial, patriarchal family and replaced it with a sensible, sentimental, and carefully planned family of beloved daughters and sons that freed women to pursue other interests. This was a different American Revolution, one invented and implemented by wives.

Explaining Transitions in Fertility

The reasons for the now worldwide shift from lifetime to limited childbearing have been much debated by economists, sociologists, anthropologists, demographers, and, to a lesser degree, historians. Explanations for the relatively sudden switch from abundant to restricted childbearing have included the effects of diminishing land availability or rising land prices in agricultural regions; industrialization, the market revolution, or modernization and its many effects; the greater availability of hired or enslaved laborers;

8. See the important study by Main, "Rocking the Cradle," *JIH*, XXXVII (2006), 35–58, who finds fertility and family size falling from the late eighteenth century and explores a number of possible means and motivations for the decline. For the South, see Cashin, "Households, Kinfolk, and Absent Teenagers," *Jour. Fam. Hist.*, XXV (2000), 141–157. See also Ansley J. Coale and Melvin Zelnik, *New Estimates of Fertility and Population in the United States* (Princeton, N.J., 1963), table 2, 36; U.S. Bureau of the Census, *The 2009 Statistical Abstract*, table 82, "Total Fertility Rates by Race and Hispanic Origin," http://www.census.gov/compendia/statab (accessed April 2009).

urbanization; the growing costs of childrearing in the nineteenth century; decreasing productive contributions by children in the shift from agriculture to manufacturing; heightened expectations for children's futures; increasing literacy or educational levels, especially for women, both as a cost of childrearing and as a factor providing options for individuals; new class formations and social identities, particularly for the middle class; the consequences of finite wage rates and salaries on family income and planning for the future; increasing female participation in the labor force; domestic feminism; religious influences, especially the divorce between sexuality and reproduction accepted by some Protestants or the self-control advocated in early-nineteenth-century evangelicalism; growing secularization; rising life expectancy and falling infant mortality levels; expanding social services or other governmental programs that replace kin-based care; numerical thinking and investment strategies; shifting intergenerational wealth flows; the invention of more reliable birth-control technologies and greater access to abortion providers, and more. In all these attempts to explain the shift to lower fertility, almost no one has asked what people at the time thought of family size, marital relationships, contraception, abortion, sons, and daughters. They have not explored the law codes or the implementation of the law or looked at what doctors, pharmacists, and midwives were advocating. In particular, scholars have not consulted the writings of contemporary women. The existing formulations, many based on English experience, fail to explain the idiosyncratic behavior of late-eighteenth-century French and American couples. None of the current explanations is entirely satisfactory.[9]

9. The classic formulation is Frank W. Notestein, "Population—the Long View," in Theodore W. Schultz, ed., *Food for the World* (Chicago, 1945), 36–57. This theory has since been much debated, complicated, modified, augmented, or rejected. A few overviews of the debates in the field include Karen Oppenheim Mason, "Gender and Family Systems in the Fertility Transition," *Global Fertility Transition,* supplement of *Population and Development Review,* XXVII (2001), 160–176; Ronald Lee, "The Demographic Transition: Three Centuries of Fundamental Change," *Journal of Economic Perspectives,* XVII (2003), 167–190; Diane Macunovich, "Economic Theories of Fertility," in Karine S. Moe, ed., *Women, Family, and Work: Writings on the Economics of Gender* (Malden, Mass., 2003), 105–124; John C. Caldwell, "The Delayed Western Fertility Decline: An Examination of English-Speaking Countries," *Population and Development Review,* XXV (1999), 479–513; George Alter, "Theories of Fertility Decline: A Nonspecialist's Guide to the Current Debate," and Michael R. Haines, "Occupation and Social Class during Fertility Decline: Historical Perspectives," both in John R. Gillis, Louise A. Tilly, and David Levine, eds., *The European Experience of Declining Fertility, 1850–1970: The Quiet Revolution* (Cambridge, Mass., 1992), 13–27 (esp. 18), and 193–226 (esp. 194); Dov Friedlander, Barbara S. Okun, and Sharon Segal, "The Demographic Transition Then and Now: Processes, Perspectives, and Analyses," *Jour. Fam. Hist.,* XXIV (1999), 493–533; John Cleland and Christopher Wilson, "Demand Theories of the Fertility Transition: An Iconoclastic View,"

In addition, periodization is a problem in the existing literature. American birthrates, among the highest in the world through the 1760s, began a steady decline in the last third of the eighteenth century even though frontier conditions continued to favor high fertility on the borderlands of the West and far North well into the nineteenth century, and European immigration, especially after 1820, brought individuals with more traditional fertility goals to American shores, slowing patterns of fertility reduction in those cities and regions where immigrants settled. Most studies of fertility levels in the United States have focused on the mid-nineteenth century, not on the beginning of the decline at about 1763, in part because detailed census reports with precise age and sex data become available only after 1830 and make data collection, research, and analysis thereafter relatively easy, and in part because it was assumed that the experience of England should be the pattern for other industrializing nations.

On the whole, it is not so much that previous economic, demographic, and sociological studies of the American fertility transition are inapplicable as they are incomplete. Perhaps not surprisingly in a research field dominated by demographers and economists, nearly all explanations for the fertility transition have sought direct, quantifiable correlations between economic change, wages, and land availability and the fiscal well-being of heads of households—that is, of men. The prevailing assumption has been that men make fertility decisions and that they make these decisions based entirely on simple cost-benefit economic analyses. Women's perceptions and goals have largely been ignored in the demographic and economic literature on fertility or have been explored primarily in third world countries. Scholars have generally neglected to consider cultural and political as well as economic transformations. Economic assumptions do help to explain, however, why the revolutionary fervor of women to reconfigure their lives expanded and intensified in the nineteenth century and beyond, even as the ideals of the Revolution fossilized into Fourth of July platitudes. They do not address the question of when and why couples first attempted, even if with little success at times, to limit family size.[10]

Population Studies, XLI (1987), 5–30; E. A. Wrigley et al., *English Population History from Family Reconstitution, 1580–1837* (Cambridge, 1997), esp. 507–511. See also Robert A. Ferguson, *The American Enlightenment, 1750–1820* (Cambridge, Mass., 1997); and Ned C. Landsman, *From Colonials to Provincials: American Thought and Culture, 1680–1760* (New York, 1997).

10. There are exceptions. See Alison MacKinnon, "Were Women Present at the Demographic Transition? Questions from a Feminist Historian to Historical Demographers," *Gender and History,* VII (1995), 222–240; Nora Federici, Karen Oppenheim Mason, and Sølvi Sogner, eds., *Women's*

Historians of women have explored the immediate experiences of child-birth in early America. They have discovered some of the superstitions, dietary advice, bloodlettings, and medications associated with pregnancy. Historians know how the construction of women's clothing allowed bellies to expand and contract without major alterations to garments. They have recovered dramatic accounts of the onset of labor, the calling of friends and neighbors (called gossips), and the arrival of the midwife. There are descriptions of the birthing chairs and stools and of the groaning boards laden with food and drink that sustained the gossips during the woman's labor (at least if she was neither enslaved nor poor). The postpartum period of lying in, breast-feeding, and the use of wet nurses have been recovered and analyzed. There are calculations of maternal mortality rates, of the income of mid-wives, of the cost of doctors' visits. The gradual insinuation of male physi-cians into the birthing chamber in the late eighteenth century has been much debated. So we know a great deal about the experience of birth and about obstetrics, but little on the social meanings attached to childbearing by both the wider public and by women themselves as they thought about the course of their lives. How did birthing change from procreation to reproduction? Why would women want large families at one point in time and then decide to limit the size of their families at another?[11]

Position and Demographic Change (Oxford, 1993); John R. Gillis, "Gender and Fertility Decline among the British Middle Classes," in Gillis, Tilly, and Levine, eds., _European Experience_, 31–47; Anita Ilta Garey, "Fertility on the Frontier: Bringing Women Back In," _Nineteenth-Century Contexts,_ XI (1987), 63–83; Daniel Scott Smith, "'Early' Fertility Decline in America: A Problem in Family History," _Family History at the Crossroads: Linking Familial and Historical Change,_ special issue of _Jour. Fam. Hist.,_ XII (1987), 73–84; Carl N. Degler, _At Odds: Women and the Family in America from the Revolution to the Present_ (New York, 1980), 189; and Nancy Folbre, "Of Patriarchy Born: The Political Economy of Fertility Decisions," _Feminist Studies,_ IX (1983), 261–284.

11. Phillis Cunnington and Catherine Lucas, _Costume for Births, Marriages, and Deaths_ (London, 1972); Catherine M. Scholten, _Childbearing in American Society, 1650–1850,_ American Social Experience, II (New York, 1985); Sylvia D. Hoffert, _Private Matters: American Attitudes toward Childbearing and Infant Nurture in the Urban North, 1800–1860,_ Women in American History, IV (Urbana, Ill., 1989); Marie Jenkins Schwartz, _Birthing a Slave: Motherhood and Medicine in the Antebellum South_ (Cambridge, Mass., 2006); Richard W. Wertz and Dorothy C. Wertz, _Lying-In: A History of Childbirth in America_ (New York, 1979); Judith Walzer Leavitt, _Brought to Bed: Childbearing in America, 1750 to 1950_ (New York, 1986); Adrian Wilson, _The Making of Man-Midwifery: Childbirth in England, 1660–1770_ (London, 1995); Laurel Thatcher Ulrich, _A Midwife's Tale: The Life of Martha Ballard, Based on Her Diary, 1785–1812_ (New York, 1990); Mary E. Fissell, _Vernacular Bodies: The Politics of Reproduction in Early Modern England_ (New York, 2004); Lisa Forman Cody, _Birthing the Nation: Sex, Science, and the Conception of Eighteenth-Century Britons_ (New York, 2005); Barbara Duden, _The Woman Beneath the Skin: A Doctor's Patients in Eighteenth-Century Germany,_ trans. Thomas Dunlap (Cambridge, Mass., 1991); Ludmilla Jordanova, _Nature Displayed: Gender, Science,_

This study examines the circumstances, motivations, and desires of married women and men at the initial point when limited fertility was seen as a positive good rather than as a personal and social misfortune. What France and the United States shared in the late eighteenth century that England and other countries did not was the experience of political and social revolution based on life, liberty, and happiness or liberty, equality, and fraternity. This book will not examine the French case, but will explore the many ways in which America's revolutionary experience allowed women and men, rich and poor, rural and urban, to reimagine marriage, procreation, reproduction, and responsibilities to children.[12]

---

and Medicine, 1760–1820 (New York, 1999); Amanda Carson Banks, Birth Chairs, Midwives, and Medicine (Jackson, Miss., 1999); Daniel Scott Smith and J. David Hacker, "Cultural Demography: New England Deaths and the Puritan Perception of Risk," JIH, XXVI (1995–1996), 367–392; Janet Golden, A Social History of Wet Nursing in America: From Breast to Bottle (New York, 1996); and Patricia R. Ivinski et al., Farewell to the Wetnurse: Etienne Aubry and Images of Breast-Feeding in Eighteenth-Century France (Williamstown, Mass., 1998).

12. Other scholars have identified revolutions as crucial in changing individual perceptions, an argument made most forcefully by Rudolph Binion in "Marianne au foyer: Révolution politique et transition démographique en France et aux États-Unis," Population, LV (2000), 81–104, and translated by Godfrey I. Rogers as "Marianne in the Home: Political Revolution and Fertility Transition in France and the United States," Population: An English Selection, XIII (2001), 165–188, but see also the responses by Jean-Pierre Bardet, Etienne van de Walle, and Rudolph Binion in "Commentaires," Population, LV (2000), 387–396. Etienne van de Walle and Virginie de Luca, "Birth Prevention in the American and French Fertility Transitions: Contrasts in Knowledge and Practice," Population and Development Review, XXXII (2006), 529–555, looks only at the period after 1800. See also Norton, Liberty's Daughters, 80–83, 232; J. William Leasure, "Mexican Fertility and the Revolution of 1910–1920," Population Review, XXXII (1988), 41–48; Jan Lewis and Kenneth A. Lockridge, "'Sally Has Been Sick': Pregnancy and Family Limitation among Virginia Gentry Women, 1780–1830," Journal of Social History, XXII (1988), 5–19; and Cashin, "Households, Kinfolk, and Absent Teenagers," Jour. Fam. Hist., XXV (2000), 141–157. England had no revolution in the eighteenth century and a very different experience. See, for example, E. A. Wrigley, "Explaining the Rise in Marital Fertility in England in the 'Long' Eighteenth Century," Economic History Review, n.s., LI (1998), 435–464.

Certain small populations were limiting fertility at roughly the same time as the Americans and French. But the goal of family limitation did not spread beyond these groups and did not affect national fertility levels. See Massimo Livi-Bacci, "Social Group Forerunners of Fertility Control in Europe," in Ansley J. Coale and Susan Cotts Watkins, eds., The Decline of Fertility in Europe: The Revised Proceedings of a Conference on the Princeton European Fertility Project (Princeton, N.J., 1986); and Klein, Population History, 99–104. For the situation in France, see David R. Weir, "New Estimates of Nuptiality and Marital Fertility in France, 1740–1911," Population Studies, XLVIII (1994), 307–331; and Weir, "Fertility Transition in Rural France, 1740–1829," Journal of Economic History, XLIV (1984), 612–614. Binion, in "Marianne au foyer," Population, LV (2000), 81–104, and "Marianne in the Home," Population: English Selection, XIII (2001), 165–188, identifies the link between revolution and family planning but does not explain it except by reference to Susan Klepp, "Revolutionary Bodies: Women and the Fertility Transition in the Mid-Atlantic Region, 1760–1820," JAH,

This emphasis on revolutionary thought and experience does not imply a simple equivalence between political ideology and fertility goals. It is not the case that the most radical of Americans were leaders in family limitation, nor that more conservative supporters of a republic of wealthy property-owners lagged behind supporters of early forms of democracy. Many of the most radical democrats favored universal rights—but for men (and usually white men) only. Overthrowing a king might only elevate the authority of male heads of households, not liberate the traditionally subordinated members of that household from some of the crassest forms of oppression. Other radicals might have been adamantly in favor of expanded property rights but less interested in human or civil rights. Nationalists could clash with states' rights advocates without considering the health and well-being of women and infants. More conservative politicians might favor greater inclusion of women, African Americans, Catholics, or Jews—so long as they were sufficiently urbane, wealthy, and presumptively conservative. Women's political stances are often difficult to determine. Denied access to political office, the bench, or partisan caucuses, many women failed to leave a record of their political beliefs. Nonetheless, the Revolution forced conservatives, moderates, radicals, and the indifferent to reevaluate or, at the least, defend their assumptions on rights and the individual. People across the political spectrum had to cope somehow with challenges to the status quo. Restricted childbearing was never embraced by all women or men. Birth control was, and has remained, controversial, primarily because it transformed and continues to transform women's traditional maternal and procreative role by opening up alternatives to a life of continual childbearing and constant childrearing. Not everyone embraced family limitation, but it was among the radical ideas in the air.

Recovering the very personal decisions individuals made about sexual expression, birth control, their future, and their children's future is difficult. In the eighteenth and early nineteenth centuries (and, indeed, for at least another century), topics touching on sexuality were considered private and, at least among those striving for respectability and refinement, rather indelicate. These subjects were not often broached openly, nor were individual intentions relating to family planning commonly preserved—either

---

LXXXV (1998), 911–945. See also Thomas A. Mroz and David R. Weir, "Structural Change in Life Cycle Fertility during the Fertility Transition: France Before and After the Revolution of 1789," *Population Studies,* XLIV (1990), 61–87; and Lee, "The Demographic Transition," *Jour. Econ. Persp.,* XVII (2003), 170.

by eighteenth-century contemporaries or by their even more censorious Victorian descendents. The very language used to describe pregnancy, birth, and childrearing has so changed over the last three hundred years that meanings are sometimes lost. What exactly did Elizabeth Drinker mean in 1780 when she wrote in her diary, "I have expected for some time to be confin'd — am thankful it is so far over"? Did she think herself pregnant? There was no subsequent birth (when a woman is "confined"). What happened and how could it be "so far over"? Was a reversal possible? Drinker, like most women whose writings have survived, was elliptical, obscurantist, or silent at key points when discussing the gynecological issues faced by herself, her daughters, her friends, and her servants.[13]

Diaries, correspondence, newspaper and magazine articles, legal, medical, religious, and political writings, and images of women provide some hints of thoughts and actions. Humor is a fruitful source of insight into contemporary thought: satire expresses the subversive intentions of those innovators who often lack other avenues of expression at the same time that laughter gives vent to the anxieties of those transgressing existing values. Benjamin Franklin's very popular almanacs both shaped and reflected middling values and provide scarce evidence of the beliefs of nonelites, particularly in the first half of the eighteenth century when few firsthand accounts by common folks survive. Women were fans of Poor Richard as well as men. In New York City in 1735, Abigaill Franks quoted some of Franklin's "Ra[i]llery" on marriage from the previous year's almanac. In 1759, Hannah Callender recorded one example of "Ben: Franklins droll humour" in her diary, and in 1773 Sallie Eve's "Mama [lamented that] we have no such almanacks as what his was." Franklin's Poor Richard proved to be a useful resource, especially at midcentury when he was concerned with population issues.[14]

Advertisements in local newspapers also suggest commonplace values. Statistics provide some clues about behavior, if not about perception or intention. Changes in birthrates, age-specific marital fertility rates, and child-

13. This passage is astutely analyzed in Stephanie N. Patterson Gilbert, "Childbearing Cycles and Family Limitation in an Eighteenth-Century, Affluent Household: The Fertility Transition of Elizabeth Sandwith Drinker and Her Daughters" (master's thesis, Pennsylvania State University, Harrisburg, 2005), 49–50.

14. Leo Hershkowitz and Isidore S. Meyer, eds., *The Lee Max Friedman Collection of American Jewish Colonial Correspondence: Letters of the Franks Family (1733–1748)*, Studies in American Jewish History, V (Waltham, Mass., 1968), 47; Susan E. Klepp and Karin A. Wulf, eds., *The Diary of Hannah Callender: Sense and Sensibility in a Revolutionary Age, 1758–1788* (Ithaca, N.Y., 2009), Jan. 15, 1759; and Sallie Eve, Diary, Apr. 4, 1773, 30, Special Collections Department, William R. Perkins Library, Duke University, Durham, N.C.

woman ratios can be tracked through local censuses, genealogies, church records, and other quantifiable sources. Portraits and prints convey symbolic keys to the cultural constructions of fertility and femininity that are often less obvious in other sources. This study therefore goes beyond the usual emphasis on numbers to look at the contemporary opinion expressed in diaries, correspondence, and print. It explores legal and medical writings on the subjects of marriage, sexuality, and fertility. It borrows from the disciplines of art history and demography as well as from history.

Given the breadth of sources that must be mined to discover attitudes and practices concerning fertility, most analysis in this study focuses on the Mid-Atlantic colonies and states—Pennsylvania, New York, New Jersey, and Delaware. Statistical evidence suggests that, although married couples in all regions of what is now the eastern United States began to limit fertility at roughly the same time, the pace of decline was most rapid in New England, followed by the Mid-Atlantic, the South, and finally the newly acquired areas to the west. The Mid-Atlantic colonies and states contained a mix of the urban, rural, and frontier settings that formed the national experience, and the area's religious and ethnic diversity allows for a comparative perspective difficult to recover in other regions. When the evidence is thin for the Mid-Atlantic alone, however, as it is for individual portraits of women, for example, then the evidentiary net is cast more widely.[15]

This study is primarily interested in legitimate fertility, that is, with the behavior and intentions of courting and married women and men. In this period of American history, nearly all free persons married at some point in their lives (Quakers were exceptional in their high rates of celibacy around the turn of the nineteenth century). Marriage was expected and was usually an economic necessity for both free men and women. The discrete tasks assigned to males and those assigned to females were equally essential. Apprentices, indentured servants, redemptioners, servants hired by the year, those placed in service by the Overseers of the Poor were not to marry during their fixed terms of service. The prevalence of bound labor was one reason why the poor, particularly the urban poor, had small families—the freedom to marry came late. But even though bound labor systems for European immigrants were in serious decline by the end of the eighteenth century, allowing many poorer women and men to marry and start families as much

15. Sources for regional rates are listed in Susan E. Klepp, "*The Swift Progress of Population*": *A Documentary and Bibliographic Study of Philadelphia's Growth, 1642–1859* (Philadelphia, 1991), 16–25. See also Alice P. Kenney, "Patricians and Plebeians in Colonial Albany, Part II—Aggregation," *Halve Maen*, XLV, no. 2 (July 1970), 9–11.

as ten years earlier than had been possible in the colonial era, total fertility rates were still falling.

An exception to the concentration on legitimate childbearing will be to investigate, insofar as scanty sources permit, the fertility goals of those permanently in bondage. Enslaved women and men could not legally marry but formed extralegal unions. They would never be free. Enslaved women's fecund potential, as Jennifer Morgan has pointed out, placed them in a terrible bind. On the one hand, their pregnancies were sources of profit to their masters: the children were both a future labor supply and a commodity to be sold, while each successive generation assisted in the process of creolization and the diminution of African cultural heritage. Pregnancy could bring unwelcome intervention by white physicians, who were employed to treat or to experiment on bondwomen. On the other hand, fertility could create the familial connections for enslaved women and men that countered the social death and physical isolation that the slave system attempted to impose upon human beings.[16]

Unwed female servants of European descent also bore children, but they had few options and little control over the outcome. Most bastard-bearers neither planned nor welcomed their pregnancies. Bastardy was not uncommon, but the social consequences were grave. An illegitimate child lengthened a servant woman's term of service and brought whippings and the mandated sale or fostering of the child by the Overseers of the Poor. Humiliation through local gossip or through admonitions in church was designed to discourage illegitimacy. Most bastard-bearers would presumably have liked to prevent having an illegitimate child—despite commonplace jokes about serving women who seduced wealthy men to get the courts to force marriage.

Prostitutes seem to have borne few unwanted children. They had access to technologies such as condoms that were little used by the respectable because of condoms' close association with illicit sex and venereal disease. Prostitutes also faced the possibility of sterility through venereal disease, a risk that other women were somewhat less exposed to.

Some important groups of women cannot be included in this study be-

16. Sharla M. Fett, *Working Cures: Healing, Health, and Power on Southern Slave Plantations* (Chapel Hill, N.C., 2002); Schwartz, *Birthing a Slave*; Jennifer L. Morgan, *Laboring Women: Reproduction and Gender in New World Slavery* (Philadelphia, 2004). In the antebellum period, doctors attempted "scientific" experiments on black bodies, while both in that period and earlier untrained doctors honed their skills by attending enslaved women (ibid., esp. 107–143).

cause of the paucity of sources. It would have been instructive to compare the attitudes and experiences of colonial women, both free and enslaved, to native American women. Although the contrast between Eastern Woodland and Western European attitudes was presumably great, evidence is even sparser for native Americans than for enslaved or servant women. A rare exception comes from a single letter, written in 1787 during treaty negotiations. Katteuha, The Beloved Woman of the Chota (Cherokee), wrote to Benjamin Franklin, justifying her political stance on the grounds that "woman is the mother of All—and that woman Does not pull Children out of Trees or Stumps nor out of old Logs, but out of their Bodies, so that they [American officials and other men] ought to mind what a woman says." She has a cultural valuation of childbearing, political influence, and femininity very different from the biblical condemnation of all women for Eve's transgression that underlay Western thought: "In sorrow thou shalt bring forth children; and thy desire shall be to thy husband, and he shall rule over thee." There are, apparently and unfortunately, too few such comments, statistics, or other sources of information to pursue such a comparison.[17]

Most free American women eventually married—even if they had borne one or more illegitimate children at some earlier moment in their lives. Most enslaved Americans created, whenever humanly possible, strong family ties. They are the subjects of this study.

The original intentions of revolutionary-era American women concerning fertility and family planning will be approached from a number of angles. Chapter 1 is an overview of the changes in experiences of married free women and enslaved women. It compares existing statistical studies of fertility and adds several new analyses, particularly for African Americans. Residential, social, religious, and ethnic differences in fertility are explored. Statistics measure behavior, however, not meaning. Subsequent chapters explore those social and cultural constructions of fertility and family relationships. Chapter 2 traces the religious, political, and economic realities that had long supported large families and high fertility. It looks, too, at the religious and economic changes in the eighteenth century that began to undermine the old ways of thinking and behaving. Chapter 3 turns to revolutionary-era women's innovative recasting of the meanings of femininity, fertility, family, and the future. These new ideals were communicated to friends and daughters at the same time that Americans, both men and women, renounced

17. "Cherokee Indian Women to Pres. Franklin, 1787," *Pennsylvania Archives*, 1st Ser., XI (1855), 181; Gen. 3:16 (1611).

slavery for themselves and proclaimed their independence from Great Britain. Chapter 4 argues that there was an aesthetic of high fertility as well as one of limited fertility that helped both to define colonial pro-natalism and to diffuse new standards of feminine beauty, virtue, and ideal family size. Chapter 5 recovers some of the techniques of birth control and abortion available to women and to men in the eighteenth century. Chapter 6 asks, by looking at the law and law enforcement, how women were able to begin to seize control over reproduction in a still-patriarchal age. Chapter 7 looks both at those Americans who resisted or did not fully adopt family limitation strategies or who employed those new ideas in defense of old hierarchies. The Conclusion highlights some of the book's findings and traces a few of the continuities and discontinuities in Americans' conceptions of family planning, birth control, and gender from the early nation to the present. Detailed statistical evidence is found in the Appendix.

THE SIGNERS OF THE Declaration of Independence came from large families. Those who were delegates to the Second Continental Congress in 1776 came from families with an average of 7.3 children. The first response of these Revolutionaries to rising expenses was to demand local control over tax and land policies; their next step was to fight a war against a recalcitrant Parliament and king for failing to heed those demands. That it might have been less costly to have fewer children did not immediately occur to either voters or politicians. Those same founders who risked their lives, their fortunes, and their sacred honor in publicly breaking from Great Britain in 1776 would also eventually break from the childbearing pattern of their parents' generation, fathering in their turn an average of only slightly more than 6 children over their lifetimes (even with the 18 children of Virginia's Carter Braxton).

And, just eleven years later, those founding fathers who met once more at Philadelphia, this time to draw up the Constitution of 1787, produced an average of just 4.9 (legitimate) children over the course of their lives, quite similar to the record of the members of the first Supreme Court (who had an average of 4.8 children) and the first president, vice-president, and Cabinet secretaries (who averaged 5.1 offspring). Who was behind these changes? These politicians were nearly completely mute and perhaps clueless on the subject. Pregnancy, birth, and the regulation of monthly cycles were still largely in the world of women, politics in the world of men, and only the rarest of circumstances brought gynecological issues into the purview of the government. We need to look beyond the founders to find another revolution in eighteenth-century America, one that would begin to transform women's lives first and, soon after, the nation as a whole.[18]

18. The figures represent legitimate marital fertility only, combining offspring from first and any subsequent marriages. They are calculated from biographies in Robert G. Ferris, ed., *Signers of the Declaration of Independence* (Washington, D.C., 1975); and John A. Garraty and Mark C. Carnes, eds., *American National Biography Online,* http://anb.org (accessed June 2006). Unmarried delegates are not included. Of course, this is not a scientific study. Not all biographies include counts of the congressional delegates' siblings, and childless couples in the parental generation would not produce any sons who might grow up to be delegates to Congress. If childless men are excluded from the delegates to the Constitutional Convention in 1787, the average would rise from 4.9 to 5.6 children, still well below the 7.3 children of the parental generation.

Starting, Spacing, and Stopping

THE STATISTICS OF BIRTH

AND

FAMILY SIZE

The radical French émigré J. P. Brissot toured the new United States in 1788 eager to locate the tangible benefits of enlightened revolution. He was especially concerned with population because he, like the majority of contemporary thinkers, thought that free societies grow rapidly and oppressive regimes stagnate. For the most part, Brissot found the rapid population growth in the former British colonies that convinced him of the advantages of republicanism, liberty, and independence. Yet, when he tallied the births in Philadelphia's Lutheran church, he discovered a discrepancy. "You will also note," he wrote, "that during the war years there were fewer births" (Figure 1). He decided that this "was natural," perhaps referring to the marital separations caused by military service or to the fears of couples about the wisdom of bearing children during wartime. It was, he intimated, only a temporary setback, and the numbers seemed to bear him out: the number of births in this congregation rose as the war wound down.[1]

Dr. Benjamin Rush was also a staunch supporter of the Revolution, but he reached a very different conclusion in that same year. He asserted, "The

1. J. P. Brissot de Warville, *New Travels in the United States of America, 1788*, ed. Durand Echeverria, trans. Mara Soceanu Vamos and Durand Echeverria (Cambridge, Mass., 1964), 293.

FIGURE 1.
Births among Philadelphia Lutherans, 1774–1787

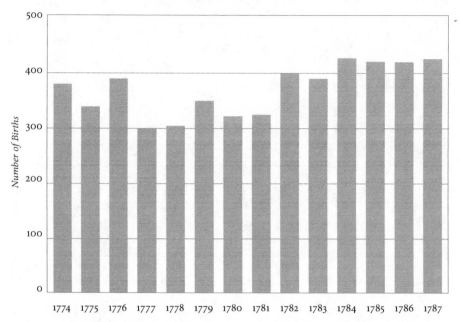

Drawn by Kimberly Foley. J. P. Brissot de Warville, *New Travels in the United States of America, 1788*,
ed. Durand Echeverria, trans. Mara Soceanu Vamos and Durand Echeverria (Cambridge, Mass., 1964), 292.

population in the United States was more rapid from births during the war, than it had ever been." This increase was not natural, but was due to the "quantity and extensive circulation of money, and to the facility of procuring the means of subsistence during the war." It was the encouragement to marriages caused by high employment that Rush assigned as the reason for rising birthrates. Who, if either of the two, was right? No one in the eighteenth century had a clear idea.[2]

Scholars have been seeking ways to compensate for the absence of eighteenth-century birth registrations by creating estimates of fertility from local censuses, family histories, wills, church records, and related sources. These often-ingenious attempts to estimate childbearing patterns have yielded interesting, but quite incompatible, results. The wills of Lutherans and Moravians in York County, Pennsylvania, for example, mentioned an average of 6.7 children before 1789, but only 5.9 thereafter. Quakers living in

2. Benjamin Rush, "Influence of the American Revolution," in Dagobert D. Runes, ed., *The Selected Writings of Benjamin Rush* (New York, 1947), 330–331.

that county apparently experienced a much sharper decline, from 7.0 to 3.9 children, according to their wills, yet Presbyterian families reversed these trends as average family size went from 5.0 to 5.6 children. According to church registers, family size among the Schwenkfelders rose from 5.5 to 7.3 over the course of the eighteenth century as the descendants of the first immigrants adapted to conditions in the New World. The genealogical records of the extended Haring family in Bergen and Rockland counties, close to New York City, saw family size fall from an average of 10 to 7.6 children between the second and third generations, and then fall even further to 5.4 in the fourth generation (not counting childless marriages), although averages rose very slightly to 5.5 for the fifth generation at the end of the eighteenth century. Mean family size in rural Chester County, Pennsylvania, fell from 9.0 children at the beginning of the eighteenth century to 6.1 during and after the Revolution. Welsh families living in Radnor Township in Chester County averaged 3 surviving children in 1798 and 3.8 in 1823. Their non-Welsh neighbors had an average of 6 surviving children in the earlier period and a quarter century later had 5, all according to analyses of wills. In Newtown, New York, 59 percent of fathers born in the late seventeenth century had fewer than 8 children, rising to 70 percent in the early eighteenth century and then falling slightly to 67 percent for those born at midcentury. In Germantown, Pennsylvania, the proportion of families having only 2 children rose from 26 percent in the middle of the eighteenth century to 45 percent at the end of the century. At the Reformed church in Albany, New York, births per marriage peaked at more than 6 in the 1730s and fell to just over 3 by the 1790s.[3]

Philadelphia probate records analyzed by Jean Soderlund indicate that enslaved women had too few surviving daughters to reproduce the parental generation. Between the founding of Pennsylvania in 1682 and the beginning

3. Daniel Snydacker, "Kinship and Community in Rural Pennsylvania, 1749–1820," *Journal of Interdisciplinary History*, XIII (1982–1983), 41–61, esp. 54; Rodger C. Henderson, "Eighteenth-Century Schwenkfelders: A Demographic Interpretation," in Peter C. Urb, ed., *Schwenkfelders in America: Papers Presented at the Colloquium on Schwenckfeld and the Schwenkfelders, Pennsburg, Pa., September 17–22, 1984* (Pennsburg, Pa., 1987), 25–40, esp. 31; Firth Haring Fabend, *A Dutch Family in the Middle Colonies, 1660–1800* (New Brunswick, N.J., 1991), 86–89; D. E. Ball and G. M. Walton, "Agricultural Productivity Change in Eighteenth-Century Pennsylvania," *Journal of Economic History*, XXXVI (1976), 102–117, esp. 109; Katharine Hewitt Cummin, *A Rare and Pleasing Thing: Radnor Demography (1798) and Development* (Philadelphia, 1977), 92; Jessica Kross, *The Evolution of an American Town: Newtown, New York, 1642–1775* (Philadelphia, 1983), 246, 314; Stephanie Grauman Wolf, *Urban Village: Population, Community, and Family Structure in Germantown, Pennsylvania, 1683–1800* (Princeton, N.J., 1976), 270; Alice P. Kenney, "Patricians and Plebeians in Colonial Albany, Part II—Aggregation," *Halve Maen*, XLV, no. 2 (July 1970), 9–11, esp. 10.

of gradual abolition in 1780, each generation of slaves would have shrunk by an average of 40 percent because of a combination of low fertility and high childhood mortality. Only the importation of fresh human stock permitted the growth of this enslaved population.[4]

Slave and free, rural and urban, and multiple faiths, ethnicities, and occupations are represented in these studies. What to make of these various attempts to pinpoint changes in fertility levels? The overall trend in these local studies is for the large average family sizes of the colonial period to fall early in the Republic, with an occasional small and temporary uptick in birthrates late in the century, perhaps a post–Revolutionary War baby boom. There were, however, many variations on these themes.

A difficulty is that these simple averages or percent distributions of births, baptisms, or surviving offspring might be influenced by factors other than fertility levels. Did the fertility of the majority really decline at all? These numbers, so laboriously collected, do not indicate whether the cause of smaller families was family planning, later marriages, higher death rates, changes in inheritance practices, more mobility, theological disputes about the necessity of infant baptism, greater secularism, random deviations caused by small numbers, or any number of other potential explanations. One possible cause of smaller numbers can generally be ruled out—it was not a consequence of sloppier documentation of births and baptisms. Record keeping and record survival were by and large far better for the years at the end of the eighteenth century than they had been earlier. Still, the statistics generated by these local studies are more suggestive than conclusive.[5]

There are three standard measures of fertility that either allow larger populations to be studied or that control for possible differences in sex ratios, mortality, marriage, and age distributions: the crude birthrate, or the number of births per thousand population (called *crude* because only the total population size is known; the ages, sex ratios, and marital status of these people are unknown); the child-woman ratio, defined here as the number of children from birth to age four per thousand women ages fifteen to forty-nine; and the age-specific marital fertility rate, or the number of children born to currently married women in five-year age categories between ages fifteen and forty-nine.

4. Jean R. Soderlund, "Black Importation and Migration into Southeastern Pennsylvania, 1682–1810," American Philosophical Society, *Proceedings*, CXXXIII (1989), 144–153, esp. table 4.

5. In New England, on the other hand, the accuracy and completeness of town records declined in the late eighteenth and early nineteenth centuries. See Gloria L. Main, "Rocking the Cradle: Downsizing the New England Family," *JIH*, XXXVII (2006–2007), 35–58.

Fertility Measured by Crude Birthrates

From 1670 through 1729, birthrates in England were stable; then, between 1730 and 1760, rates began to rise (Figure 2). By the 1790s, the average annual birthrate in England had stabilized at just under forty births per thousand. French rates can be computed only from the 1740s and indicate a steady decline, with rates dropping below English averages around the time of the French Revolution and continuing to fall through the nineteenth century. In the overwhelmingly rural British American colonies as a whole and in rural areas of the Mid-Atlantic region, birthrates began to fall in the wake of the American Revolution. Crude birthrates in Philadelphia exhibit a decline a decade or more earlier, starting as early as the 1760s. American and French declines tracked fairly closely, although from quite different starting points, and urban rates continued to outpace rural rates through the nineteenth century and well into the twentieth century. Most African Americans, overwhelmingly enslaved people living in the southern colonies, did not share in the revolutionary moment but experienced continued enslavement and rising fertility rates until the Civil War. Then, as freedom became possible for the first time, birthrates began to fall.[6]

The colonial American rise in crude birthrates was likely primarily brought about by changes in the composition of the underlying population — the early settlements had large numbers of bound servants who were forbidden to marry, a surplus of males and a scarcity of females, and, perhaps, the persistence of Old World attitudes and habits. Gradually, over the late seventeenth and early eighteenth centuries, the sex ratios evened as births outpaced immigration. More individuals married, and married earlier, than had been the norm in Europe. Marital fertility throughout the colonial period was high and families large, even if substantial portions of the earliest settler populations were unmarried and, presumably, celibate.

An approximation of the age structure in the colonies can be gleaned from the handful of early censuses that allow calculation of age distributions (Figure 3). These numbers support contemporary impressions that the colonies had very youthful populations. More colonists than Englishmen were in their late teens or early twenties, the years in which people are most free to immigrate. These young women and men were soon to marry or were

6. See J. Potter, "The Growth of Population in America, 1700–1860," in D. V. Glass and D. E. C. Eversley, eds., *Population in History: Essays in Historical Demography* (Chicago, 1965), 631–688, esp. table 10, 674–676.

FIGURE 2.

Crude Birthrates, 1670–1879

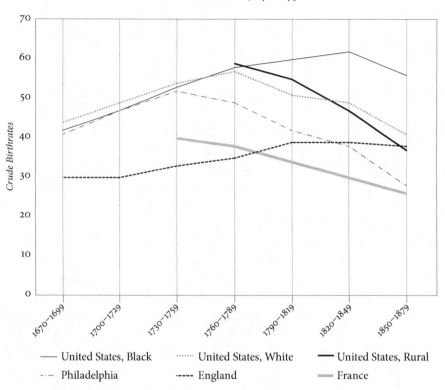

— United States, Black   ⋯⋯ United States, White   — United States, Rural

–·– Philadelphia   ---- England   ▨ France

Drawn by Kimberly Foley. Estimates of white or Euro-American population are based on the life table rates implied in Robert W. Fogel et al., "The Economics of Mortality in North America, 1650–1910: A Description of a Research Project," *Historical Methods*, XI (1978), 99. Estimates for the total African American population are from Robert W. Fogel, "Revised Estimates of the U.S. Slave Trade and the Native-Born Share of the Black Population," in Robert W. Fogel et al., eds., *Without Consent or Contract: The Rise and Fall of American Slavery; Evidence and Methods* (New York, 1992), calculated from table 6.1, 62. The life tables (model west) are in Ansley J. Coale and Paul Demeny, *Regional Model Life Tables and Stable Populations* (Princeton, N.J., 1966). My thanks to Robert W. Fogel for confirming these calculations. For Philadelphia, see Susan E. Klepp. "Demography in Early Philadelphia, 1690–1860," in Klepp, ed., *The Demographic History of the Philadelphia Region, 1600–1860*, American Philosophical Society, *Proceedings*, CXXXIII (Philadelphia, 1989), table 2, 103–107, as revised by the author. For rural U.S. counties, see Morton Owen Schapiro, "Land Availability and Fertility in the United States, 1760–1870," *Journal of Economic History*, XLII (1982), table 3, 594. For England, see E. A. Wrigley and R. S. Schofield, *The Population History of England, 1541–1871: A Reconstruction* (Cambridge, 1989), table A3.3, 531–535. For France, see David R. Weir, "New Estimates of Nuptiality and Marital Fertility in France, 1740–1911," *Population Studies*, XLVIII (1994), table B2, 329.

FIGURE 3.

Age Distributions

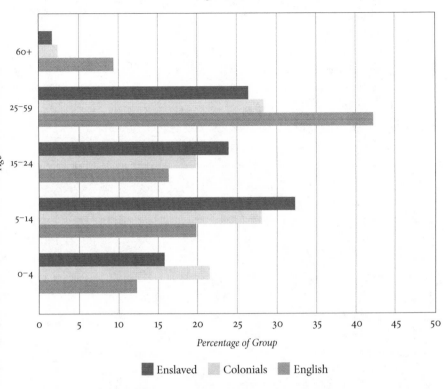

Percentage of Group

■ Enslaved ▨ Colonials ■ English

Drawn by Kimberly Foley. English (1701–1751): E. A. Wrigley and R. S. Schofield, *The Population History of England, 1541–1871: A Reconstruction* (Cambridge, 1989), table A3.1, 529. Colonials: Jeffrey L. Sheib, "A 1688 Census of Kent County, Delaware," *Pennsylvania Genealogical Magazine,* XXXVII (1991), 135–156; G. B. Keen, "Early Swedish Records—Extracts from Parish Records of Gloria Dei Church, Philadelphia," *Pennsylvania Magazine of History and Biography,* II (1878), 224–228; John Rodgers, "Census of Northampton, Burlington County, 1709, Extracted from the Minutes of the Town Meeting . . . ," New Jersey Historical Society, *Proceedings,* IV (1850), 33–36; "Census, 1783/4," in Gloria Dei Lutheran Church Records, I (MS transcription by E. D. McMahon, 1934), 755–772, Historical Society of Pennsylvania, Philadelphia; Slave registry (1780), in Henry Graham Ashmead, *History of Delaware County, Pennsylvania* (Philadelphia, 1884), 203–205, and at http://www.afrolumens.org/slavery/index.html (accessed December 2004).

recently married and about to start families; if they were enslaved, they were starting families without being legally married. Compared to England, the colonies had proportionally fewer individuals in their prime childbearing years (between twenty-five and forty-nine), a finding that explains how the relatively low crude birthrates of the early colonies could coexist with consistently high marital fertility rates—the population was heavily weighted toward children, adolescents, and young adults. Sex ratios were uneven. Mid-Atlantic censuses for 1688, 1697, 1709, and 1783/4 indicate a sex ratio of 120 men ages twenty to forty-four for every 100 women of the same age.

The rising crude birthrate of African Americans between 1670 and 1879 also occurred because theirs was a young population—there were very few elderly slaves. The market in human beings favored youth. Masters preferred the presumed malleability of twelve- to fourteen-year-olds, so slave traders imported boys and girls in that age range whenever possible. Forced migration helped produce a higher proportion of African American children between five and fourteen than appeared among the free and fewer infants and very young children. Similarly, there was a paucity of individuals above sixty, even after a century of habitation in the New World—two of many indications that this was not the benign system that owners liked to claim in their own defense.

What about fertility in the countryside where the vast majority of free colonists lived? Morton Owen Schapiro's calculation of crude birthrates by decade for rural counties in the United States (the white population only) reveals the early lead of the New England states in fertility reduction (Figure 4). The Mid-Atlantic region, which stretched farther into the western frontiers than did New England, had a slower rate of decline. Maryland, the only southern state for which rates were calculated, followed a quite different path. Here, birthrates were virtually identical to New England's from the 1760s through the 1790s, but, starting in the early nineteenth century, the rate of fertility decline stagnated, falling much more slowly than in any of the northern states. Other measures of fertility in the nineteenth century upper South show a similar reluctance among inhabitants to decrease fertility before the 1850s. It seems that the free, white residents of the slave states resisted the demographic and familial implications of family limitation because white security rested in part on maintaining patriarchal households and white mastery.

In the far West, meanwhile, the newly colonized areas in the Ohio and upper Mississippi River valleys were settled by easterners and immigrants in sizable numbers only after 1790. Despite a later start, settlers in the old

FIGURE 4.

Rural Crude Birthrates by Region, 1760–1849

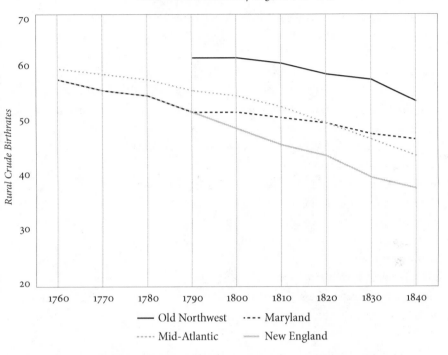

Legend:
— Old Northwest   ···· Maryland
····· Mid-Atlantic   ～ New England

Drawn by Kimberly Foley. Derived from Morton Owen Schapiro, "Land Availability and Fertility in the United States, 1760–1870," *Journal of Economic History,* XLII (1982), 577–600.

Northwest would soon mimic the earlier patterns established in the northern states—fertility was initially high but then fell every decade thereafter. There was no equilibrium or stasis in the Northeast or in the Northwest: once birthrates began falling around the time of the Revolution, they continued to fall. If Benjamin Rush was wrong about birthrates rising in Philadelphia during the war, he was closer to the truth about rural rates. There was no dramatic drop in birthrates during the Revolution as there was in Philadelphia. Rural rates simply exhibited a slow, steady, and initially imperceptible decline from the 1760s. Overall, rural northern and western decadal birthrates declined by a quarter, from fifty-eight to forty-four births per thousand population, between the 1760s and 1840s; Philadelphia rates fell by more than a third, from fifty-six to thirty-five births per thousand population in that ninety-year period. These were major changes.

The records used to calculate crude birthrates primarily track the free, white portion of the population, yet from 1788 through 1801 Philadelphia printer Zachariah Poulson collected baptismal figures from the African Episcopal and African Methodist churches and the number of births among the poorest, unchurched residents, both black and white (tallied separately). This was a significant period in the history of race relations: Pennsylvania had provided for the gradual abolition of slavery in 1780 and strengthened the law in 1788. By 1800, the majority of African Americans were nominally free, which usually meant that they were indentured for a period of years and their time could still be bought and sold. They faced considerable racial discrimination and found themselves at the mercy (if such there was) of kidnappers from the slave states. Yet, despite these formidable obstacles, African Americans founded their own churches and established the first large, free black community in the North. Philadelphia became a beacon. Former bondmen and bondwomen from the upper South and rural Delaware Valley found freedom by absconding from masters, by buying themselves, or by private emancipation. The city's black population numbered 2,150 in 1790 and 6,083 in 1800.[7]

Poulson's accounts of births by race show that African Americans initially had birthrates comparable to the first waves of western settlers and to southern slaves. In the first seven years of this record, birthrates were fifty-six per thousand (compared to forty-nine for whites). In the last seven years, the birthrates of urban, free African Americans had already fallen to forty-seven per thousand (compared to a proportionally similar drop to forty-one for whites). Almost certainly, these newly arrived residents were, like other immigrants, largely young adults. They embraced the opportunity to legally marry and to establish families, as the marriage registers of several churches show. Once free, African Americans also began limiting births. Poverty was a factor. A strong desire to provide education, apprenticeships, and other opportunities for their children was certainly a related concern. Community uplift through church and benevolent associations engaged African American women. As Erica Armstrong Dunbar has found, African American conceptions of motherhood "blurred the distinction between the public sphere and the private." Limited childbearing could allow women to tend to their children, their church, and their community.[8]

---

7. Susan E. Klepp, "The Demographic Characteristics of Philadelphia, 1788–1801: Zachariah Poulson's Bills of Mortality," *Pennsylvania History*, LIII (1986), table 9, 216.

8. Ibid., table 10, 217; Erica Armstrong Dunbar, *A Fragile Freedom: African American Women and Emancipation in the Antebellum City*, Society and the Sexes in the Modern World (New Haven, Conn., 2008), 51. The efforts of the Society for the Propagation of the Gospel to baptize slaves in Philadelphia produced a rough census of the men, women, and children owned by Anglicans. The

After 1760, crude birthrates fell for the free population, both black and white, decade after decade. Rates fell more sharply in the cities than in the country, earlier in the East than the West, and approximated an equilibrium only in the upper South (and perhaps the rest of the South). Fertility was becoming independent of immediate economic, political, or military circumstances (see Appendix, below). Family planning, with its emphasis on anticipating the future, was replacing short-term decision making. By the last third of the eighteenth century, Mid-Atlantic women were finding continual pregnancies unacceptable. As their surviving writings reveal, they wanted to control their fertility and not entrust childbearing to blind fate.

The turn to family limitation has often been preceded by unusually high fertility, as demographers have long been aware. The exuberant fertility levels of the 1740s through 1760s might have urged a retreat, especially in the face of the limits on westward expansion in the Proclamation Line of 1763 as well as the rising taxes proposed by Parliament, from the Stamp Act through the Townshend Acts. What happened after the Revolution? The decadal crude birthrates show a steady decline. What was going on according to censuses or in individual families?[9]

Fertility Measured by Census Counts

When demographers write about fertility, they expect to base their findings on the analysis of large numbers—provinces, regions, and nations. These numbers are most commonly available from national censuses, but there was no federal census before 1790. In the American colonies, settlements were widely scattered over a vast countryside. Travel was difficult, even for those familiar with the terrain. Roads, maps, and sometimes even paper and ink were scarce, especially outside the largest towns on the East Coast. The bureaucracies and trained clerks needed to collect data systematically were in short supply. The inhabitants of the colonies were more heterogeneous than those of Europe in race, language, religion, ethnicity, and bound or free legal statuses, and they were often mistrustful of the relatively small elite that dominated officialdom. Many householders feared that censuses were a pre-

---

estimated crude birthrate for 1742–1744 and 1745–1748 is forty-one to forty-nine per thousand at a time when white rates were forty-five—an unusually low figure for the colonial period. See the baptismal records for Christ Church, held at the Genealogical Society of Pennsylvania, Philadelphia.

9. Karen Oppenheim Mason, "Gender and Family Systems in the Fertility Transition," *Global Fertility Transition*, supplement of *Population and Development Review*, XXVII (2001), 160–176, esp. 168.

lude to taxation, so officials seeking to ensure domestic tranquillity were wise to avoid riling citizens by asking pointed questions about family members, occupations, and possessions.[10]

Still, knowledge of the size and characteristics of towns, districts, and colonies would have been useful to officials in London as well as America and was often requested. Pennsylvania seems never to have complied with these requests, except in the most general of terms, but there were frequent censuses taken in New York and New Jersey. These censuses offer few details. Because the number of men available for military service was crucial for war and diplomacy, colonial and early national censuses provided only two age categories: men of military age (sixteen years of age and older) and boys under sixteen. All females were either lumped together or, less often, divided along the same lines as the men. A very few scattered local censuses give the exact ages of every resident. These reveal that early census takers routinely undercounted infants, particularly girls. This omission reflects a widespread habit of mind: infants and girls were simply less important than males and older children. Such omissions became less common by the last decades of the eighteenth century, one indication of more inclusive visions of the importance of children. Presumably, the colonywide censuses also undercounted the very young. The first censuses of the United States provided no information on the age or sex of enslaved individuals.[11]

Even when these colonywide censuses are reasonably complete, the numbers might vary according to factors other than fertility or childbearing patterns; age distributions, marital status, mortality levels, and in- and out-migration can all affect child-woman ratios. Not all children were the offspring of resident women. From age twelve, and sometimes earlier, European boys and girls commonly left home for service or apprenticeships, but, if their parents were too poor to pay a master to take on their child, if they

---

10. Evarts B. Greene and Virginia D. Harrington, *American Population before the Federal Census of 1790* (1932; rpt. Gloucester, Mass., 1966); Stella H. Sutherland, *Population Distribution in Colonial America* (1936; rpt. New York, 1966); Robert V. Wells, *The Population of the British Colonies in America before 1776: A Survey of Census Data* (Princeton, N.J., 1975).

11. In Kent County, Delaware, and Burlington, New Jersey, the census failed to count infants and had suspiciously low counts of one- and two-year-olds. In the records of the Swedish Lutherans, there was some underrecording of infants, particularly under six months, but most noticeably a marked absence of young girls. The sex ratio in the late seventeenth century from birth to age four was 132 males for every 100 females; for birth to age nineteen, it was 130. In the 1780s, the sex ratio in the Lutheran census was 147 from birth to age four, a dismal performance. At older ages, girls were no longer ignored, something of an improvement in female visibility.

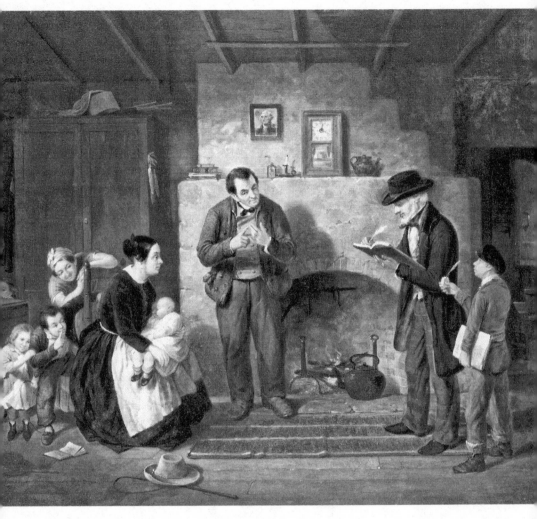

PLATE 1.

Taking the Census. By Francis William Edmonds, 1854.
Private Collection. Permission, The Brooklyn Museum, New York.

The befuddled head of this farm household struggles to calculate the
ages, and perhaps even the number, of family members. His wife looks
blankly on, offering no assistance, and the children do not help by shyly
hiding behind their mother or behind a blanket chest. A century earlier,
families were even less likely to be accustomed to thinking numerically.

were "fatherless and friendless," or if they simply had a taste for adventure, emigration to the New World or other colonies beckoned.[12]

The handful of local censuses that give exact ages provide the best information. It is possible to calculate the number of children from birth to age four per every one thousand women ages fifteen to forty-nine based on seven censuses (Table 1). These census counts confirm that child-woman ratios were rising as settlements matured but that the trend was reversed, at least for the Swedish Lutherans in Pennsylvania and New Jersey, after the Revolution. These counts, however, are flawed. All the censuses undercount infants, and most undercount toddlers. Generally, fewer girls are recorded than boys, at least among the free. These sources are suggestive, but they must be used carefully.

The enslaved population grew only slowly at first. The initial response of seventeenth-century neophyte slaveowners was to return pregnant bondwomen to the seller as damaged property. Soon, however, the economic value of slave reproduction became apparent, and women were acceptable purchases. Yet family formation was difficult. Large slave quarters were rare. A northern slave was far more likely than a southern slave to be the only person of African descent in the household or neighborhood. Once rural areas were more densely populated in the middle of the eighteenth century, informal marriages became more feasible, causing the enslaved population to grow through births as well as through importation.[13]

The Pennsylvania slave registrations of 1780 allow a rare, detailed look at this more mature, rural enslaved population. The Pennsylvania Assembly passed a bill providing for the gradual abolition of slavery in 1780; the legislation freed no person who was currently a slave but provided for the future children of those slaves to be freed after twenty-eight years of servitude.

---

12. Farley Grubb, "Fatherless and Friendless: Factors Influencing the Flow of English Emigrant Servants," *JEH*, LII (1992), 85–108; Aaron S. Fogelmen, "From Slaves, Convicts, and Servants to Free Passengers: The Transformation of Immigration in the Era of the American Revolution," *Journal of American History*, LXXXV (1998), 43–76; Marianne S. Wokeck, *Trade in Strangers: The Beginnings of Mass Migration to North America* (University Park, Pa., 1999). For two case studies, see Susan E. Klepp, Farley Grubb, and Anne Pfaelzer de Ortiz, eds., *Souls for Sale: Two German Redemptioners Come to Revolutionary America; the Life Stories of John Frederick Whitehead and Johann Carl Büttner* (University Park, Pa., 2006).

13. Darold D. Wax, "Quaker Merchants and the Slave Trade in Colonial Pennsylvania," *Pennsylvania Magazine of History and Biography*, LXXXVI (1962), 143–159, esp. 149 and 152; Edward Raymond Turner, *The Negro in Pennsylvania: Slavery—Servitude—Freedom* (Washington, D.C., 1911), 24n; Kenneth E. Marshall, "Work, Family, and Day-to-Day Survival on an Old Farm: Nance Melick, a Rural Late Eighteenth- and Early Nineteenth-Century New Jersey Slave Woman," *Slavery and Abolition*, XIX, no. 3 (December 1998), 22–45.

TABLE 1.

Ratio of Children from Birth to Age 4 per 1,000 Women Ages 15–49

Census	Date	Community Type	Child/ Woman Ratio
Kent, Delaware	1688	Recently settled	541
Swedish Lutherans	1697	Recently to long settled	1,194
Burlington, N.J.	1709	Recently settled	637
Morris, N.J.	1771	Long settled	913
Enslaved Pennsylvanians	1780	Recently to long settled	668
Swedish Lutherans	1783/4	Long settled	462
Recently emancipated African Americans, Salem, N.J.	1797	Long settled	857

Sources: Jeffrey L. Sheib, "A 1688 Census of Kent County, Delaware," *Pennsylvania Genealogical Magazine,* XXXVII (1991), 135–156 (total population with known ages, 226); G. B. Keen, "Early Swedish Records — Extracts from Parish Records of Gloria Dei Church, Philadelphia," *Pennsylvania Magazine of History and Biography,* II (1878), 224–228 (Swedish Lutherans in Pennsylvania and New Jersey, 1697, total population, 533); John Rodgers, "Census of Northampton, Burlington County, 1709; Extracted from the Minutes of the Town Meeting . . . ," New Jersey Historical Society, *Proceedings,* IV (1850), 33–36 (total population, 312); William A. Ellis, "Census of Morris Township, Morris County, N.J., 1771–2," ibid., LXIII (1945), 24–36 (with estimates for two missing pages, total population, 1,453); Henry Graham Ashmead, *History of Delaware County, Pennsylvania* (Philadelphia, 1884), 203–205 (Delaware County slave register). Slave registers for other Pennsylvania counties from www.afrolumens.org/slavery/index .html (accessed December 2004) (total registry population, 3,173); "Census, 1783/4," in Gloria Dei Lutheran Church Records, I (MS transcription by E. D. McMahon, 1934), 755–772, Historical Society of Pennsylvania, Philadelphia (total population, 340); Clement Alexander Price and M. M. Perot, ed., *After Freedom* (Burlington N.J., 1987), 69–72 (Salem, N.J., total population, 79).

It was, as Robert W. Fogel and Stanley L. Engerman have noted, "philanthropy at bargain prices," placing the property rights of slaveholders above the human rights of the enslaved. To hold on to their human property, however, slaveowners were required to register their slaves. If they failed to do so, the offending slaveowner's bondmen, bondwomen, and children were to be immediately freed. Cupidity was a strong motivating force for heads of households to accurately and completely count and record an entire population, including infants and girls. Still, few infants were recorded, indicating, despite the economic interests of the owners of human chattel, a persistent disregard for newborns (only about half the number of infants as one-year-olds were recorded, and very few were under six months old). On the other hand, the small number of newborns recorded in 1780 may mean that enslaved couples were carefully delaying childbearing, aiming for birthdates after July 4, 1780, when the law provided that their children would eventually be freed. These numbers might well be another example of family planning (but not necessarily family limitation) among African Americans.[14]

The age and sex pyramids formed from the information in the surviving 1780 slave registers are similar in their broad bases and their sharp setbacks as ages rise from birth to sixty-plus. These formations are typical of populations with high fertility and high mortality. Yet there are significant differences across the state. The oldest-settled areas in southeastern Pennsylvania, including Bucks, Chester, Delaware, and Lancaster counties, had the highest child-woman ratios (Figure 5). Tied to Philadelphia and containing sizable populations of Quakers, this region was a stronghold of antislavery opinion, so slaveowners were especially careful to register their chattel slaves. In an environment relatively hostile to slavery, masters sometimes might have been shamed into treating their bound laborers with more humanity than was normal, producing better conditions for enslaved families. The eastern enslaved population was more mature than those in more recently settled areas, and the sex ratio was closely balanced at 103 males per 100 females. Child-woman ratios were higher for those enslaved in the east than those in other regions, with 709 children from birth to age four per 1,000 women ages fifteen to forty-nine, and well above the revised child-woman ratio of 550 estimated—by adding more girls—among neighboring Swedish Lutherans in 1783/4.[15]

The far western region of Pennsylvania, Washington and Westmoreland counties, was recently settled by newcomers looking for agricultural and commercial opportunities in trade along the Ohio and Mississippi rivers (Figure 6). The overall sex ratio was 99 males per 100 females, an indication of investments in laborers of both sexes, but with important age differences. The preferred slaves were of two sorts. One was quite young girls ages five to fourteen. They were less expensive to purchase and were prized as domes-

14. Robert W. Fogel and Stanley L. Engerman, "Philanthropy at Bargain Prices: Notes on the Economics of Gradual Emancipation," in *Without Consent or Contract: The Rise and Fall of American Slavery*, II, *Conditions of Slave Life and the Transition to Freedom: Technical Papers* (New York, 1992), 587–605.

15. Because the Lutherans undercounted girls, it was assumed for this calculation that the number of girls equaled the number of boys. The Swedish Lutheran census of 1783/4 is the only one from early America to record ethnicity. It was a heterogeneous population: 50 percent were of Swedish descent, 32 percent were British, 14 percent were other Europeans, and 4 percent were African.

FIGURE 5.

Age and Sex Distributions of Enslaved Persons, Eastern Pennsylvania

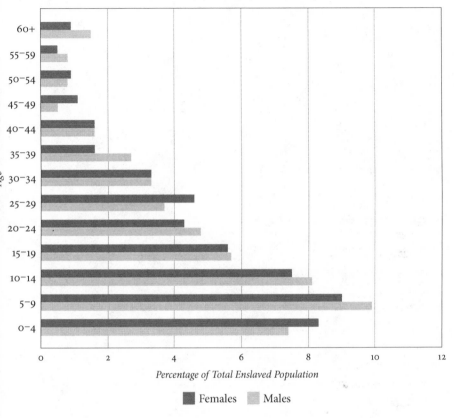

Percentage of Total Enslaved Population

■ Females ▓ Males

Drawn by Kimberly Foley. Slave registry (1780) for Delaware County in Henry Graham Ashmead, *History of Delaware County, Pennsylvania* (Philadelphia, 1884), 755–772. All other Pennsylvania county registries from http://www.afrolumens.org/slavery/index.html (accessed December 2004).

tic workers because they were old enough to be useful but too young to be starting families; at these ages, the sex ratio was 84 males per 100 females. These western settlers also purchased young adult men. A large proportion of males were ages twenty to thirty-four, prime hands for undertaking the hard labor of clearing the land; at these ages, the sex ratio was 126. Given the youth of many of the enslaved females, the differences in age, and the distances between farmsteads on this frontier, the child-woman ratio in the west was only 616 children from birth to age four per 1,000 women of child-bearing age. Slaves were isolated, marriage partners scarce, and family formation most difficult in the far west.

In contrast to both eastern and western Pennsylvania were the three south

FIGURE 6.

Age and Sex Distributions of Enslaved Persons, Western Pennsylvania

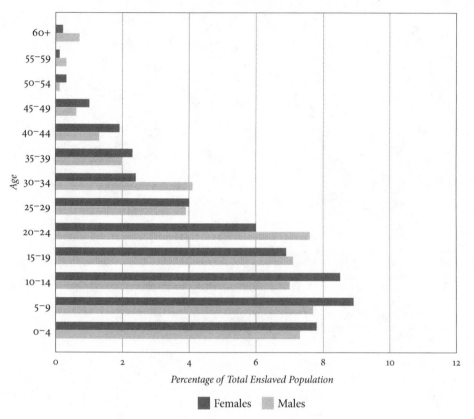

Percentage of Total Enslaved Population

■ Females   ▨ Males

Drawn by Kimberly Foley. Pennsylvania county registries from
http://www.afrolumens.org/slavery/index.html (accessed December 2004).

central Pennsylvania counties, Bedford, Cumberland, and Dauphin (Figure 7). Settled for nearly two generations by 1780, the local economy was linked via the Susquehanna River to the slave state of Maryland and the slave markets of the port city of Baltimore. These counties were among those that "held on to their slaves most persistently" even after the gradual abolition act was implemented. That 1780 law "could not, however, foresee all the abuses and subterfuges to which the forces of greed would resort," as Brissot observed in his *Travels.* Central Pennsylvania farmers participated actively in the slave trade, unloading unwanted humans to the markets in Baltimore and elsewhere—a trend most evident in the striking shortage of girls under the age of ten. In 1780, there were 112 males per 100 females of all ages in these

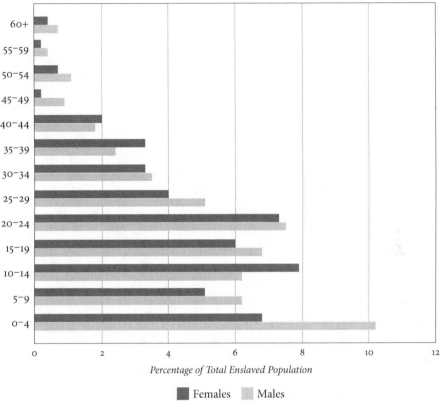

FIGURE 7.

Age and Sex Distributions of Enslaved Persons, Central Pennsylvania

Percentage of Total Enslaved Population

■ Females   ▨ Males

Drawn by Kimberly Foley. Pennsylvania county registries from
http://www.afrolumens.org/slavery/index.html (accessed December 2004).

counties. Among the youngest, the sex ratio was far more skewed. There
were 141 males per 100 females from birth to age nine, suggesting that these
farmers were keeping the baby boys born to their enslaved women but sending young female babies and toddlers to western Pennsylvania or into the
Chesapeake—already a slave-exporting region. These "barbarous" slaveowners, as Brissot called them, were also already circumventing the law by re-
moving pregnant women from Pennsylvania and into slave states so that the
babies would be born slaves for life (note in Figure 7 the shortage of women
ages twenty-five to twenty-nine, prime childbearing years). Sometimes both
mother and child were sold, and sometimes the mother was returned to her
Pennsylvania owner until she was again pregnant. These technically legal

ploys were so common that the state legislature strengthened the abolition law in 1788 to block these loopholes. Thereafter, the export of enslaved individuals was illegal, but not always enforced. This region of central Pennsylvania had a comparatively low child-woman ratio, even though it bordered the eastern counties and was no longer on the frontier. There were 652 children from birth to age four per 1,000 slave women of childbearing age. The intent of the 1780 statute was already being thwarted by masters who continued to profit from slavery through the legal or illegal export of selected types of human commodities.[16]

Some of the lowest effective fertility rates for the eighteenth and early nineteenth centuries come from free African American families in the urban North. In 1820, Lancaster City, Pennsylvania, officials feverishly imagined that local African Americans were an immediate danger to public safety and required all black residents (even a newborn not yet named) to register with authorities. Nearly all the 307 inhabitants complied within the first two months. The resulting list shows 42 individuals who had "no family." Most of these were live-in servants in white households. Of 63 family groups living in their own or someone else's household, virtually all with both husband and wife present, 17 marriages were childless, and 15 households had only a single child—so just over half of these families were failing to reproduce the parental generation. The largest family consisted of 7 children, but the average number of own children of all ages was just 1.8. This number compares to the approximate average of 2.4 minor children in European American families in Lancaster City. Even including foster children and apprentices in the calculation brings the average only to just below 1.9 children per African American household. Nominal freedom for African Americans was accompanied by severe economic, social, and political discrimination, the strong probability of shorter life spans than the European American population, and, it appears, by severely limited childbearing.[17]

16. Brissot, *New Travels*, ed. Echeverria, trans. Vamos and Echeverria, 228; Gary B. Nash and Jean R. Soderlund, *Freedom by Degrees: Emancipation in Pennsylvania and Its Aftermath* (New York, 1991), 4, 127–128.

17. These calculations are from the initial entries, May to June 1820, in Leroy T. Hopkins, "The Negro Entry Book: A Document of Lancaster City's Antebellum Afro-American Community," *Journal of the Lancaster County Historical Society*, LXXXVIII (1984), 142–180. Only the ages of heads of household were recorded. The white family size is estimated from the fourth U.S. census (*Census for 1820* [Washington, D.C., 1821]).

Fertility Measured by Age-Specific Marital Fertility Rates

A more sophisticated measure of fertility addresses how fertility levels fluctuated. What did married women experience when birthrates were high? How did the behaviors of married couples change as fertility levels fell? What happens if differing mortality levels and ages at marriage are eliminated from the calculations? Age-specific marital fertility rates measure the childbearing experiences of married women in five-year age categories over the course of their reproductive years (births per one thousand woman years from ages fifteen to forty-nine through ages forty-five to forty-nine). These calculations avoid the pitfalls of the previous measures of fertility by assuming that all women married either on their fifteenth or twentieth birthday and remained married until the day before their fiftieth birthday and that they all bore children at the observed rates. Differences in death rates, sex ratios, and immigration have no direct impact on these numbers.

These calculations require a great deal of information: a woman's age, the date of marriage, the exact birthdates of all children, and, in most studies, the dates of death for children and spouses. These details must first be collected for individual nuclear families either from genealogies or from religious records through a process known as family reconstitution, the collation of birth, marriage, and burial records to provide an outline of the behavior and experiences of these families. Once the family's history is reconstituted, childbearing experiences can then be explored. The summation of the experiences of many reconstituted families provides a detailed look at the average experience of those under study and, presumably, of the larger population from which the study group of families is drawn.

Age-specific marital fertility rates have been calculated for a number of early American communities. The oldest of these studies, upon which many later investigations were modeled, is Robert V. Wells's study of 216 Quaker families in New York, New Jersey, and Pennsylvania, most from rural areas or small towns. Louise Kantrow investigated 149 families living between 1680 and 1900 who descended from a handful of wealthy colonial forebears. These interrelated families were largely of British origin and Quaker or Anglican in religion and selected by sociologist Digby Baltzell as members of the Philadelphia elite. Another study of Philadelphia, covering the period from 1720 to 1830, includes Anglican, Quaker, Presbyterian, German Lutheran, German Reformed, and Swedish Lutheran families, cross-classified by the husband's occupation. The upper sorts were merchants and professionals, some few as wealthy as Kantrow's gentry, but most not. The middling sorts were artisans and shopkeepers, and the lower sorts were laborers and the poor. In total, there were 744 married couples and 4,286 births. Reconstituted from genealogies by Robert Cohen are 300 Ashkenazi and Sephardic Jewish families residing in Philadelphia, New York, Newport, Charleston, and Savannah, circa 1700–1860. The Jewish population was a tiny proportion of the total during these years. Another tiny group was the 29 free Afro-Dutch families living in New York and northern New Jersey between 1650 and 1774, who can be studied thanks to a careful genealogy prepared by Henry Hoff. It was an unusual population: free, Dutch-speaking, Calvinist, and of African heritage. Rodger C. Henderson has reconstructed the life histories of 1,378 families in rural Lancaster County, Pennsylvania, between 1710 and 1840, most Moravian, Lutheran, Reformed, Quaker, or Presbyterian. In addition, Kristin Senecal has studied 301 Presbyterian, Episcopalian, and United Church of Christ congregants from Cumberland County, Pennsylvania, between 1800 and 1859.[18]

Because of the strict evidentiary requirements, these studies cover relatively small populations (in total, more than twenty-five hundred marriages) and may not be representative of the total regional or American population (this is especially true for nineteenth-century urban population rates), nor are they comprehensive investigations of whole communities or of the region. Some faiths are not included. Many individuals did not belong to a church or did not baptize their children as infants and are therefore difficult to track. Poorer people were often unable to pay for baptisms or burials and were sometimes hesitant to ask for charity. Highly mobile families were

18. Robert Vale Wells, "A Demographic Analysis of Some Middle Colony Quaker Families of the Eighteenth Century" (Ph.D. diss., Princeton University, 1969); Wells, "Family Size and Fertility Control in Eighteenth-Century America: A Study of Quaker Families," *Population Studies*, XXV (1971), 73–82; Louise Kantrow, "Philadelphia Gentry: Fertility and Family Limitation among an American Aristocracy," *Population Studies*, XXXIV (1980), 21–30; Susan E. Klepp, *Philadelphia in Transition: A Demographic History of the City and Its Occupational Groups, 1720–1830* (New York, 1989); and Robert Cohen, "Jewish Demography in the Eighteenth Century: A Study of London, the West Indies, and Early America" (Ph.D. diss., Brandeis University, 1976). Afro-Dutch rates were calculated by the author from Henry B. Hoff, "A Colonial Black Family in New York and New Jersey: Pieter Santomee and His Descendants," *Journal of the Afro-American Historical and Genealogical Society*, IX (1988), 101–134; and Hoff, "Additions and Corrections to 'A Colonial Black Family in New York and New Jersey: Pieter Santomee and His Descendants,'" ibid., X (1989), 158–160. See also Rodger C. Henderson, "Demographic Patterns and Family Structure in Eighteenth-Century Lancaster County, Pennsylvania," *PMHB*, CXIV (1990), 349–383; Henderson, *Community Development and the Revolutionary Transition in Eighteenth-Century Lancaster County, Pennsylvania* (New York, 1989); and Kristin Senecal, "Marriage and Fertility Patterns in Cumberland County, 1800–1859," *Pennsylvania History*, LXXI (2004), 191–211.

less likely to be captured by researchers than families with strong roots in a particular place. Illegitimate or enslaved children were rarely counted, and their births usually went unrecorded. Childless couples left fewer tracks in the records. There is no easy way of weighting these studies to provide for the possible unrepresentativeness of these samples; too little is known of the characteristics of the whole population. Yet, despite the shortcomings of the surviving record, the pooling of individual calculations of age-specific marital fertility rates gives valuable details not available in other sources and illuminates trends that larger-scale studies can only suggest.

In the colonial period, age-specific birthrates were not so very far from the highest ever recorded—the women in the Hutterite religious community of the early-twentieth-century northern Great Plains, who, if they married at fifteen and lived to fifty, bore fourteen children on average. No other large population is known to have equaled these rates. If a colonial woman had married on her fifteenth birthday and if she bore children at the observed rates, she would have had just over eleven children if she lived in the city, twelve in the country—two or three fewer than Hutterite women (Figures 8 and 9, Tables 6–13). Most colonial women did not marry at so early an age. Marrying at age twenty instead of fifteen meant two fewer children on average in all groups. Still, even nine or ten births are a considerable number. Colonial women did not match Hutterite women in part because eighteenth-century women were far less healthy. Sterility-inducing diseases like tuberculosis and syphilis were common. Women's medical practices (discussed in Chapter 5) also influenced fertility rates.[19]

In real life, although bearing nine or more children was not uncommon and not even cause for comment, the average Philadelphia woman gave birth six times during her life; the farm woman, seven times. She was able to do so in part by marrying for the first time at an average age of twenty-one and a half years, not at twenty. In addition, in real life, as opposed to statistical reconstructions, not all marriages lasted until the eve of the woman's fiftieth birthday; death or desertion might intervene.

From the individual community studies that make up the colonial statistics (see Appendix), it appears that Philadelphia's gentry, the largely urban Jewish communities, and the chiefly German inhabitants of Lancaster County had the largest families. In these groups, marriage age was one factor. Gentry, German, and Jewish women married earlier than the average

---

19. Charles Wetherell, "Another Look at Coale's Indices of Fertility, I_f and I_g," *Social Science History*, XXV (2001), 589–608.

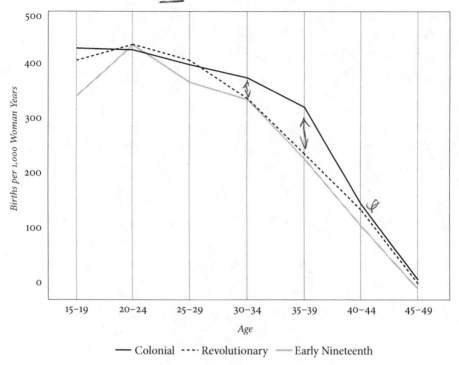

FIGURE 8.

Urban Age-Specific Marital Fertility Rates

Births per 1,000 Woman Years

Age

—— Colonial ---- Revolutionary ——— Early Nineteenth

Drawn by Kimberly Foley. See Appendix, Tables 6, 8, 9, 10, 11, 12.

and, therefore, spent a larger portion of their lives bearing children. Among the very wealthy, the use of wet nurses probably also served to raise fertility, since the period of postpartum subfecundity produced by breast-feeding would be reduced. Shortened periods of breast-feeding might have been another cause of higher fertility in the colonies. The villagers in Colyton, England, managed to wait an average of thirty months between the births of their first and second child; the French, twenty-four months. Yet, for colonial American Jews and American Quakers, the interval was only twenty-one months; for Philadelphia gentry, it was twenty-two months.

Minority groups in a sometimes hostile environment, like the Jews and the Germans, might have promoted higher fertility to redress the imbalance in numbers. Abigaill Franks worried that there were no eligible marriage partners for her daughters, finding "noe prospect of it here." She was devastated when, soon after, a daughter and a son married outside the faith. Other families faced similar problems. Small numbers, scattered settlements,

FIGURE 9.

Rural Age-Specific Marital Fertility Rates

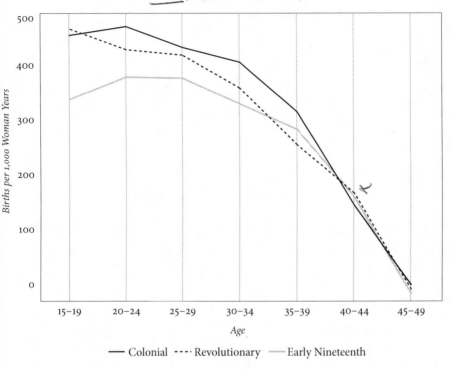

Drawn by Kimberly Foley. See Appendix, Tables 6, 8, 9, 10, 11, 12.

threats from the Spanish and French empires and from native Americans, linguistic barriers, and, perhaps, cultural conservatism might have encouraged pro-natalism.[20]

Surprisingly, given popular beliefs to the contrary, it was the poorest urban couples who had the smallest families. A number of factors might have been involved. In general, those in comfortable circumstances were healthier than poorer people. Those who could not easily afford firewood, tightly chinked houses, adequate clothing, fresh milk, meat, vegetables, and other practical stuffs were unable to weather the many endemic and epidemic diseases prevalent in the eighteenth century. Impoverished women could not call on

20. John Bongaarts, "Why High Birth Rates Are So Low," *Population and Development Review*, I (1975), 289–296; Cohen, "Jewish Demography," table 7.3, 123; Kantrow, "Philadelphia Gentry," *Population Studies*, XXXIV (1980), table 8, 28; Leo Hershkowitz and Isidore S. Meyer, eds., *The Lee Max Friedman Collection of American Jewish Colonial Correspondence: Letters of the Franks Family (1733–1748)*, Studies in American Jewish History, V (Waltham, Mass., 1968), 110.

TABLE 2.

Urban and Rural Age-Specific Marital Fertility Rates:
Summaries and Supplemental Data

	URBAN			RURAL		
Category	Colonial (N=230)	Rev. (N=572)	19th Century (N=201)	Colonial (N=346)	Rev. (N=428)	19th Century (N=963)
Total fertility (no. of births) at ages 20–49	9.2	8.6	8.1	9.7	9.0	8.4
% births by age 35	69.8%	73.7%	75.2%	71.9%	72.1%	69.6%
Actual no. of children	6.2	5.9	5.8	7.0	6.5	6.3
Mean age, first marriage	21.5	22.4	21.9	21.6	22.4	22.7
Mean age at last birth	40.0	38.5	37.6	38.9	37.3	37.6
Childbearing years	18.5	16.1	15.7	17.3	14.9	14.9

Note: Total fertility is the number of births married women might have had if they all married on their twentieth birthdays and remained married until the eve of their fiftieth birthdays, giving birth at observed rates. It allows fertility to be studied independently of differences in nuptiality and mortality. The actual number of births does not attempt to compensate for earlier or later marriages or for the early deaths of wives or husbands. Childbearing years indicates the number of years from marriage to last birth.

Sources: See Note 18. Barbara A. Anderson and Brian D. Silver, "A Simple Measure of Fertility Control," *Demography,* XXIX (1992), 343–356. For details, see Tables 6–13.

the services of doctors, midwives, nurses, pharmacists, servants, washer-women, and others to tend to the sick and to women in labor or to clean their houses and apparel. They could not afford to summer in the country, away from the heat and stench of city streets. The poor suffered from inadequate diets, exposure to the elements, and heavy labor. Miscarriages must have been common. Perhaps most important, the poorest city residents married late because many had been bound servants in their youth—indentured servants, redemptioners, apprentices, or slaves. Husbands were often absent, either tramping about searching for work or working as sailors, fishermen, draymen, farmhands, soldiers, or casual laborers on infrastructure projects such as cutting roads, digging canals, or ditching and draining swamps. Poorer women, both black and white, might also have been the earliest to deliberately limit births to better provide for a few children. A study of rural New York State found that agricultural workers' families had low fertility levels compared to the families of craftsmen and white-collar and blue-collar workers in the first half of the nineteenth century. Still, limited evidence suggests the poorest women and men were situated like Americans during the Great Depression of the 1930s: miserable conditions and anxiety about the future forced birthrates below desired levels. By the second half of the nineteenth century, the poor had the highest birthrates. How this change occurred needs more study.[21]

Although the base numbers are small for the poorer sort of colonists, the results correspond to Gregory King's 1688 census for England: English merchants, officeholders, and lawyers, the equivalents of the colonial elite, are estimated to have had households of 6 to 8 persons, including servants. Farmers and shopkeepers, the backbone of the middling sort of people, had 4.5 to 5.5 persons in the average household. The families of laboring people, seamen, and soldiers contained only 2 to 3.5 persons. When contemporaries equated children with wealth, they were correct. Wealthier women married younger, were more likely to employ wet nurses, and were healthier. The rich had many children, both their own and, as servants, those of poorer families. Poor parents often spent their youth in service, were physically stressed, and were often unable to feed the children that they did bear. Those children were placed in other situations, usually as servants. Small families also resulted from low fecundity, high mortality, and fragile family ties. This association of plentiful children with wealth and of small families with poverty was a powerful disincentive to the adoption of family limitation practices. Who would want to be associated with penury?[22]

High fertility rates began to moderate and then decline during the upheavals of the Revolution. Age-specific fertility rates show how that happened. Couples can employ three main strategies to limit the number of offspring: "starting," "spacing," and "stopping." They can reduce childbearing

---

21. Billy G. Smith, The "Lower Sort": Philadelphia's Laboring People, 1750–1800 (Ithaca, N.Y., 1990); Simon P. Newman, Embodied History: The Lives of the Poor in Early Philadelphia (Philadelphia, 2003); Michael R. Haines and Avery M. Guest, "Fertility in New York State in the Pre–Civil War Era," Demography, XLV (2008), 345–361, esp. 358.

22. "Gregory King's Scheme of the Income and Expense of the Several Families of England Calculated for the Year 1688," reproduced in Peter Laslett, The World We Have Lost (New York, 1965), 32–33.

by delaying marriage for one or many years. They therefore delay the start of family formation. They can lengthen the intervals between all births, or they can concentrate childbearing into the first few years of marriage. These are spacing tactics. Or, they can stop childbearing well before menopause forces an end to childbearing careers. Most demographers consider the third strategy, ending childbearing early, as the only real evidence of deliberate family planning, because it implies that couples have agreed upon an ideal family size and have planned accordingly. No longer is fertility left to chance (what demographers misleadingly call "natural" fertility), but, rather, conscious decisions are made concerning reproduction. Others, however, give more credit to spacing and timing behaviors as forms of rationalized family limitation.[23]

The evidence from the revolutionary and postrevolutionary era in the Mid-Atlantic region shows that all three strategies were being employed. Both in the city and in the countryside, childbearing was delayed as marriage ages rose for women in the early Republic. Women were entering motherhood somewhat later, often spending more time in school or earning wages in domestic service. By the postwar period, average marriage ages rose by nearly a full year in the city and in the countryside by almost half a year. (The marriage ages for the nineteenth century are unrepresentative.)

Moreover, Philadelphia women were clearly planning their childbearing careers by concentrating childbearing in the early years of marriage (particularly the poorest residents) and by reducing childbearing in their thirties through both spacing and stopping behaviors, quite modern tactics that demographers have traditionally regarded as proof of family planning. Rural women did not follow the same pattern. Rather than having most of their children in their early twenties, they reduced fertility in every age category. The age at which women had their last child, both in the city and in the countryside, fell by a year and a half to thirty-eight and a half. The amount of time between a woman's marriage and her last child fell by two years in the new Republic.

Despite these innovative alterations in childbearing, neither the total fer-

23. A few examples of studies that emphasize starting and stopping behaviors are Jan Van Bavel, "Detecting Stopping and Spacing Behaviour in Historical Demography: A Critical Review of Methods," *Population* (English ed.), LIX (2004), 117–128; Alfred Perrenoud, "Espacement et arrêt dans le contrôle des naissances," *Annales de démographie historique 1988* (Paris, 1989), 59–78; and Wally Seccombe, "Starting to Stop: Working-Class Fertility Decline in Britain," *Past and Present*, no. 126 (February 1991), 151–188. But not all agree; see, for example, Simon Szreter and Eilidh Garrett, "Reproduction, Compositional Demography, and Economic Growth: Family Planning in England Long before the Fertility Decline," *Population and Development Review*, XXVI (2000), 45–80.

tility rate (the number of children born to women ages fifteen to forty-nine or twenty to forty-nine) nor the actual number of children fell as much as the age at last birth or the amount of time devoted to childbearing between marriage and the last child. City women were still bearing around six children, and rural women, six and a half. These numbers may indicate the limitations of the available methods of birth control as well as ignorance or inaccessibility of effective birth-control techniques. Yet, as two demographers have argued, "an increasing trend in the proportion of births that occur by age 35 can signal increasing control even before the total fertility rate falls substantially." By this standard, more married couples in the city were practicing family planning. The proportion of births under age thirty-five increased from 68 to 74 percent. There was only a slight increase among rural women. Either fewer rural women were limiting births, or they were unable or unwilling to concentrate childbearing into the early years of marriage, preferring spacing strategies across their childbearing years.[24]

In this composite view of multiple studies of age-specific fertility, it appears that wives and husbands in the era of the American Revolution were employing an indirect approach to family limitation by delaying marriage. Some were also taking a gradualist approach by spacing births farther apart, especially in the countryside, and, at least in the city, by clustering births before age thirty-five. These strategies, accompanied by the more radical policy of stopping childbearing earlier (up to a decade before menopause), thus curtailed the number of years women spent in childbearing. Women, especially urban women of middling or upper-middling ranks, were moving toward making birthing and infant care a life stage rather than the commitment of a full lifetime.

Not all inhabitants behaved alike in the new nation. Resistance to new fertility practices appears strongest among the gentry, those wealthiest Philadelphians who, ironically, left the bulk of contemporary commentary on personal family matters. The extant written record may well underestimate the interest in new fertility strategies. The urban elite might have been reluctant to reduce fertility because they could easily afford many children and had nursemaids to do the most laborious (and smelly) tasks of infant care, because an interest in maintaining a lineage was stronger among this segment of the population (sociologist Digby Baltzell certainly thought so), or because this group was socially and politically more conservative than others.

24. Barbara A. Anderson and Brian D. Silver, "A Simple Measure of Fertility Control," *Demography*, XXIX (1992), 343–356, esp. 353.

It was, not the elite, but the urban middling sort that led the way in fertility reduction.

Other groups adopted some, but not all, of these techniques to reduce fertility. Jewish women, many of whom were the wives of merchants and petty traders, were waiting substantially longer to marry than had previous generations, perhaps because of a shortage of eligible partners or perhaps to reduce fertility, but they continued to bear children later than any other group. The upper sorts in Philadelphia, the wives of lesser merchants and professionals, also delayed marriage. In addition, these women had their last birth a year and a half earlier than colonial women of similar status. They combined a truncated childbearing career with a dramatic increase in the proportion of births before age thirty-five. Both Jewish and upper-sort women managed to reduce the average number of births by one and a half, whereas the gentry averaged a decline only half as large.

The behavior of the poor ran in the opposite direction during and after the Revolution. The very poorest urban residents married more than two years earlier than their colonial counterparts and slightly increased the number of actual births from 4.2 to 4.4. The waning of bound labor was a major factor and affected some of the middling sort as well. No longer were the poor so likely to be indentured during adolescence and early adulthood. Wage labor was just beginning to replace the strictures of bound servitude, giving young adults enough income to form an independent household, but not much opportunity for later advancement or economic independence through shop-ownership, a phenomenon that affected some middling-sort Philadelphians as well as the poor. Still, high death rates among the least-advantaged adults shortened marriages and kept actual family size well below the hypothetical experience of the woman who married at age fifteen and remained married until fifty. A similar but more moderated pattern characterized rural Cumberland County in the nineteenth century. Merchants and professionals averaged 6.7 children ever born, whereas farmers, artisans, and laborers averaged 6.4. Social status certainly affected fertility.[25]

The experience of the urban poor bears a passing resemblance to that of their English contemporaries. In England, marriage ages were falling and fertility and family sizes were rising as more food, more pregnancies carried to term, wage labor, imperial ventures, and the early stages of industrialization were transforming social relations and encouraging higher fertility. To a lesser degree, the same forces were at work in the northern cities of the early

25. Senecal, "Marriage and Fertility Patterns," *Pennsylvania History*, LXXI (2004), table 6, 206.

Republic. Indentured servitude was less common for whites, apprenticeships were more flexible, and journeyman (wage) labor was more often a permanent condition than a brief transitional status before becoming a master. Many of the middling and poorer sort also were English immigrants who brought late-eighteenth-century English ways to the colonies. As Thomas Robert Malthus observed in England, when "the situation of the labourer [becomes] tolerably comfortable, the restraints to population are in some degree loosened." Probably true, at least early in the lives of young married couples. In middle age, however, large families, sickness, and economic downturns could easily tip families into a miserable poverty. But the poorest Philadelphians did not, for the most part, have large families. They were as adept as their wealthier contemporaries in spacing births and in concentrating births before age thirty-five. If these small numbers are roughly accurate indicators of a high-fertility gentry class and a low-fertility lower-class system, what does it mean that in early America the urban poor were incapable of reproducing themselves? With low reproductive rates and high mortality, the growth or even the persistence of poverty must have come from some combination of downward mobility and immigration.[26]

Free Afro-Dutch families had the lowest fertility of any group so far studied in the early United States. They married later than every group but the Jews. They bore their last child at age thirty-eight and a half—later than most contemporaries. They did not concentrate childbearing into the earliest years of marriage, but achieved long intervals between births across a woman's childbearing years. African customs of lengthy breast-feeding might have been employed by these women. Slave masters often resented or forbade any activity, like childcare, that interfered with women's labor, but these free women could have revived the customary practices. Nursing was a continual point of contention between southern slave women and masters and probably was for their counterparts in the North as well. Like poor whites, former slaves and free people of African descent had few children, but those of African descent were less likely to employ stopping behaviors. Instead, they proved to be the most adept of any Americans at maintaining long intervals between births. The scattered information available on Afri-

26. E. A. Wrigley, "Explaining the Rise in Marital Fertility in England in the 'Long' Eighteenth Century," *Economic History Review*, n.s., LI (1998), 435–464; David Levine, *Family Formation in an Age of Nascent Capitalism* (New York, 1977); Jona Schellekens, "Nuptiality during the First Industrial Revolution in England: Explanations," *JIH*, XXVII (1996–1997), 637–654; Thomas Robert Malthus, "An Essay on the Principle of Population [1798]," in Scott W. Menard and Elizabeth W. Moen, eds., *Perspectives on Population: An Introduction to Concepts and Issues* (New York, 1987), 100.

can Americans in the middle states points to high fertility under slavery and rapidly falling fertility in the state of semifreedom that was the lot of people who were generally the poorest of Americans.[27]

In rural areas, one group was behaving like the urbanites. Quakers were relatively prosperous, but few of those studied by Robert Wells lived in Philadelphia or New York City. Women Friends from small towns and farms in New Jersey and New York surpassed even urban women in increasing the proportion of births before age thirty-five. Indeed, these women had their last birth earlier than any of their contemporaries. As a consequence, childbearing took up a smaller portion of Quaker women's lives than it did with that of any other women of their time. The independent position of Quaker women within the faith was undoubtedly a factor—it seems to have been especially strong in New York during the war, causing "a significant increase in the number of mavericks, particularly women, who defied parent and religious community to follow their own inclination." Quaker women also enjoyed an institutionalized space in the monthly, quarterly, and yearly meetings for business. They met together to supervise marriages, to dispense charity, and, increasingly, to run schools. These formal roles contributed to an active sociability that expanded women's opportunities and contacts and facilitated the diffusion of innovative ideas. Non-Quakers in the countryside had a very different experience. Lancaster County women exhibited little change in childbearing between the colonial period and the early nineteenth century.[28]

The question of ethnic differences is unaddressed in the literature on early American fertility, but the evidence from these scattered studies suggests that it was an extremely significant factor: dominant groups were more likely to adopt innovative ideas on procreation; minorities were reluctant. For example, there is some evidence that German-speaking women did not participate in the diffusion of new ideas on reduced family size. Among the Moravians in Bethlehem, Pennsylvania, total marital fertility rates followed a very different path from that exhibited by other groups. Women ages twenty to forty-nine averaged 8.0 children in the colonial period, falling to 6.5 during the Revolution and rising to 7.6 in the early Republic and then to 7.8 in the

27. Sharla M. Fett, *Working Cures: Healing, Health, and Power on Southern Slave Plantations* (Chapel Hill, N.C., 2002), 194; Marie Jenkins Schwartz, *Birthing a Slave: Motherhood and Medicine in the Antebellum South* (Cambridge, Mass., 2006), 94–95, 224–225.

28. Judith L. Van Buskirk, *Generous Enemies: Patriots and Loyalists in Revolutionary New York* (Philadelphia, 2002), 68.

first three decades of the nineteenth century. Postwar Moravian fertility rates never quite reached colonial levels, but the postwar rise was far more sustained than a transient baby boom would have been. Moravian experiences are not easily translated into general practice, since the increase in fertility coincides with a shift from communal, sex-segregated living arrangements to nuclear families.[29]

The studies of nineteenth-century age-specific marital fertility rates suffer either from being even more unrepresentative of the total population than the studies of the eighteenth century or from using assumptions that make them incompatible with other studies. Urban fertility rates show a decrease across all age categories and an especially pronounced rise in the proportion of births occurring before age thirty-five. These figures are, however, based on two minority populations. Neither the gentry nor the Jewish populations are likely to have been typical. What the average woman was experiencing over the course of her childbearing years has yet to be investigated. Figures for the rural population include Kristin Senecal's study of Cumberland County, Pennsylvania. The author has counted children from the husband's first marriage as well as those from subsequent marriages. Other studies consider only the wife's first marriage. Since people embarking on a second or third marriage behave like other newlyweds and commonly start expanding their families as soon as they are married, the Cumberland fertility rates may exaggerate births in later-age categories and make the proportion of births by age thirty-five appear regressive. Still, total marital fertility levels fall in these studies of nineteenth-century rural fertility. Senecal's study of Cumberland County offers the most sophisticated analysis of birth intervals by birth parity. She found that spacing strategies were employed from the first birth in low-fertility families and not employed at any stage in households with many children. Couples were either actively restricting births or they were not.

Married couples in the countryside were restricting fertility with increasing success, and by the nineteenth century more couples than ever were practicing family limitation. The scattered studies of rural areas suggest that ethnic and linguistic differences were a major factor affecting marital fertility, but there was no single path to lower fertility, nor was fertility reduction in-

---

29. Beverly Prior Smaby, *The Transformation of Moravian Bethlehem: From Communal Mission to Family Economy* (Philadelphia, 1988), calculated from table 2-6, 74. Age-specific rates are not available.

evitable. Most studies suggest a multiplicity of behaviors and strategies behind the decline in birthrates, child-woman ratios, and marital fertility.

SIMPLE AVERAGES OF FAMILY size from wills and baptismal records, crude birthrates, child-woman ratios, age-specific marital fertility rates, the proportion of births before age thirty-five: each calculation has its problems, and each has certain strengths. But, as various as these results are, they point to similar conclusions. On the whole, most married women bore large numbers of children in the colonial era, even if overall birthrates and child-woman ratios were relatively low because substantial segments of the population were too young to have children, were bound laborers required by contract to remain celibate, or, if male, were unable to find a spouse. Sex ratios became more even by the mid-eighteenth century as the population matured. A greater proportion of the population was free, adult, and married. Family size remained large. The peak in fertility occurred during the last years of the Seven Years' War, bringing international attention to the fecundity of colonial women and men.

Then, during and after the Revolution, average family sizes began shrinking. Crude birthrates were trending downward in Philadelphia by the 1760s and in rural areas after the 1770s. African Americans reduced fertility levels substantially in the shift from enslavement to freedom. For many free Americans in the early national period, the proportion of births before age thirty-five was rising. Among those women who did embrace the new ideal, the evidence strongly suggests that they were using every tactic available to accomplish family limitation. The majority were putting off childbearing by marrying somewhat later than colonial women. They were spacing births both to limit childbearing and, particularly in the city, to concentrate childbearing into the earliest years of marriage. Almost all women were stopping childbearing at ever earlier ages.

It was the moderately wealthy and middling sort in the city, and the Quakers in the countryside, who appear to have been the leaders in adopting family-planning strategies. English-speakers, members of mainstream religious groups, easterners, and city dwellers were most amenable to innovation. The very poorest Americans, both free white and free black, had very low fertility, perhaps depressed below their own goals. Certain minorities, including the very wealthiest Philadelphians, slaves, and the rural German and urban Jewish communities, nineteenth-century immigrants, and isolated settlers on western frontiers all lagged behind other groups in implementing family planning in the wake of the American Revolution.

Too little is known about the language, ethnicity, religious affiliation, or status of the majority of early Americans. The statistics are intriguing and give some hints about the behavior, if not the goals, of individuals who otherwise left little record of their thoughts and hopes. German, Dutch, Swedish, and African women in the Middle Colonies left almost no indication of their thoughts on fecundity, family limitation, or birth-control practices. Even among English-speakers little has survived, especially from the poorer sort or rural women. But as protests against taxes and representation roiled the Middle Colonies, almanacs, letters, diaries, paintings, and more indicate that women's fecundity was being rethought. J. P. Brissot and Benjamin Rush both might have wanted to affirm high fertility in the revolutionary Republic, but increasing numbers of American women and men had other ideas. It is to those ideas that we will now turn.

2

Old Ways and New

"Colonies," wrote proprietor and promoter William Penn in 1681, "are the Seeds of Nations . . . best for the increase of Humane Stock." According to Penn, Europe was hovering on the brink of ruin because unemployment levels were rising and wages were falling. Far too many men could not afford to marry. Private morality was being undermined by the poverty and rootlessness of these miserable men. The prevalence of vice caused population to stagnate, since many men "chuse rather to vend their Lusts at an evil Ordinary [tavern] than honestly Marry." The "great Debauchery in this Kingdom" even "rendred many unfruitfull when married." But all was not lost. In coming to the colonies, those "that were but low here [in England], if not poor; [become] now Masters of Families," thereby increasing population, trade, and wealth for themselves and for the entire Empire. Colonies would not drain population from the mother country. Instead, imperial ventures would provide opportunities for underemployed and desperate men to become masters of households and to breed both valuable commodities and hardworking children.[1]

From the very beginning of European exploration, proprietors and entrepreneurs enticed settlers to the Middle Atlantic region by touting the fertility of the land; it was, for example, "very good and fruitfull and withall very healthfull." Plentiful, flourishing land was made redolent of an expansive

---

1. "Some Account of the Province of Pennsilvania, by William Penn, 1681," in Albert Cook Myers, ed., *Narratives of Early Pennsylvania, West New Jersey, and Delaware, 1630-1707,* Original Narratives of Early American History (New York, 1912), 202–206, esp. 202, 205, and 206.

abundance in all facets of life. Promotional tracts generally targeted men, but several enticed women to cross the ocean. "Barrenness among Women," wrote Gabriel Thomas at the end of the seventeenth century, was "hardly to be heard of, nor are old Maids to be met with; for all commonly Marry before they are Twenty Years of Age, and seldom any young Married Woman but hath a Child in her Belly, or one upon her Lap." A half century later, another writer made virtually the same observation: every household "is full of children" and, "whenever one meets a woman, she is either pregnant, or carries a child in her arms, or leads one by the hand." The promoters of empire promised young women an escape from the dismal possibility of years of servile drudgery in the households of strangers. They could instead move to the colonies and become the mistresses of large families. Of course, this idyllic account ignores the enforced celibacy and labor of the intermediate step of indentured servitude that most young immigrants faced.[2]

The emphasis on American fertility persisted beyond the founding. A slippage between the productivity of women and the productivity of agriculture can be seen in Israel Acrelius's 1756 account of Pennsylvania: "The country is undeniably fruitful, as may be judged from the following examples: Joseph Cobern . . . had the blessing to have his wife have twins, his cow two calves, and his ewe two lambs, all on one night." His wife, his cow, his ewe: all redounded to the blessing of their owner and the reputation of the country. In the city, a Lutheran minister remarked that "a favorite bitch in the house had three puppies and a catt three kittens" and that a robin's egg hatched just before his daughter was born. This "singular" and "mysterious" abundance was worth recording (although the state of his wife was not). When William Logan replied to his brother-in-law's teasing in 1764, "I am Obliged to thee for thy desires of my hav[in]g more Children as I am for thy Banter about my Great Estate," both men assumed the equivalency of children and wealth. Before the Revolution, women "produced" children, and childbearing was labeled generation or procreation. Women's bodies had created abundance and a symbolic, if not always actual, form of wealth.[3]

2. "Relation of Captain Thomas Yong, 1634," in Myers, ed., *Narratives of Early Pennsylvania*, 31–49, esp. 48; "An Historical and Geographical Account of Pensilvania and of West-New-Jersey, by Gabriel Thomas, 1698," ibid., 307–352, esp. 333; Gottlieb Mittelberger, *Journey to Pennsylvania*, ed. and trans. Oscar Handlin and John Clive (Cambridge, Mass., 1960), 81.

3. Israel Acrelius, *Description of the Former and Present Condition of the Swedish Churches, in What Was Called New Sweden . . .* (1759), in Acrelius, *A History of New Sweden* (1874; rpt. Ann Arbor, Mich., 1966), 156; Rev. Andrew [Anders] Goeransson, Baptism of Mary and Elizabeth Goeransson, Aug. 14, 1777, Gloria Dei Lutheran Church Baptismal Records, I, 186, Historical Society of

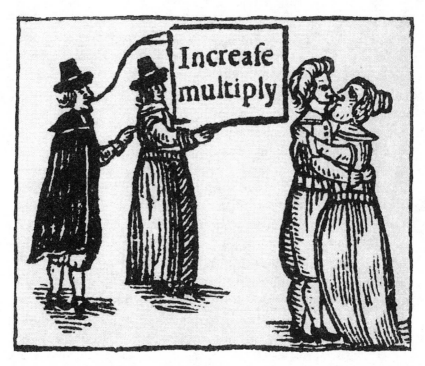

PLATE 2.

Increase multiply. A seventeenth-century woodcut
from an unknown source, reproduced in Mary Cable, *American
Manners and Morals: A Picture History of How We Behaved
and Misbehaved* (New York, 1969), 24.

Traditionally, high fertility was encouraged.

Even before substantial European settlement had occurred, Englishmen imagined a future where procreative restraints would be removed and population would flourish. They were not far from the truth. Colonial American crude birthrates were substantially higher than those in Europe, and almost double those in England. Benjamin Franklin followed Penn in pointing to the importance of land availability in encouraging both marriage and America's population growth. The more facetious laughed at the differences between the Old World and the New. Rosalie Stier Calvert urged her childless brother and his wife back in Germany to pay her a visit because "I am sure he would

Pennsylvania, Philadelphia; William Logan to John Smith, 5th day morning, circa 1764, John Smith Correspondence, 1740–1770, HSP.

not return without a young American." Yet American fertility rates began to fall by the end of the eighteenth century. What were the economic, religious, and political contexts in which women and men reassessed family size?[4]

Women and Gender

British colonists might have imagined a wealth of children, but they did not intend to otherwise change familiar cultural patterns in settling the New World. Colonists reproduced, as much as possible, the traditional, subordinate feminine roles of servant, wife, mother, and mistress over servants that dominated in the Old World. Religious belief, ethnicity, and status provided many variations within these roles for women in the Middle Colonies. Quaker women might be called to preach, but other women could not. Married women under Dutch law and custom had greater property rights than the English. A few German women's medical talents earned them the title of "Doctor." The only title free or enslaved African American women were granted was the demeaning term "wench": they were not considered respectable goodwives, let alone ladies, no matter what their condition. German and most enslaved women did fieldwork, which was considered unsuitable among the English except at harvest time. Women of the middling sort tended to have skills that could support a meager economic independence; poor women did not. However various tasks might be gendered as male or female in specific subcultures, and however belief, geography, and settlement patterns might alter experience, the similarities in women's lives were greater than the differences.[5]

4. Alfred Owen Aldridge, "Franklin as Demographer," *Journal of Economic History*, IX (1949), 25–44; Margaret Law Callcott, ed., *Mistress of Riversdale: The Plantation Letters of Rosalie Stier Calvert, 1795–1821* (Baltimore, 1991), 122. More negative analyses of American population growth are discussed in Gilbert Chinard, "Eighteenth Century Theories on America as a Human Habitat," American Antiquarian Society, *Proceedings*, XCI (1947), 27–57.

5. Cathy Matson, ed., "Special Forum: Women's Economies in North America before 1820," *Early American Studies*, IV (2006), 271–470; Rebecca Larson, *Daughters of Light: Quaker Women Preaching and Prophesying in the Colonies and Abroad, 1700–1775* (New York, 1999); Marilyn J. Westerkamp, *Women and Religion in Early America, 1600–1850: The Puritan and Evangelical Traditions* (New York, 1999); Karin Wulf, *Not All Wives: Women of Colonial Philadelphia* (Ithaca, N.Y., 2000); Marla R. Miller, "The Last Mantuamaker: Craft Tradition and Commercial Change in Boston, 1760–1845," *Early American Studies*, IV (2006), 372–424; Diane Rothenberg, "Mothers of the Nation: Seneca Resistance to Quaker Intervention," in Mona Etienne and Eleanor Leacock, eds., *Women and Colonization: Anthropological Perspectives* (New York, 1980), 63–87; Brendan McConville, "Conflict and Change on a Cultural Frontier: The Rise of Magdalena Valleau, Land Rioter," *Pennsylvania History: Supplement*, LXV (1998), 122–140; Lucy Simler, "'She Came to Work':

By the eighteenth century, women from the territory of Maine to the colony of Georgia were under English governance. English law stipulated that a married woman was a feme covert: she had no legal existence separate from that of her husband. Her wages, inheritances, clothes, children, even her body belonged to her husband, her lord and master. Husbandless women (spinsters, servants, slaves, widows, the abandoned) were also supposed to be under the authority of men (fathers or guardians, masters, executors or grown sons, the Overseers of the Poor) even though widows and heiresses could in fact have considerable economic independence. Older women could achieve some local authority in supervising community sexual norms by reporting transgressions to the sheriff or by giving expert testimony in criminal cases.[6]

Free and bound women engaged in gender-specific chores, especially food preparation and preservation, local marketing, gardening, poultry raising, dairying, textile and clothing production, domestic medicine, neighborhood charity, midwifery, and undertaking. They cared for their family, turned raw materials into finished products, and exchanged goods and services with neighbors. If free and of comfortable means, their "family" included servants, slaves, and day workers as well as kin. Many women took in paying boarders or travelers or sold butter, eggs, pies, jam, thread, salves, or other items, or helped neighbors at harvest to earn cash. The majority of adult women were active in raising children: for free women, as wives, or, for many enslaved women, as partners in insecure relationships likely to be sundered at any time by sale. Procreation fit with the tasks of childcare, the practical education of older daughters and servants, and the production of food and clothing, or, rather, it was the reverse: the constraints of pregnancy and nursing delimited the scope of women's lives, whether married or enslaved, rich or poor, to what could be accomplished with big bellies, swollen

---

The Female Labor Force in Chester County, 1750–1820," *Early American Studies*, V (2007), 427–453; Joan M. Jensen, *Loosening the Bonds: Mid-Atlantic Farm Women, 1750–1850* (New Haven, Conn., 1986); Alice Miler Wiles, "Susannah Rohrer Muller and Her Ancestry," Lancaster County Historical Society, *Publications*, XLI (1937), 168–172; "Mrs. Anna Maria Iserloh," in Louis A. Meier, *Early Pennsylvania Medicine: A Representative Early American Medical History* (Boyertown, Pa., 1976), 136–137. African American women did not necessarily acquiesce to insulting addresses: Elizabeth Hood and her husband filed a defamation suit against a neighbor in Bucks County, Pennsylvania, in 1745. See Rosemary Radford Ruether and Rosemary Skinner Keller, *Women and Religion in America*, II, *The Colonial and Revolutionary Periods* (San Francisco, 1983), 251–252.

6. Wulf, *Not all Wives*. For a particularly violent episode in Easton, Pennsylvania, in the 1760s, see Elizabeth F. Ellet, "The Fate of a Flirt in the Olden Time: A Real Incident," *Godey's Lady's Book*, XLIII (July 1851), 13–17.

breasts, and crying babies. Women's lives were centered on procreation and childrearing. In the language of the day, they were "the Sex," an inferior subset of humanity ideally meek, obedient, and mild, but ruled at bottom, not by reason, but by their procreative physiology.

Childbearing was welcomed throughout the Empire. Procreation, it was widely believed, produced wealth for both families and nations, particularly since children were an important source of labor and, therefore, of potential income. Women gained their husbands' approval as well as local renown by bearing as many sons as possible, even if being continually "barefoot and pregnant" foreclosed many other options and was often counterproductive—women were weakened from vitamin, calcium, and iron deficiencies after repeated pregnancies. They suffered debilitating injuries or infections during and after childbirth, and they more often died young than did men—in Lancaster County, Pennsylvania, for example, women were 40 percent more likely to die between ages fifteen and forty-five, their childbearing years, than were men—even when the battlefield casualties incurred during the wars of the second half of the eighteenth century are included. Babies were stillborn or failed to thrive when born to physically exhausted women. Infants sickened because they were weaned too early or passed on to wet nurses when their mothers were once again pregnant. Infant losses were more than one-third higher in Philadelphia's large families than in medium-sized families, even though it was the wealthiest families with the most resources that tended to have the largest number of children. Despite these serious costs of multiple pregnancies, many factors and beliefs promoted a high-fertility regime.[7]

Patriarchal assumptions and masculine identity were at stake in attitudes about fertility. Exceptionally prolific fathers gained fame. Richard Buffington, who died in 1739 at Chester, Pennsylvania, was "a patriarch indeed, [and] had assembled in his own house 115 persons of his own descendants, consisting of children, and grand and great grand children, he being then in his 85th year, in good health, and doubtless in fine spirits among so many of his own race." The ability to produce male offspring was considered particularly indicative of the strength of both a country and its men; William Penn

7. Calculations by the author from the life tables in Rodger C. Henderson, *Community Development and the Revolutionary Transition in Eighteenth Century Lancaster County, Pennsylvania* (New York, 1989), 99, 100, 185, 186, 237, 238. Completed families of 4, 5, or 6 children (considered here as medium-sized families) in Philadelphia's richest and poorest congregations (Christ Church [Episcopalian] and Gloria Dei Lutheran Church) between 1780 and 1830 experienced an infant mortality rate of 163 stillbirths or deaths in the first year of life per 1,000 births. The death rate was 224 per 1,000 persons in families of 9 or more children (large-sized), even though few of the poor had large families.

complimented Pennsylvania Swedes in 1683 by noting, "They have fine children, and almost every house full; rare to find one of them without three or four boys, and as many girls; some, six, seven, and eight sons." Conversely, it was an insult to aver low fertility. Hessian doctor Johann David Schoepff had little good to say about America in 1780 as his British allies faced losing the war, so that he found that "American women are not very prolific" is hardly surprising. "They are amazed at the fourteenth pregnancy of the queen, and, when I tell them that I know mothers with eighteen and twenty-four living children, those who accept the story at all cannot help betraying envy in the expression of their countenances." Undoubtedly people made strange faces, but Schoepff had to stretch to come to his conclusion, which was not supported elsewhere in his own writings. His comment does point to the competitive element in male attitudes on women's reproductive capacities, a competition that helped to shape local, national, and imperial identities. In private, as in public, large families were sources of pride and proof of virility for men, especially when they contained a number of sons.[8]

Having many children was ideal—Samuel Johnson's great dictionary defined the word "fertility" as abundance, not as it is currently, the capacity to reproduce, or, more technically, the actual, quantifiable rate of reproduction. Not all children were equally valuable or valued, however. Daughters were trained in housewifery and soon became valuable adjuncts to their mothers, but they would eventually leave to marry. Most women, like their husbands, favored their sons over their daughters, giving them more and better food, more clothing, and more education and other opportunities. Early in the eighteenth century, Jane Colden congratulated her son on the occasion of his wife's second pregnancy. She hoped that "by this time [her daughter-in-law is] the Joyful mother of another son" and expressed her pride that in only two years her son "should thous multiply and increas o bless the Lord." The daughter-in-law was not dignified by name, and only the birth of sons was deemed worthy of congratulation. Heads of household routinely forgot to report their youngest daughters to census takers. Even in seventeenth- and eighteenth-century family portraits, depictions of boys outnumbered those of girls by 50 percent.[9]

8. John F. Watson, *Annals of Philadelphia, and Pennsylvania, in the Olden Time* (Philadelphia, 1899), I, 599; William Penn, "Letter to the Free Society of Traders [1683]," in Jean R. Soderlund, ed., *William Penn and the Founding of Pennsylvania: A Documentary History* (Philadelphia, 1983), 317; Johann David Schoepff, *The Climate and Diseases of America*, trans. James Read Chadwick (Boston, 1875), 11 n. 1.

9. Jane Colden to Cadwallader Colden, Oct. 11, 1717, *The Letters and Papers of Cadwallader*

For both women and men in the Atlantic world, male offspring were preferred. Sons continued the family line, they might improve the family's status through an advantageous marriage, and they were expected to provide for their widowed mothers. So Francis Jones "was enriched . . . by the birth of a little son" in 1749. Of course, not even all sons were equal. The first-born son, often symbolically named after his father or paternal grandfather, headed the lineage of descendants. He commonly received a larger share of the family's estate, a better education, and more opportunities, especially in courtship and marriage. Redundant boys, then daughters, then stepchildren, then orphaned kin reflected the inequalities of a hierarchical society through their lower ranks in the family. Mothers as well as fathers endorsed this system. Colonial women and the family were not "at odds" over reproduction. Colonial women supported high fertility and were rewarded for upholding patriarchy.[10]

In the seventeenth century, a dying pregnant woman elaborated her hopes for a son and then briefly addressed her future child by asking rhetorically, "If thou beest a Daughter, thou maist perhaps thinke I have lost my labour?" That is, daughters are not worth the pains of childbearing. They were less likely to reimburse their parent's investment in their rearing because they would serve the interests of their future husband's family, and their weaker minds and passionate nature might lead them into sin and familial disgrace. But it was not just the British gentry who were concerned with maintaining patrilineal succession. Even relatively poor men sought to maintain their lineage through the birth of sons. Joseph Price, a struggling farmer, carpenter, and unsuccessful innkeeper, frequently noted the social and personal consequences of the failure to sire male offspring. An uncle "Lived and dyed in Celebacy and of Course not much Lamentations after him." Only if a man left descendents would his passing be mourned and his life memorialized. Men were also obligated to their ancestors to preserve their surname. When the last of four local brothers died in 1804, Price observed that, because they had "never married, the name [was] Lost." A few weeks later, another, more prominent neighbor's surname became "extinct" because "he had no Mail Childern nor his Brother Jos [who] had but 3 daughters . . . the hole of an

Colden, 7 vols., New-York Historical Society, *Collections,* L–LVI (New York, 1917–1923), I, 17–19; Karin Calvert, "The Family in Early American Portraiture, 1670–1810," *William and Mary Quarterly,* 3d Ser., XXXIX (1982), 89, table 1.

10. William N. Schwarze and Ralf Ridgway Hillman, trans., *The Dansbury Diaries: Moravian Travel Diaries, 1748–1755* (Camden, Maine, 1994), 68; Carl N. Degler, *At Odds: Women and the Family in America from the Revolution to the Present* (New York, 1980).

Large family has Lost the name." Personal identity and familial obligations were tied to the preservation of surnames through the male line. Political standing was also grounded in fertility. Price connected good government and good citizenship to the "Meritt" achieved by "Maintain[ing] a large family by industry." And it seemed to Price that some unmarried men behaved oddly. His comment on one "Batchlor" was that he was "ver[y] Quear and Drole." Hannah Callender concurred. She reported going to "see General Forbes funeral, a poor old Batcheler who seemed alone in a Croud, no tender ties broken, not one to drop the Funeral Tear." Marriage was expected and brought prestige as well as bonds of affection. As Bruce Dorsey has observed about free white men's notions of masculinity in the eighteenth century, "The greater number of those dependent on him, of course, the greater the independence, and hence manliness, of the man." Childless bachelors as well as sonless fathers were thus put in peculiar positions—just as George Washington was, to the consternation of "Old Lydick." Masculine success was predicated on family and fertility in general and on the production of sons in particular.[11]

The focus on procreation and large family size was also reflected in the contemporary vocabulary of pregnancy and birth. Before the American Revolution, common descriptive terms for pregnant women, used by women and men alike, were agricultural or botanical (for example, "flourishing" women, "breeding" women, "teeming" women, and, most commonly, "fruitful" women). These descriptions were suggestive of a bountiful, domesticated natural order in which agricultural production and human reproduction merged into a single vision of welcome abundance. German and Swedish speakers in Pennsylvania, as well as English speakers, employed analogous adjectives, many of which are biblical in origin.[12]

Women's writings also linked abundance in agricultural productivity and human procreation. Abigail Adams was more consciously metaphorical

11. Elizabeth Joceline, *The Mother's Legacy to Her Unborn Child* (1622; rpt. London, 1894), 8–9; Susan E. Klepp and Karin A. Wulf, eds., *The Diary of Hannah Callender: Sense and Sensibility in a Revolutionary Age, 1758–1788* (Ithaca, N.Y., 2009), Mar. 6, 1759; Bruce Dorsey, *Reforming Men and Women: Gender in the Antebellum City* (Ithaca, N.Y., 2002), 35. See also the Joseph Price Diary, esp. Sept. 7, 1794, Aug. 24, 1795, May 19, 1798, June 29, Aug. 4, Aug. 10, 1804, www.lowermerionhistory .org/texts/price/index.html (accessed October 2004).

12. Traditional metaphors were themselves unstable and had become more patriarchal in the seventeenth century. See Mary Fissell, "Gender and Generation: Representing Reproduction in Early Modern England," *Gender and History*, VII (1995), 433–456. The longevity of the basic concepts is suggested in Etienne van de Walle, "Flowers and Fruits: Two Thousand Years of Menstrual Regulation," *Journal of Interdisciplinary History*, XXVIII (1996–1997), 183–203.

(and ironic) when she commented in 1775, as war followed years of escalating conflict: "Philadelphia must be an unfertile soil, or it would not produce so many unfruitful women. . . . [but] they are certainly freed from the anxiety every parent must feel for their rising offspring." For Adams, childlessness might have been a rational response to wartime anxiety, but it was also selfish and reflected badly on both the environment and the women of the city. In 1805, Sally Hastings chastised a friend for turning down a proposal of marriage. Her friend, she asserted poetically, was getting old and would be barren like the trees of winter if she did not change her ways and marry. The husband-to-be was unimportant; the chance to have children, to bear fruit, was. Sample stanzas link seasonal cycles of fertility and infertility to women and the married state.

> Oh! hadst thou, in thy April dress,
>   Secur'd thy shining store, [that is, marriage]
> Thy fragrant shade [home] we would not miss;
>   Thy fruit [children] would charm us more!
>
> . . . .
>
> Then do not spend your spring in vain,
>   Nor let your blossoms fade,
> 'Till you secure a fruitful gain,
>   And leaves for future shade.
>
> . . . .
>
> 'Then, in old age, when others fade,'
>   Like barren leafless trees,
> You still will bloom, yield fruit and shade;
>   You'll profit, shine, and please.[13]

Hastings's assumption of profitability, rather than primitive accumulation, or the simple amassing of resources, in childbearing and in fruited trees was new, but her linkage of children, wealth, and fruitfulness was traditional. Her poem was one of the last times these metaphors would be employed, and it appeared in far western Washington County, not urban Philadelphia, where such sentiments were already old-fashioned. In 1776, Annis Boudinot Stockton's primary wish for her newlywed daughter's birthday was, "May prattling

---

13. Charles Francis Adams, ed., *Familiar Letters of John Adams and His Wife Abigail Adams, during the Revolution, with a Memoir of Mrs. Adams* (New York, 1876), 129; Sally Hastings, "To Miss Jane C——; September 29, 1805," *Poems, on Different Subjects; to Which Is Added, a Descriptive Account of a Family Tour to the West; in the Year, 1800; in a Letter to a Lady* (Lancaster, Pa., 1808), 88–90.

infants round you smile / And pay with love their mother's toil." An abundance of children was the ideal. Children's future rewards to their parents were couched in terms of love and duty, not hard cash or productive labor, and were perceived as an exchange for a mother's toil, or, more commonly, for paternal cares. Women attained consequence through their productive powers, especially as harnessed in their husbands' interests.[14]

These images of teeming, flourishing, and fruitful trees, soils, crops, livestock, and women were partially rooted in the Bible and partially in a close familiarity with agricultural production. Opposed to fertility, both for women and for farms, were barrenness, unfruitfulness, and infertility. Pregnancy was the "natural" condition of married women (although hardly without dangers and needing careful management); barrenness was unnatural. As these images related to women, they evoked an organic unity of women and pregnancy. The normative condition of women, the center of housewifery, was procreation. Sally Logan Fisher worried over every indication that she might not be pregnant and welcomed each of her nine pregnancies as a blessing despite increasing difficulties in labor and delivery. Elizabeth Coates Paschall recalled around 1750 that she "Never Expected health again" until she had cured herself "after So Long a habit of Miscarriage." Childbearing was welcomed as a sign of health and well-being. Other common terms for late pregnancy included being "lusty," in a "thriving way," or Esther Edwards Burr's self-description: "very comforttable state of helth—I suppose more Fleshey an Fresh than ever you saw me."[15]

14. Ludmilla Jordanova, "Interrogating the Concept of Reproduction in the Eighteenth Century," in Ginsburg and Rapp, eds., *Conceiving the New World Order*, 369; "To Mrs Rush on Her Birth Day" (Mar. 2, 1776), in Carla Mulford, *Only for the Eye of a Friend: The Poems of Annis Boudinot Stockton* (Charlottesville, Va., 1995), 96. Cash flows seem to have gone from parents to children even before the fertility transition, at least in some segments of the population. Among rural Quaker farmers, child-centered families meant that children were expenses, rather than sources of income. See Barry Levy, *Quakers and the American Family: British Settlement in the Delaware Valley* (New York, 1988). Among Lutherans, farmers on small holdings (twenty to ninety-nine acres) were likely to keep adult sons working on the family farm, but they were a minority: most farmers had more acreage and had servants or cottagers as laborers. See Susan Klepp, "Five Early Pennsylvania Censuses," *Pennsylvania Magazine of History and Biography*, CVI (1982), 494. Formal education was increasingly necessary by the end of the eighteenth century and into the nineteenth. Textile mills in the nineteenth century rewarded families that could provide child labor, but only the most desperate immigrants accepted such employment. See Cynthia J. Shelton, *The Mills of Manayunk: Industrialization and Social Conflict in the Philadelphia Region, 1787–1837* (Baltimore, 1986), 61–63.

15. For a brief notice of similar adjectives as they applied to colonial women and farm animals but that are analyzed as "straightforward" descriptions rather than as metaphors, see Catharine M. Scholten, *Childbearing in American Society: 1650–1850* (New York, 1985), 15. See also Sylvia D. Hoffert, *Private Matters: American Attitudes toward Childbearing and Infant Nurture in the Urban*

For women as well as men there was an element of competition with regard to fertility. Burr was invited to a forthcoming lying-in in 1757 and commented, "This is quick work for her Child is near two Months younger than mine." Elizabeth Drinker observed in 1795 that her daughter-in-law's first labor was "severe," but "I have been accustomed to severer labours." Mary Boyd Simm wrote to her Scottish sister-in-law in 1778, "I also rejoice with you in being the Mother of So large a family." But she bemoaned the "calamities of War" in America that make "we Women . . . Say blessed is the Womb that beareth not," adapting Luke 23:29 to the dire consequences of the Revolutionary War. Women took pride in their large families of children, they enjoyed calling friends together to assist at the birth, they regaled each other with heroic tales of survival from difficult labors, they remembered tragic cases of suffering and death, they poked fun at men and male pretension, and they welcomed the gifts and cash bestowed on the new mother in the weeks after the baptism. There was, by and large, no latent demand for an end to childbearing. To flourish as a childbearer was to have health, prosperity, and success.[16]

Abundance was welcome and children were undoubtedly loved, but the botanic imagery was quite unsentimental, both as it related to wives and to children. Women could be as callous toward children as men could be about women or children. If parents have "a crop both feeble and redundant," wrote Anne Grant, "they must carefully weed and prop." Grant articulated the prevailing social inequalities in an attitude that was evident in the behavior of many parents. Some family members were more important than others. James Tilghman introduced a discussion of his six sons in 1766 by noting in passing that "Breeding has almost destroyed" his wife after bearing ten children. He was not dismayed by the toll on his wife, and his four daugh-

North, 1800–1860 (Urbana, Ill., 1989), 15; Laurel Thatcher Ulrich, *Good Wives: Image and Reality in the Lives of Women in Northern New England, 1650–1750* (New York, 1982), 159–162; Marylynn Salmon, "The Cultural Significance of Breastfeeding and Infant Care in Early Modern England and America," *Journal of Social History*, XXVIII (1994), 247–269; Norton, *Liberty's Daughters*, 80–83; Elizabeth Coates Paschall, Recipe Book, circa 1745–1767, 10L, College of Physicians of Philadelphia; Randolph Shipley Klein, *Portrait of an American Family: The Shippens of Pennsylvania across Five Generations* (Philadelphia, 1975), 134, 277; Carol F. Karlsen and Laurie Crumpacker, eds., *The Journal of Esther Edwards Burr, 1754–1757* (New Haven, Conn., 1984), 287.

16. Karlsen and Crumpacker, eds., *Journal of Esther Edwards Burr*, 253; Elaine Forman Crane et al., eds., *The Diary of Elizabeth Drinker*, 3 vols. (Boston, 1991), I, 741–742; Barbara De Wolfe, ed., *Discoveries of America: Personal Accounts of British Emigrants to North America during the Revolutionary Era* (New York, 1997), 148. At least one European thought cash gifts to new mothers rather extravagant: "Politeness required that a gratuity of four or five shillings or even a dollar, be given," wrote Peter Kalm. See Adolph B. Benson, ed., *Peter Kalm's Travels in North America: The English Version of 1770* (New York, 1964), 677.

ters did not merit a mention. Even more solicitous husbands assumed masculine superiority. In 1761, James Read planned to give his wife "the last Ride, perhaps, She will get ere she rejoices, with me, that a Son is born." A son was the great desideratum. So Elias Boudinot bemoaned the "rage of Girls" born in his family but congratulated his colleague on "having an addition to your Family, especially as it is of the Male kind." Sallie Eve in 1772 was "not a little laught at as I had pronounced that both the Ladies would of had males instead of fefales [sic] however I was mistaken," and Sarah Logan Fisher noted her cousin's "favorite Son and 4 of her other Children" in 1778. Eliza Chadwick, a redundant girl born on a New Jersey farm in 1784, later recalled, "My father was no doubt disapointed as to my sex and oftimes wished me a boy." A brief comment by Edward Shippen in 1760 sums up the tangle of values: "My Peggy this morning made me a Present of a fine Baby, which tho' of the worst Sex, is yet entirely welcome. You see my Family encreases apace; I am however in no fear by the Blessing of God but I shall be able to do them tolerable Justice." Wifely sacrifice, male preference, pride in a large family of children, and a fatalistic hope for the future are combined in this notice of Peggy Shippen's birth. The bountiful births and agricultural imagery might envoke health and prosperity but, like a farmer at work in his fields, could also allow a ruthless picking, weeding, and sorting of superfluous or disappointing offspring, especially daughters, and lead to the natural exhaustion of the fertile soil of the female body.[17]

These agricultural motifs were not the only conceits employed to describe pregnancy. To first "be with child" or to "go with child," and then to "be big with child," and finally to be "great with child" were common self-referential terms used by women, especially in informal conversations with family and friends. Relatively little of daily conversation survives, and it may well be that these terms would have loomed even larger in the eighteenth-century. These terms stressed the existential state of the woman, "being with," or the process, "going with," as much as the end of the pregnancy, "child." "Child"

---

17. Anne M. Grant, *Memoirs of an American Lady* (1808; rpt. New York, 1970), I, 274; James Tilghman to Mr. Anderson, Sept. 10, 1766, box 1764–1769, Miscellaneous Manuscripts Collection, American Philosophical Society, Philadelphia (my thanks to Konstantine Dierks for this citation); James Read to John Smith, undated, circa 1761, John Smith Correspondence, 1740–1770, HSP; Elias Boudinot to Lewis Pintard, Apr. 17, 1783, in Paul H. Smith et al., eds., *Letters of Delegates to Congress*, 25 vols. (Washington, D.C., 1976–2000), XX, 196; Sallie Eve, Diary, Feb. 1, 1772, 18, Special Collections, William R. Perkins Library, Duke University, Durham, N.C.; Sarah Logan Fisher Diary, 1 mo. [January] 1778, V, 4, HSP; Eliza Chadwick Roberts Scott, "The Ocurances of Life," circa 1814, 12, Monmouth County Historical Association, Library and Archives, Freehold, N.J.; Edward Shippen quoted in John T. Feris, *The Romance of Old Philadelphia* (Philadelphia, 1918), 214.

itself could be used to objectify the fetus, and its etymology is rooted in the Old English word for womb, not infant or person. The vocabulary of process measured the progression of the pregnancy through the growth of the woman's body developing in tandem "with child." As Barbara Duden has pointed out, the seventeenth- and eighteenth-century pregnant female body was viewed externally, and the assessment of the viability of the pregnancy was made by the woman herself. The womb provided a matrix in which life might or might not finally develop. The use of the term "life's porch" for the birth canal was another indication of the ambiguous status of the fetus prior to birth, especially given the high rate of stillbirths and neonatal deaths. Mary Wollstonecraft concurred, "With respect to the formation of the fetus in the womb, we are very ignorant." Only at birth did the child become a distinct entity. A crude term for childbirth was that women "fell apart." What had been unified became two. Women did not give birth but were "brought to bed," "confined to their chamber," or they "lay in," sometimes "with child." The woman remained at the center of the images of pregnancy, and process was stressed over end; the future child was an uncertain, hazily conceptualized possibility. Even after birth, women's offspring were frequently referred to only as "my little flock"—the undifferentiated, but now animate, products of fruitfulness.[18]

This view of pregnancy as organic and natural could encompass a wide range of responses to a suspected or self-diagnosed pregnancy. It might engender passivity in some women, who could see their bodies only as the fields on which men's heirs were born, all according to the will of God. Hannah Callender wrote in 1758, "There can be no greater felicity on this side [of] the grave than that of a Man who has a good Wife and large family of Promising children, to think that he has been one means of fitting so many inhabitents for the region of Eternal Happiness." This extreme example of feminine passivity, written by a young woman before her marriage, attributed all creation to the actions of a patriarch. (It caused a descendant, probably in 1888, to pencil three exclamation marks in the margin, an indication of how foreign this particular opinion had become.) Women sometimes commented on the inevitability and indeterminacy of multiple pregnancies. Esther Edwards Burr wrote in 1755 after her second child's birth, "How I shall get along when

18. Mary Wollstonecraft, *A Vindication of the Rights of Woman*, ed. Charles W. Hagelman, Jr. (New York, 1967), 118; Norton, *Liberty's Daughters*, 85; Barbara Duden, *Disembodying Women: Perspectives on Pregnancy and the Unborn* (Cambridge, Mass., 1993), esp. 62–66, 79–93; Crane et al., eds., *Diary of Elizabeth Drinker*, I, 872, and 872 n. 132; Margaret Morris, *Private Journal Kept during the Revolutionary War* (1836; rpt. New York, 1969), 6, 11, 21.

I have got ½ dzn. or 10 Children I cant devise." But obviously she knew that she would, somehow, get along, even if she could not anticipate the frequencies within the course of her lifetime of childbearing.[19]

On the other hand, these views of organic unity could also give women a measure of control over their bodies. Eighteenth-century medical texts, herbals, and home guides to health contained instructions on how to apply abdominal pressure or how to prepare herbal medicines to restore menstruation. Women's recipes intended to prevent miscarriage were as frequent as those for inducing menstruation. Women did have some control over their reproductive lives, but that control focused on immediate circumstances rather than lifetime goals. Public and private pressure to conform to contemporary standards of high fertility was intense, and women who failed to produce children could find themselves the objects of pity or censure. Their private failure became a source of public comment. It was a reflection of their abilities, of their husband's masculinity, and of the country's prosperity.[20]

Although a range of behaviors was possible under the fruitful images of the early eighteenth century, what could not apparently be imagined was an alternative to the reproductive cycle. Women were physical beings whose lives conformed to biological rhythms.

There were very practical as well as patriarchal reasons for high fertility in the eighteenth and nineteenth centuries. Given the high death rates among children — both in the countryside and in the city, nearly one in five children died in the first year of life — having many offspring helped ensure that a few would survive to care for their parents in sickness and old age. And at a time when only minimal, and degrading, social services existed for the sick, the disabled, or the elderly, offspring provided the best insurance against destitution, warning out, or incarceration in the local almshouse. Married daughters were expected to nurse their infirm parents, a function especially impor-

19. Klepp and Wulf, eds., *Diary of Hannah Callender,* Oct. 30, 1758. Similar sentiments were expressed by Hannah Harkum Hodge concerning a daughter's birth and death in 1754: "A christian parent possesses an unspeakable privilege, who gives birth to an immortal being, and is permitted to give it away to God" ("Memoirs of Mrs. Hannah Hodge, Who Died in Philadelphia, Dec. 17th, 1805, in the 85th Year of Her Age," *General Assembly's Missionary Magazine; or, Evangelical Intelligencer,* II, no. 1 [1806], 44–46, II, no. 2, 92–96, esp. 93). See also Karlsen and Crumpacker, eds., *Journal of Esther Edwards Burr,* 192. It is interesting that all these cases of extreme passivity date from the 1750s, a decade not only of peak fertility rates in the Mid-Atlantic but also of religious revivalism. Burr and Hodges were New Light Presbyterians; Callender was a Quaker.

20. Susan E. Klepp, "Colds, Worms, and Hysteria: Menstrual Regulation in Eighteenth-Century America," in Etienne van de Walle and Elisha Renne, eds., *Regulating Menstruation: Beliefs, Practices, Interpretations* (Chicago, 2001), 22–38. See also Chapter 5, below.

tant in poorer families. Sons provided labor or food to elderly parents. Both daughters and sons could, through advantageous marital connections, bring important economic and social ties, although daughters required dowries that could crimp their families' fortunes.[21]

Children, if they lived, could provide first unskilled and then skilled labor and did not need to be paid: they were valuable assets. Elizabeth Ashbridge wrote that, when she turned fourteen, her mother "might reasonably have expected the benefit of her Labours, and have had Comfort in me." That is, by early adolescence, parent-child relationships were reversed, and the diligent child provided some respite from work and responsibility for the parent. So it was that in a 1752 letter Elizabeth Colden DeLancey referred to her children as "my dear little Comforts." Children would grow up to provide for their parents through their service and labor. Diaries, letters, and conduct books were filled with admonishments for children to be dutiful. As Poor Richard advised in 1739, "Let thy Child's first Lesson be Obedience, and the second may be what thou wilt." All children were debtors: when older, they were expected to work and thereby reward their parents, repaying them for their upbringing. The sentimental, child-centered family was only beginning to transform parent-child relations in the middle of the eighteenth century. Childbearing long remained overwhelmingly pragmatic and, for parents, self-interested.[22]

It did not cost much to raise children because most got minimal educations and minimal supervision when they were not at work. Except among the well-to-do, children wore cast-off clothing, slept in the same beds as siblings and servants, and ate whatever was served to the rest of the family. One more mouth did not significantly burden most family incomes, even if women bore the brunt of the care and nursing of infants and toddlers.

From the earliest settlements, and well into the nineteenth century, children were fungible. When Peggy Dow's father lost his property, "the children

---

21. Infant mortality rates are based on six studies of places in New York, New Jersey, and Pennsylvania, 1700–1830, summarized in Susan E. Klepp, "Malthusian Miseries and the Working Poor in Philadelphia, 1780–1830: Gender and Infant Mortality," in Billy G. Smith, ed., *Down and Out in Early America* (University Park, Pa., 2004), 65. Among the most destitute of the working poor in the city, there is evidence that daughters were preferred to sons. Male children often left the family early, whereas female children provided social services.

22. Daniel B. Shea, ed., "Some Account of the Fore Part of the Life of Elizabeth Ashbridge," in William L. Andrews et al., eds., *Journeys in New Worlds: Early American Women's Narratives* (Madison, Wis., 1990), 147–148; Elizabeth DeLancey to Cadwallader Colden, June 7, 1752, in *Letters and Papers of Colden*, NYHS, *Colls.*, L–LVI (1917–1923), IX, 489; Van Wyck Brooks, ed., *Poor Richard: The Almanacks for the Years 1733-1758* (New York, 1976), 67.

were scattered as a consequence." She ended up as a kind of servant for her married but childless older sister. Eliza Chadwick was given to an uncle who had "Lost three Children of an Ulcer Sore throat in a week." In times of difficulty, boys were sent to sea, and daughters were encouraged to marry at very young ages. When Ann Baker's father became ill, she was married, at age fifteen, to a forty-year-old ship's captain. Her older sister was also married, and her younger brother was sent to sea. After the death of their father in the 1760s, the Biddle boys were disposed of in accordance with their age rank. The eldest, James, was to train as a lawyer; the second son, Edward, was sent as an ensign into the army; and the next two younger boys were sent to sea to make their fortunes. Elizabeth Munro's father tried to marry her off to a forty-five-year-old man with "no teeth and gray hairs" rather than pay for his sixteen-year-old daughter's room and board in 1775. She eloped instead. The expense of rearing unneeded or unaffordable children could always be shifted to relatives, neighbors, masters, or sons-in-law. In desperation, the Overseers of the Poor might step in and auction children to local farm families. Demographers call these and similar practices "post-natal controls on family size." These rather hard-hearted customs provide necessary supports for high-fertility societies by ridding individual families of excess children while supplying the labor needs of other families. In these transactions, it was not so much that parents were uncaring; rather, they could not afford to be sentimental. In a hierarchical society, the interests of the household head superseded the interests of particular, low-ranked individuals. Hansel and Gretel had many real-life counterparts.[23]

Still, there were fewer economic constraints on children's finding a means of subsistence in early America than there had been in the Old World. In Europe, land had been scarce and costly at the same time that laborers were numerous and often poorly paid. Since custom dictated that married couples should be self-supporting, Europeans had to delay marriage while attempting to accumulate the land, goods, skills, or income necessary to maintain a

23. Peggy Dow, *Vississitudes; or, The Journey of Life,* 2d ed. (Philadelphia, 1815), 3–4; Scott, "The Ocurances of Life," 21, Monmouth County Historical Association; Susan E. Klepp and Susan Branson, eds., "A Working Woman: The Autobiography of Ann Baker Carson," in Billy G. Smith, ed., *Life in Early Philadelphia: Documents from the Revolutionary and Early National Periods* (University Park, Pa., 1995), 166; Charles Biddle, *Autobiography of Charles Biddle, Vice-President of the Supreme Executive Council of Pennsylvania* (Philadelphia, 1883), 3; Sharon Halevi, ed., *The Other Daughters of the Revolution: The Narrative of K. White (1809) and the Memoirs of Elizabeth Fisher (1810)* (Albany, N.Y., 2006), 78–83; Karen Oppenheim Mason, "Gender and Family Systems in the Fertility Transition," *Global Fertility Transition,* supplement of *Population and Development Review,* XXVII (2001), 160–176, esp. 165–166.

self-sufficient nuclear family — 5 to 15 percent never succeeded in marrying. Women in the Old World often spent many of their most fertile years as unmarried servants working in someone else's household.

The economic situation was reversed in the colonies. The expectation of economic self-sufficiency for married couples was less restrictive since landownership was widespread among those of European descent, particularly before 1760 or so. Settlers, artisans, and servants were in demand and, on the whole, comparatively well compensated. For free individuals, economic independence and marriage came earlier than in the Old World. As a consequence, childbearing took up a larger portion of women's lives in the colonies than it had in Europe, birthrates were higher, and family sizes were larger by one to two and a half children on average, even when age at marriage is held constant. Birth intervals were shorter in the colonies, and more women continued to bear children into their middle forties.[24]

Comparable data are hard to come by, but colonial-era American Quaker women bore their last child at age 38.9, almost a year and a half after their British counterparts had stopped childbearing at age 37.5. American Quakers, however, stopped childbearing a year before Irish Quaker women, who bore their last child at age 40.1. It was average family sizes that show the procreative edge of the colonists. For Quaker women who married before menopause and whose marriages remained intact until age 50, those living in Britain averaged 5.1 children, those in Ireland, 6.9, and those in America, 7.5. Earlier marriages in the colonies, shorter intervals between all births, perhaps accompanied by better nutrition or fewer endemic diseases, less economic pressure to limit family size, and less access to the herbs and pharmaceuticals that Old World women used to regulate menstrual periods are among the factors that could have influenced average family size. Benjamin Franklin estimated that the European population was stagnant, with only 2 children per married couple surviving to adulthood, while colonial America's population, based on an average of 4 surviving children per family, was doubling every twenty years. He might have exaggerated, but only slightly: the fertility of American women astounded contemporaries.[25]

24. Daniel Scott Smith, "American Family and Demographic Patterns and the Northwest European Model," *Continuity and Change,* VIII (1993), 389–415; Robert V. Wells, "The Population of England's Colonies in America: Old English or New Americans?" *Population Studies,* XLVI (1992), 85–102. See also Benjamin Franklin, "Observations concerning the Increase of Mankind, [1751]," in Leonard W. Labaree et al., eds., *The Papers of Benjamin Franklin* (New Haven, Conn., 1959–), IV, 227–234.

25. For New York, New Jersey, and Pennsylvania Quakers that married before age twenty-five and were born before 1730, see Robert V. Wells, "Family Size and Fertility Control in Eighteenth-

So long as labor was in short supply and land relatively abundant, parents could hope that all their surviving sons might acquire good livings and all their daughters might find supportive husbands who did not demand purse-draining dowries. If not, there were plenty of other options for surplus children, particularly in service to others. Governments as well as private families favored high birthrates, and so official policies were intended to enhance growth by expanding the "employment of the people, political stability, promotion of internal trade, [and] development of foreign commerce, and colonies."[26]

Economists have long argued that land prices and the cost of providing sons with a good start in life were the major factors controlling fertility levels. Because land prices were higher in the East than in the West, cost must be the controlling factor. But noneconomic conditions could influence regional differences in birthrates. Many societies have had concerns about being "outbred," so groups in "ethnically or racially diverse settings" may compete for dominance through procreation, a factor that will "retard fertility decline." The South had higher child-woman ratios than the North; the West had higher ratios than the East. In the slave states, white supremacy was maintained in part through patriarchal control over fertility, and the monetary gains expected from increasing the supply of enslaved people might have continually conflicted with the fears of domestic enemies. Staples of anti-Indian propaganda were graphic (and usually imaginary) accounts of killer Indians who would rip out fetuses from the bellies of dying wives and mothers. Savages were out to destroy not just the present generation but the future of the colonies. Perhaps the more palpable the threat from perceived enemies, whether domestic (enslaved and bound servants) or regional (native peoples, the French, and the Spanish), the more societal norms would promote high fertility.[27]

Century America: A Study of Quaker Families," *Population Studies*, XXV (1971), 75, table 2, 79, table 5, 80, table 6. The rates for English and Irish Quaker women between 1650 and 1750 are calculated from Richard T. Vann and David Eversley, *Friends in Life and Death: The British and Irish Quakers in the Demographic Transition, 1650–1900* (Cambridge, Mass., 1992), 137, table 4.3, 151, table 4.8, 153, table 4.9. The findings on last birth intervals are less definitive. American Quaker women managed a gap of 40.7 months between their penultimate and final births, whereas British Quakers, who were younger at their last birth, had an interval of 39.4 months, and Irish Quakers, who were older, had an interval of 45.6 months. See Franklin, "Observations," in Labaree et al., eds., *Papers of Benjamin Franklin*, IV, 227–234.

26. E. P. Hutchinson, *The Population Debate: The Development of Conflicting Theories up to 1900* (Boston, 1967), 66.

27. Edward M. Crenshaw, Matthew Christenson, and Doyle Ray Oakey, "Demographic Transi-

Benjamin Franklin's *Interest of Great Britain with Regard to Her Colonies,* published in London at the height of both the Seven Years' War and Philadelphia's crude birthrate, finds an ominous competition over population increase everywhere—between the British and the French in Canada and the Caribbean, between settlers and native Americans, and between the mother country and the colonies. America was a "vast wilderness thinly or scarce at all peopled, [that] conceals with ease the march of [French and Indian] troops," wrote Franklin. The French, through "frequent family alliances" with the "barbarous tribes of savages," threaten "the certain diminution of our people." If Great Britain fails to allow expansion into Canada, he argued rather hysterically, it would be better to enjoin "the colony midwives to stifle at birth every third or fourth child," because there would soon be no place for these excess children. Anyway, he added, in imitation of Jonathan Swift's *Modest Proposal,* "grief for the death of a child just born is short and easily supported." If the British Empire failed to support population growth, Franklin continued, then English men, women, and children would be overrun by savages, or at least reduced to poverty under French masters. Only the acquisition of French territories would secure the growth of Britons.[28]

Eliza Stedman reported in 1764 that a group of women "in counsel" had recognized the need for an increasing population and determined to "call to there assistance [those] whom had given over the good work such as Mrs. Bond, the elder Mrs. Plumstead and many more too tedious to mention." The production of sons was closely linked to war. The poet Richard Savage, quoted at length in *Poor Richard's Almanack* for 1752, imagined an enlightened age when public spirit and public works would end war so that "Peace o'erstocks us with the Sons of Men." Scottish novelist John Galt predicted a long American war for independence when there was an unusual preponderance of boy babies born in a fictive Scottish parish in 1778 because "it had been long held as a sure prognostication of war, when the births of male children outnumbered that of females." Procreation by patriotic women of boy babies was closely linked to military success and imperial security.[29]

tion in Ecological Focus," *American Sociological Review,* LXV (2000), 371–391, esp. 376–377; Peter Silver, *Our Savage Neighbors: How Indian War Transformed Early America* (New York, 2007), 85.

28. Benjamin Franklin, *The Interest of Great Britain Considered, with Regard to Her Colonies . . .* (London, 1760); also included was an abbreviated version of Franklin's *Observations concerning the Increase of Mankind,* which had originally appeared in 1755.

29. Simon Gratz, "Some Material for a Biography of Mrs. Elizabeth Fergusson," *PMHB,* XXXIX (1915), 277; Brooks, ed., *Poor Richard,* 207; John Galt, *Annals of the Parish,* ed. James Kinsley (1821; rpt. New York, 1986), 91.

Perhaps not surprisingly, then, colonial crude birthrates peaked during the Seven Years' War, when Americans were surrounded by French and Indian enemies—although other factors, such as a smaller proportion of indentured servants and a more even sex ratio were undoubtedly at play as well. Yet the link between war and rising birthrates was uncoupled by the time of the Revolution. As men in the Northeast became less interested in maximizing fertility in response to external threats, women, for other reasons, would become convinced of the values of liberty, equality, and future happiness that might derive from family limitation.

In colonial America, the prosperity of families, the strength of nations, and the growth of empires were guaranteed by the increase of families and measured particularly in the number of producers and potential soldiers and sailors: that is, in males. There were many reasons—personal, religious, economic, familial, and political—to choose to have big families.

Slave status and racism combined to produce very different circumstances for parents of African descent. Colonial slaveowners thought the male slave's "Business [was] to get [children] for his Master's use," and so masters often encouraged informal marriages, especially since they quickly recognized that the creation of family ties "often prevents their running away." At the end of the eighteenth century, Thomas Jefferson voiced a common assessment that "a woman who brings a child every two years [is] more profitable than the best man." But enslaved individuals had their own goals and purposes. Bearing children created kinship networks of husbands and wives, parents and children, aunts, uncles, and cousins for those in bondage. These bonds, roles, and identities might create personal spaces that were outside the master's control and contrary to the social death that the slave system was designed to impose.[30]

Yet the power imbalances in the slave system could never be fully circumvented. Those very kinship ties created by enslaved men and women could be manipulated by the master class to enforce obedience and impress the enslaved with their powerlessness. Children might be whipped, sold, or given away as presents without consulting parents. Mothers could be forced to wean their infants when their labor was needed. Fathers and husbands went unrecognized. Wives could be and were sexually exploited. Threats of separation and sale could be used to suppress resistance. When a New Jersey

30. Susan E. Klepp and Billy G. Smith, eds., *The Infortunate: The Voyage and Adventures of William Moraley, an Indentured Servant* (University Park, Pa., 2005), 58, 59; Marie Jenkins Schwartz, *Birthing a Slave: Motherhood and Medicine in the Antebellum South* (Cambridge, Mass., 2006), 68.

employer informed his hired slave that "he had an addition to his family," the employer noted the "mixed feeling in his face." "There was more pain than joy. I understood that awareness of the fate and the state of this baby was the cause for these mixed feelings . . . the inborn desire for freedom in man does not permit him to be happy without it." Or her, either. The relationship of enslaved men and women to procreation was far more complex than for those fortunate enough to be free, although little of their own beliefs and practices have survived.[31]

Changes

The emphasis on high fertility was increasingly contested by the middle decades of the eighteenth century. Benjamin Franklin, speaking in his very popular almanacs as Poor Richard, waffled in his evaluations of fertility, just as many of his readers did. He could, in a serious mood, note in 1733, "He that lives carnally, won't live eternally," reflecting the ancient tension in Christian thought between physicality and spirituality. Two decades later, Poor Richard quoted at length from Richard Savage's poem "On Publick Spirit": "Rapt I a future Colony survey! Come then ye Sons of Mis'ry come away! . . . Here live enjoying Life, see Plenty, Peace; Their Lands encreasing as their Sons increase!" This typical promoter's vision of the American colonies and the rising British Empire echoed both William Penn's promotional literature and Franklin's contemporaneous writings on the rapid natural increase of Americans. The New World offered unparalleled opportunity for downtrodden European men because easy and early marriages produced the next generation of males whose adolescent labor made possible an increase in acreage under cultivation, prosperity, and the rewards of full citizenship. Both fathers and the mother country benefited. This formulation, of course, entirely obscures the contributions and labor of the actual women who would fulfill the roles of fecund wives and prolific mothers of sons. Abundance was welcome everywhere in colonial America. That was one perspective.[32]

On the other hand, Franklin's comic sayings and didactic aphorisms were often subversive of the apparent pronatalism of his more serious pieces. One 1741 joke played on a common theme in the almanacs of the duplicitous wife

---

31. Jennifer L. Morgan, *Laboring Women: Reproduction and Gender in New World Slavery* (Philadelphia, 2004); Julian Ursyn Niemcewicz, *Under Their Vine and Fig Tree: Travels through America in 1797-1799, 1805, with Some Further Account of Life in New Jersey*, trans. and ed. Metchie J. E. Budka (Elizabeth, N.J., 1965), 280.

32. Brooks, ed., *Poor Richard*, 11, 210.

who feigns affection and loyalty to her husband. In this instance, a recent widow seems to mourn the loss of her dear departed spouse, but the real cause of her grief, according to the anecdote, is then revealed: "With the Charge of ten poor Children left; A greater Grief no Woman can know. / Who (with ten Children) — who will have me now?" The first lesson is that a husband should never trust his wife because her fickle, greedy, and sexually insatiable desire for remarriage has a good chance of turning his own off-spring into another man's despised stepchildren. The second lesson is that a brood of ten children is excessive and burdensome, at least for women and potential stepfathers. A few years later, Franklin privately touted the advantages of nonprocreative sex by advising a young man to take on an older (postmenopausal) lover, since there would be "no hazard of Children." Perhaps sex was best divorced from procreation.[33]

Poor Richard also declared, "Late Children, early Orphans," and, "The hasty bitch brings forth blind Puppies." These pointed adages criticized par-ents who continued to produce children into their forties or who failed to pace births through appropriate intervals. Franklin was particularly harsh on the "bitch," the bestial female, as the source of incapacitated offspring. Parents had obligations to their children, and wives needed to regulate the timing and spacing of births in order to produce the best possible outcome. These maxims are as much about sexual restraint as about children and family size. Still, readers might discover, as they pondered and absorbed this homely advice, that childbearing was a costly responsibility and not neces-sarily a source of wealth and prosperity. "If," chided Franklin in a serious mood, laboring men "even look far enough forward to consider how their Children when grown up are to be provided for," they will carefully time their marriages to fit economic circumstances. But it seems from Franklin's tone that most men had not yet adopted the necessary foresight or prudence to amply provide for their children (and here, perhaps, he still resented his father, who had pulled him from school because of the expense of providing for his eighteen children).[34]

There were other dissenting voices, particularly by the middle of the eigh-teenth century, chipping away at the assumptions and practices embedded in pronatalist beliefs. Some critiques, of course, were quite old: the old woman who lived in a shoe (a euphemism for the vagina and sexual intercourse)

33. Ibid., 87; Benjamin Franklin, "Old Mistresses Apologue," Jan. 25, 1745, in Labaree et al., eds., *Papers of Benjamin Franklin*, III, 27.

34. Brooks, ed., *Poor Richard*, 95, 240, 281; Franklin, "Observations," in Franklin, *The Interest of Great Britain*, 228.

had so many children that she didn't know what to do. A few early econo-mists blamed widespread poverty on excess population, although most feared underpopulation. Some middling and elite fathers were already com-plaining about the high costs of educating sons or preparing daughters for the marriage market, but most still maintained that high birthrates brought prosperity. Popular publications were offering mixed messages on fertility and family size, particularly after the 1750s, yet birthrates remained high—indeed, crude birthrates and child-woman ratios continued to rise into the 1760s in the city and the into the 1770s in the country.

The Great Awakening and Fertility

In the second quarter of the eighteenth century, the Great Awakening, the growth of the Baptists, and, to a much lesser degree, the reformation of the Quakers offered certain antiauthoritarian tenets through a return to the spiritual. The charismatic Reverend George Whitefield spread the word of a religion of the heart, and the later emergence of the Methodists con-tinued that message. Other denominations were also influenced. The spirit could move the wealthy and the downtrodden, the free and the enslaved, and men and women. Personal experience and the Bible were better guides to salvation and piety than religious authorities and obtuse theology. Only Quaker women could address the public in religious testimony, but New Light evangelicals, Methodists, and Baptists sometimes included women as leaders of Bible study groups and called upon women to spread the Gospel, to assist and support ministers, and to build new congregations. All of these religious movements renewed emphasis on personal responsibility.

Hannah Harcum Hodge was among those young people from Philadel-phia who followed the spellbinding itinerant missionary George Whitefield "on foot to Chester, to Abingdon, to Neshaminy, and some even to New-Brunswick, in New-Jersey, the distance of sixty miles." Disowned and cast out by her father for her beliefs and independent behavior, she and her sister supported themselves with their needles, attending prayer meetings and helping to found a new church dedicated to New Light Presbyterian-ism. She married a coreligionist. They opened a shop and remained active in the church. She waited eleven years before deciding to have children—how she remained childless is not known—but, suddenly inspired by the rite of baptism, she changed her mind and quickly bore a daughter and a son. Both of Hodge's children predeceased her, but she continued her business and church activities as long as health permitted, recalling as her proudest achievement, not childbearing, but the deathbed conversion of the enslaved woman who served the household. She admitted in old age: "I have not half so much comfort, not even in religion, as when I was bustling half the day behind the counter. . . . I become moped and stupified for the want of something to rouse me." Her personal strivings led to an active and independent life and to considerable control over childbearing.[35]

The impact of religious awakenings and reformations on the role of colonial women within marriage was mixed, however. Mary Cooper and Ann Whitall were among the women who had their spiritual aspirations frustrated by the demands of farmwork and unsympathetic husbands. Cooper, a Long Island Baptist, complained unavailingly about the demands on her time but never fully located the sources of her discontent. The closest she came to recording the gendered inequities of her lot in life was when her husband, in a raw display of authority, refused to let her have a turkey to celebrate their daughter's recovery from smallpox. She wrote, "I am so aflicted and ashamed about it that I feele as if I should never get over it." She was insulted, her daughter's survival was cavalierly dismissed as unworthy of note, and her standing with her neighbors, who had helped in nursing her daughter, was diminished. But, for all her complaints, Cooper shied away from probing the basis for her perceived exploitation.[36]

Ann Whitall, like Cooper, poured out her unhappiness in her diary, but she was more attuned to locating the causes of the perceived injustices that brought her so much pain. She came to identify a growing hypocrisy among Quakers: "We du pretend we are all guided by the right spirit," she wrote in 1760. But a self-selecting clique of weighty Friends, whom she called the "big wons," in fact dominated: "O it makes me ofen greve as if the leittle wons had not as much right to preech as the big wons." And when public friend John Scarborough preached that "the woman was a halp to Man," she protested in her diary: "Manoah was a gud man but [his wife] exceded [him], We dont reed of her name[, she is] only the woman, in holy rit." Unchristian social inequalities could be found even in certain biblical passages, in her analysis (see Judg. 13:2–25). Not only were the "leittle wons" ignored, but they were especially burdened. She worried that she had "such a pasal of Children." How could she support them if her husband died? Her sons' unwillingness to conform to Quakerly precepts particularly troubled her, especially since

35. "Memoirs of Mrs. Hannah Hodge," *General Assembly's Missionary Magazine*, II, no. 1 (1806), 44–46, esp. 45, no. 2, 92–96, esp. 92.

36. Field Horne, ed., *The Diary of Mary Cooper, Life on a Long Island Farm, 1768–1773* (Oyster Bay, N.Y., 1981), 26.

their father seemed to be abetting their misbehavior by frequently skipping meetings to work or play on Sundays. Whitall wanted men to conform equally with women to religious proscription, and she hoped to open up the meeting to the voices of the "leittle wons" like herself. She also came to advocate abstinence. She wrote, "Our Sensuel Appetites [must be] quite cut down, before we can attain true pleasure in Holiness," and she noted that the wicked are "Full of Sin, yet full of Children," elaborating on Psalms 17:14. She had no more control over the births of her seven children than she did over the horse that her husband sometimes denied her when she wished to go to meeting. Her bitterness lasted for decades.[37]

Revivals could produce fulfillment or frustration. A few women raised issues of gendered and other forms of inequality, but, isolated, they failed to generate any substantial redress of emerging discontent. The Bible commanded the faithful to be fruitful and multiply, at least according to a common reading, and reminded women that Eve's disobedience had forever relegated women to subordination and suffering. Still, sermons and devotional literature had little of the sociological emphasis on identity, sexuality, and social relationships that frame much of twenty-first century discourse, whether religious or not. The usual eighteenth-century gloss on injunctions to be fruitful and multiply was to advocate enhancing faith, not procreation. "We must be fruitful," George Whitefield preached in England and America; "In what? In every good word and work." New Testament, ministerial, and print sources advocated a spiritual and metaphorical understanding of these commandments to increase and multiply, but many eighteenth- and nineteenth-century Americans remained literalists. Colonial birthrates continued to rise, and average family sizes remained high.[38]

The Consumer Revolution, Markets, Wages, and Salaries

The religious intensity of the Great Awakening overlapped with gradually accelerating changes in the Anglo-American economy. From the middle decades of the eighteenth century, a flood of consumer goods was gathered from around the globe and shipped to the colonies. As Susanna Hopkins Mason noted in the 1780s, houses could be designed to be convenient.

---

37. "The Diary of Ann Whitall," typescript by Michael C. Osborne (1976), esp. B46–47, B-55, B-59, B-65, B-119, Gloucester County Historical Society, N.J.

38. Christian Classics Ethereal Library, "Selected Sermons of George Whitefield," sermon 12, "Christ the Believer's Husband," http://www.ccel.org/ccel/whitefield/sermons.toc.html (accessed June 7, 2004).

Cabins could be replaced with brick or frame houses with glass windows, stoves, carpets, and a host of other additional amenities. Tools and implements of all sorts could multiply. The prices of high-tech items like clocks and watches declined. Individual plates, glasses, and cutlery were neater than shared utensils. Even the relatively poor might assert their equality through the possession of a tea caddy and tea tray or by hanging framed prints on the wall of a twelve-by-sixteen-foot, single-room house. Chairs seated guests more comfortably than benches. Imported cotton cloth saved the labor-intensive preparation of linen and woolen yarns. Exotic medicines promised miraculous cures for common and uncommon diseases. Books opened new worlds. Children's puzzles and books could be justified as educational. Hannah Callender Sansom took her six-year-old daughter to Philadelphia's semiannual fair with its booths filled with imported and domestic goods. She "bought Sally an undressed baby [a doll]," ostensibly so Sally could practice her sewing, as well as personal copies of several favorite books, even though Sansom had written before that the noise and dazzle of the fairs "set the childrens heads crazey." Even careful parents fed consumer frenzy.[39]

Less practical purchases beckoned. Luxuries large and small were advertised weekly and displayed daily in shop windows; mirrors, rugs, mahogany veneers, ribbons, wigs, and cosmetic powders were only a few of the possibilities. Tea, sugar, coffee, wines, and spices could be purchased even by the relatively poor and served graciously to visitors. The developing "consumer culture," writes Bernard Herman, "relied on the broadest possible market for luxury goods." And, by the end of the century, there were taverns, beer gardens, balls, circuses, concerts, plays, traveling zoos, newspapers, magazines, prints, and a museum where those who could never have afforded a portrait could have their silhouettes cut. In 1758, Ben Franklin had the parsimonious Father Abraham quip, "What maintains one Vice, would bring up two Children." The vices enumerated by this thrifty character were not terribly vicious: some tea or punch, better food and clothing, and a *little Entertainment.*" If this maxim in the enormously popular, tongue-in-cheek

---

39. Bernard L. Herman, *Town House: Architecture and Material Life in the Early American City, 1780–1830* (Chapel Hill, N.C., 2005), esp. 193–202; Klepp and Wulf, eds., *Diary of Hannah Callender,* Nov. 28, 1769, June 4, 1770; Paul G. E. Clemens, "The Consumer Culture of the Middle Atlantic, 1760–1820," *WMQ,* 3d Ser., LXII (2005), 65; Judith A. McGaw, "'So Much Depends upon a Red Wheelbarrow': Agricultural Tool Ownership in the Eighteenth-Century Mid-Atlantic," in McGaw, ed., *Early American Technology: Making and Doing Things from the Colonial Era to 1850* (Chapel Hill, N.C., 1994), 328–357; John Brewer, *The Pleasures of the Imagination: English Culture in the Eighteenth Century* (Chicago, 1997).

essay "The Way to Wealth" ostensibly advises readers to avoid vice, it also equates children, not—as tradition would have it—with wealth formation, but rather with parental expenditure and consumer choice. Readers might well have reversed this equation and decided that fewer children might mean greater buying power and more clothes and food and that little bit of entertainment. "A large family," the newly married Esther de Berdt Reed wrote in 1772, would "be a heavy weight." She hoped instead to be free to visit her brother in London. Large families were costly. Other pleasures and responsibilities beckoned.[40]

As is usual in the study of the late eighteenth century, the extant evidence reveals more about the views of literate, urban, wealthy women than the illiterate, semiliterate, rural, and laboring women, or even the middling-sort farmers and artisans who were in fact the majority. Little survives of the aspirations of the average man or woman. One fruitful source for common attitudes is the advertisements written and placed in local newspapers for modest sums by job seekers, employers, potential landlords, and the buyers and sellers of real estate (Table 3). Many were undoubtedly placed by men, but women also offered houses, rooms, and employment or sought employment.

These real estate and employment advertisements provide one of the few places where family size was described, defined, and evaluated in early America. Before the Revolution, little attempt was made to distinguish the suitability of particular properties based on family size, but the distinction between properties deemed appropriate for "large" families and those for "small" families emerged around 1760 and became common between the 1770s and 1790s. Job seekers and employers also began to stress the importance of smallness at roughly the same time.[41]

Just what a "large" family might be was never defined in either the real estate or employment advertisements, although one advertiser did seek to employ three women and one man to serve in a large family (1814). Four servants would be an unusually large number, and here family is being used

<hr>

40. Herman, *Town House*, 200; Brooks, ed., *Poor Richard*, 281; William B. Reed, *The Life of Esther de Berdt, Afterwards Esther Reed, of Pennsylvania* (Philadelphia, 1853), 171. See also Richard Bushman, *The Refinement of America: Persons, Houses, Cities* (New York, 1992).

41. This and subsequent paragraphs are based on word searches for "small family" in the electronic databases of Early American Newspapers (now titled America's Historical Newspapers) and Accessible Archives, both available through Paley Library, Temple University, Philadelphia. The search was limited to advertisements in journals from Pennsylvania, New Jersey, and Delaware, 1720–1815 (accessed September–October 2006).

TABLE 3.

Real Estate Advertisements and Family Size, 1720–1815

Years	Average Acreage (Instances)		No. of Stories (Instances)		No. of Rooms (Instances)		House Footprint Square Feet (Instances)	
LARGE FAMILY								
1720–1769	687	(3)	2.0	(2)	8	(2)	—	
1770–1799	250	(15)	2.9	(8)	12.5	(8)	2,106	(2)
1800–1810	128	(12)	2.9	(15)	10.6	(22)	1,415	(11)
SMALL FAMILY								
1720–1769	100	(1)	1.5	(2)	4.0	(1)	—	
1770–1799	52.1	(13)	1.9	(9)	3.4	(18)	268	(3)
1800–1810	7.8	(10)	2.2	(11)	4.1	(12)	688	(2)

Sources: Calculated from Early American Newspapers and Accessible Archives for journals from Pennsylvania, New Jersey, and Delaware (accessed September–October 2006). The number of stories in these houses encompasses living quarters only and does not include garrets or cellars. The number of rooms does not include hallways or rooms in outbuildings or kitchens, whether or not the latter were attached to the main house. A spot-check of New York City advertisements supports these findings.

in its older sense of a household of kin, dependents, and laborers. Employing multiple servants would entail a substantial annual expense, certainly well beyond the familial income of most households. The properties deemed suitable for large families were either large farms or, increasingly over time, rural estates for the wealthy, desirable more for their views and flower beds than for their agricultural productivity.

The advertisements contain more hints about what qualified a family as "small," especially by the 1790s and after. Some advertisements placed by employers mention that the work will be in a small family, that is, in "a Batchelor's house" (1793) or a residence "where there is no woman or children" (1812). Several notices specify that the small family includes only "a Child" (1793, 1795, 1799), "a female Child" (1808), or "no Children" (1791, 1799, 1800). Alternatively, housing a small family was perceived by landlords to be the equivalent of boarding or renting to "two or three Gentlemen" (1807), "four Gentlemen" (1791), "six Gentlemen" (1801), or "a few Ladies and Gentlemen" (1792). Another real estate advertisement describes a small household "consisting of a Gentleman, his Wife, Child and Servant" (1815) who were seeking a suitable dwelling. In all these advertisements, small families and gentility were clearly linked, as in "genteel boarding" for small families (1790). Meanwhile, a large family might aspire to "grand rooms" (1803). "Small" meant a family of one to six persons, no more.

Properties for small families outnumbered those for large ones, although the advertisements for small houses, tenements, and rented rooms less often contained the quantifiable detail that is present in the longer and more descriptive advertisements for substantial houses with extensive acreage. Over time and as population density increased, there was a remarkable shrinkage of available acreage. The advertisements do not give prices, but undoubtedly the long-term trend was for land values to rise. This corresponds with what economists and demographers have found in other contexts: the pressure of population on land was growing, causing eastern farms and garden plots to shrink over time, and forcing westward migration.[42] For the wealthy, square footage also declined by the early decades of the nineteenth century: there was a shortage of grand houses. What the bare numbers do not indicate is that these large properties were primarily working farms in the colonial era and nonproductive summer residences thereafter.

The opposite trend characterized the living spaces of middling families— a phenomenon less appreciated in the scholarship on fertility. Small families expected roomier domestic spaces: there was less acreage available, certainly, but more stories and larger houses, if the few notations of square footage are indicative of actual changes. Given the idiosyncratic content and limited number of quantifiable notices, firm conclusions are impossible, but it does appear that middling-sort buyers, especially those with small families, were expecting more living space, more privacy, and more convenience by the end of the eighteenth century. The number of rooms did not increase. The advertisements show that many small families were choosing to board rather than to run their own households—a choice that freed women from housekeeping, especially food preparation. Comfortable, "genteel" surroundings could be acquired by maintaining a small family size.[43]

Servants advertised that they would only work in a small family. A woman, for example, wrote that she "Wants a place as House-Keeper, in a small Family" (1790). Potential employers were anxious to attract servants

---

42. For example, see Lee A. Craig, *To Sow One Acre More: Childbearing and Farm Productivity in the Antebellum North* (Baltimore, 1993); Richard A. Easterlin, "Factors in the Decline of Farm Family Fertility in the United States: Some Preliminary Research Results," *Journal of American History,* LXIII (1976), 600–614.

43. Carole Shammas examines evidence from the 1798 direct tax in "The Housing Stock of the Early United States: Refinement Meets Migration," *WMQ,* 3d Ser., LXIV (2007), 549–590.

by affirming that the work would only be for a small family: "Wanted in a Small Family Where there is no Children" (1791). A "Lady of Character with a small family" sought boarders (1795). A landlord made clear that same year that his premises were "Only for a Small Family." Employers insisted that only good recommendations and a small family would find men positions as tenant farmers, artisans, or shopkeepers. A very early example was quite specific: "WANTED A MAN with a small Family, that understands Gardening and Plantation Work: Likewise, a Man, with a small Family, that understands a Grist Mill. Such Persons, that can be well recommended, may meet with Encouragement" (1760). Increasingly, large families were a luxury, and those with small families found expanding opportunities in housing and employment.

If the standard date of 1750 is accepted as an accurate marker of England's emergence as the world's first industrial economy, then America lagged behind. Conventionally, it would not be until 1815–1820, some seventy years — or almost three generations—later, that industrialization and market relations would come to be the driving force. Still, the early United States, particularly the Northeast, was in advance of most of the world in transforming labor, production, consumption, and finance and in coping with the promises, uncertainties, and dislocations of the new economy, whether the tipping point came in 1815 or a few decades earlier or later. By the last years of the eighteenth century, many Americans, particularly those living in or near cities, would find economic reasons to favor small families.

But how did the preference for small families emerge? A very few signs of discontent and rebelliousness had appeared during the religious upheavals, wars, and commercial expansion of the 1750s and early 1760s, yet by the 1790s the ideal of limited family size was so widespread, so unremarkable, that it saturated the public prints and the common language of average Americans.

Looking Ahead

Women were at the center of these developments. Some were converted to evangelical faiths, and others maintained traditional beliefs. Many women cultivated the new sensibilities that could be found in novels and poems, but the poor and the enslaved experienced a harsh world that offered little scope for fine feelings. Women, like men, were patriotic, which might mean adherence to an expanding empire, a locality, a dissident faction, or, soon, a new nation. Women ran away from masters whenever possible. Other women relished their status as mistresses of social inferiors, and some of these were harsh taskmasters. Women stood on both sides of store counters, buying and selling or producing many of the goods flowing into new markets. Their lives, like everyone else's, would be transformed by a flood of goods and an expanding cash and wage labor system. Women read, if they could, both fact and fiction and absorbed or worried about novel ideas. Nothing might have come of all this but for the American Revolution.

Amid calls for liberty and rights and the experience of independence and privation came an additional, if less immediately apparent, change. Starting around 1765, concomitant with the first rumblings of American independence and expanding with the rebelliousness and radicalism of a social as well as political upheaval, first women and then men began another revolution, the one demographers call the fertility transition: the shift from lifetime, abundant childbearing to family planning and limited childbearing. This transition was neither simple nor easy and required overturning centuries of beliefs and practices.

WILLIAM PENN HAD WRITTEN that the colonies promised an "increase of Humane Stock," as if women were the equivalent of cows or sows or ewes producing animate wealth for their owners. By 1770, Susanna Hopkins had rejected that image of ever-producing, bovine females, mindlessly absorbed in their procreative physicality: "Do not you, my friend, think the person very contracted in his notions who would have us [women] to be nothing more than domesticated animals?" The striking novelty of the family-planning intentions of the first generations of founding women and men drew on the religious, political, and economic transformations of the eighteenth century. Susanna Hopkins's query was just one indication of the radically original intentions of the founding generation of American women.[44]

44. Susanna Mason, *Selections from the Letters and Manuscripts of the Late Susanna Mason: With a Brief Memoir of Her Life, by Her Daughter* (Philadelphia, 1836), 30.

3

Women's Words

Martha Bowen lived much of her life in and around Williamsport in central Pennsylvania. In 1855, she composed a family history for her granddaughter and namesake, gathering tales of success and failure, marriages and religious conversions, amusements and deathbeds. Prominent in her history was a depiction of her paternal grandmother, a woman who was unusually well educated for her day. She "wrote beautifully, and was an Arithmetician." Married at age sixteen around 1770, Grandmother Walton became "the mother of *twelve* Children." This striking and underlined aspect of her grandmother's life provided an object lesson for Bowen, since "having the care of a large family, and residing on a Farm—her [grandmother's] sphere of operation was limited." Walton's considerable talents were little appreciated, and, with the double burden of a very large family of children and the isolation and drudgery of farmwork, she had little or no opportunity to use those talents to improve society at large. Yet, despite these limitations, Grandmother Walton certainly had some influence, since, as Bowen reconstructed the tale, several of her children possessed her love of numbers, and, more important, her daughters and sons acquired a critique of traditional marriage.[1]

Bowen's father, one of Martha Walton's sons, married in 1799. Jane Huston was an accomplished seamstress but lacked any other housekeeping skills. Her "conversational gifts were brilliant," however, and the "rational enjoy-

1. Virginia Slate Orton and George Slate, eds., "The Journal of Martha Lewis Walton Grier Bowen," undated typescript, circa 1965, of unlocated MS, 1855–1856, in the author's possession, 4–5.

ment" of agreeable discourse suited Ellis Walton: "I don't want a wife for a drudge," he said in proposing, "but for a companion—I have been too much grieved seeing my Mother toil." During their companionate marriage, Jane and Ellis Walton had four children, spaced three years apart, just as statistics indicate many other rural women were doing. The children were raised with the help of Beck Brown, "a colored woman—who had been [Bowen's] nurse," but who eventually became "free—married—and gone" to her own home and family. Her life, too, was transformed in the early Republic.[2]

Like her grandmother, Bowen herself excelled in mathematics. She also founded and taught in Sunday schools and assisted her second husband's career as an itinerant Methodist minister. She had only one child, a daughter, and one grandchild. In three generations, over some fifty years, the women in this family escaped the cycle of repeated pregnancies and birth in part by communicating lessons and ideals from mothers to daughters, in part by instilling sons with new values, and in part by having more options, including the freedom from bondage that Beck Brown embraced. Women ran prayer meetings and missionary societies; they read novels, poetry, and plays; they traveled; and they had many fewer children than the colonial generations. Northern bondwomen like Beck Brown, who herself had one daughter, went from being chattel to becoming wives and mothers. There were many fewer limitations on women's "sphere of operation," especially if family limitation was practiced.[3]

The American Revolution and Fertility

The American Revolution, as an intellectual, social, and cultural phenomenon, began with protests in 1764 and lasted at least through the political debates of the 1790s. Revolutionary challenges to the status quo were reinforced by news and refugees from subsequent revolutions in France, Haiti, and South America. Colonial grumbling about "hard Times, heavy Taxes, and chargeable Families" soon gave way to protests. Issues of tyranny, slavery, liberty, and individual pursuits of happiness were raised and debated in the street and in print. The Declaration of Independence promoted rights in universal terms: Americans are "entitle[d]" as "one people" to cast off bonds and assume a "separate and equal station" among nations. This entitlement derives from the fact that "all men are created equal," just pos-

2. Ibid., 54–56, 75.
3. Ibid., 4.

sibly meaning mankind rather than males, and all have "unalienable rights." Only America's barbarous enemies have failed to protect "all ages, sexes, and conditions."[4]

The reception of these ringing statements was broader than the representatives to the Second Continental Congress expected. The defenders of the Revolution raised issues of liberty, individual rights, and independence, but for whom? How these ideals might be implemented was a matter of considerable debate and a good deal of anxiety among men. As Benjamin Rush observed in 1788, the Revolution led some people, particularly those who had been appropriately dependent, to what he considered an "excess of the passion for liberty," a physical "disease" that he labeled "*Anarchia*." Even those hesitant to expand the body politic had to grapple with the potential of an enlarged social and political order, if only to reject as absurd any such outcome. New ideas were circulating.[5]

Liberty and Restraint

Revolutionaries were taken aback by the extent to which subordinates, including women, adopted the language of liberty. Some women sagely considered their political stance. "I have retrenched every superfluous expense in my table and family," wrote Sarah Mifflin in an anonymously published 1775 letter to a British officer. "I know this, that as free I can die but once, but as a slave I shall not be worthy of life. I have the pleasure to assure you that these are the sentiments of all my sister Americans." Frugality, restraint, and self-assertion were promoted by Mifflin and many others, but the rhetoric of the American Revolution raised questions that few were willing to pursue to their logical conclusions. If slaves, by definition, had no control over their bodies, what did it mean for women to refuse to be slaves? How would such a stance affect husbands, marriages, propertyownership, citizenship, pregnancy, and more?[6]

An undercurrent in the rhetoric of the Revolution was the noxious effect of the British Empire on America's population growth. The Declaration of

4. Benjamin Franklin, "The Way to Wealth" [1758], in Van Wyck Brooks, ed., *Poor Richard: The Almanacks for the Years 1733–1758* (New York, 1964), 277–285, esp. 281.

5. Benjamin Rush, "Influence of the American Revolution," in Dagobert D. Runes, ed., *The Selected Writings of Benjamin Rush* (New York, 1947), 325, 333.

6. Alden T. Vaughan, ed., *Chronicles of the American Revolution* (New York, 1965), 172. Attribution of authorship to Sarah Mifflin in Mary Heaton, "Bucks County Women in Wartime," Bucks County Historical Society, *Papers*, V (1926), 135.

Independence chastised George III for "endeavor[ing] to prevent the Population of these States" by discouraging immigration. The Declaration did not repeat the fecund hopes of the colonial founders for each American woman to have "a Child in her Belly, or one upon her lap" as the basis for natural increase. Instead, Tom Paine asserted, "Our present numbers are . . . happily proportioned to our wants." There was no exuberant cry to increase and multiply as an act of patriotism as there had been during the Seven Years' War. Women were both less central to victory in the revolutionary era and more prominent in seizing opportunities and self-definitions that were based, not on their fecundity, but on their roles as consumers and producers of American manufactures, as protectors of home and hearth while acting in their husbands' steads, and as republican, thoughtful wives and mothers.[7]

American women, wrote Esther de Berdt Reed in her 1780 broadside, are "born for liberty, disdaining to bear the irons of a tyrannic Government." Women, in Reed's interpretation, had innate natural rights that limited overbearing authority in both marriage and politics. In her own marriage, Reed wished to limit her family to two children, a girl and a boy. She saw the connection between women's limitation of births and their personal and political independence. In politics, Reed proposed a de facto shadow government of female "treasuresses" who would collect money voluntarily raised by local women and who were linked to the de jure government through their husbands' positions on the county, state, and federal levels. She knew that money was power in politics, and so did George Washington, who stubbornly insisted that the women sew shirts instead. Reed lost this battle, just before her untimely death in 1780. She might not have achieved all she hoped for, but her ideas and organizational techniques spread from Pennsylvania to New Jersey, Maryland, and Virginia. Women like Mifflin and Reed posited a political role for women that might be achieved, at least in part, through self-control, self-mastery, and restraint.[8]

Not all women embraced Revolution, but few could avoid getting caught

7. Thomas Paine, "Common Sense," in Harry Hayden Clark, ed., *Thomas Paine: Representative Selections* (New York, 1961), 35; "An Historical and Geographical Account of Pensilvania and of West-New-Jersey, by Gabriel Thomas, 1698," in Albert Cook Myers, ed., *Narratives of Early Pennsylvania, West New Jersey, and Delaware, 1630–1707,* Original Narratives of Early American History (New York, 1912), 333.

8. [Esther de Berdt Reed], "The Sentiments of an American Woman," *Pennsylvania Magazine of History and Biography,* XVIII (1894), 361–366; William B. Reed, *The Life of Esther de Berdt, Afterwards Esther Reed, of Pennsylvania* (Philadelphia, 1853); Mary Beth Norton, "The Philadelphia Ladies Association," *American Heritage,* XXXI, no. 3 (April-May 1980), 102–107.

up in the turmoil of the times. Hannah Griffitts supported the early protests but balked at war. As a loyalist, she lambasted Tom Paine and defended tory womanhood against his aspersions:

> Of female Manners never scribble,
> Nor with thy Rudeness wound our Ear,
> Howe'er thy trimming Pen may quibble,
> The Delicate—is not thy Sphere.

Hers was a robust public defense of delicate, domestic femininity. Even traditionalists had to grapple with changed circumstances as they defended their political stances.[9]

At other times, declarations of independence emerged only in the heat of the moment. Christopher Marshall, who was disowned by the Quakers for his own radical activities, was nonetheless shocked to hear his daughter-in-law throw off all male authority in the course of a family dispute. She angrily said that even "if her own father was liveing she would not be Controuled nor dictated what Company she should keep and [be] entertaining, much less to be directed by a Father in law[.] She would not put up with [it], besides said she[,] I am independent." These attitudes persisted well beyond the war. Rachel Van Dyke differed with a local judge about marriage: "I said I would never promise to *fear* and *obey*—and if ever I got married I would omit that part of the ceremony or else my husband should say the same." A New York City woman reacted furiously at being asked to announce her "mistress's" English visitor: "My *mistress,* Sir! I tell you I have no mistress, nor master either. . . . In this country there is no mistresses nor masters; I guess, I am a woman citizen." The emphatic use of the first person singular by these women, even if the outbursts were rare and much criticized, suggests the assertive and self-aware identities made possible by revolutionary rhetoric. Independence and citizenship could be claimed even by those legally excluded from those civic categories. Anger at persistent inequalities might lie just below the surface of otherwise conventional relationships and interactions. The Revolution provided the language that made it possible to articulate that anger in ways that resonated with widely espoused values.[10]

9. Hannah Griffitts, "On Reading a Few Paragraphs in the Crisis, April, 1777," in Catherine La Courreye Blecki and Karin A. Wulf, eds., *Milcah Martha Moore's Book: A Commonplace Book from Revolutionary America* (University Park, Pa., 1997), 299–300.

10. Christopher Marshall Diary, July 26, 1775, Historical Society of Pennsylvania, Philadelphia; Lucia McMahon and Deborah Schriver, eds., *To Read My Heart: The Journal of Rachel Van Dyke,*

Women's adoption of revolutionary rhetoric was sometimes playful: "My God! if this nonsense should [fall] into your husband's hands, I should die," wrote one woman to a friend in 1778, before insisting that the two women run the country. In but "a week or two," she laughingly proposed, the friends could "settle the nation, as we are most profound politicians." Unwilling or unable to stage a frontal assault on male dominance, women used humor to undermine its basic assumptions, if only for the moment.[11]

Humor was also employed in defense of women's bodily integrity. Several young women protested men's excessive kissing. Sallie Eve wrote in a light, mocking manner of an older man's visit, "One hates to be always kissd especially as it is attended with so many inconveniences, it discomposes the economy of ones hankerchife, it disorders ones high roll, and it ruffles the serenity of ones countanance." How serious these complaints were cannot be recovered, but changes in women's posture in portraits at the same time indicate a wider interest in bodily self-control and privacy (see Chapter 4). Philadelphia's nineteenth-century chronicler, John F. Watson, looked back with amazement at the 1760s when brides were kissed by all visitors: "Even to one hundred [men] in a day, kissed her! Even the plain Friends submitted to these things." But, after 1770, this promiscuous kissing faded away, along with all mentions of the bride's "large or handsome fortune." Women's bodies had become private and less commodified.[12]

More censorious than humorous was Sally Hastings's poetic advice to a friend:

SWEET Delia, draw your tucker close
And do not needlessly expose
Your bosom . . . to vulgar eyes.

1810–1811 (Philadelphia, 2000), 68; Paul A. Gilje and Howard B. Rock, eds., *Keepers of the Revolution: New Yorkers at Work in the Early Republic* (Ithaca, N.Y., 1992), 254.

11. Anonymous "Lady in Philadelphia" to Mrs. Theodorick Bland, n.d., in Charles Campbell, ed., *The Bland Papers*, 2 vols. (Petersburg, Va., 1840), I, 90–94, esp. 91–92.

12. Sallie Eve Diary, Feb. 26, 1773, Special Collections, William R. Perkins Library, Duke University, Durham, N.C. For other examples, see Lucinda Lee, who complained in 1787 of "two horred Mortals . . . who seized me and kissed me a dozen times in spite of all the resistance I could make," in Sharon M. Harris, ed., *American Women Writers to 1800* (New York, 1996), 60, 297; and Kathryn Zabelle Derounian, ed., *The Journal and Occasional Writings of Sarah Wister* (Rutherford, N.J., 1987), 63. See John F. Watson, *Annals of Philadelphia, and Pennsylvania, in the Olden Time*, rev. ed., 3 vols. (Philadelphia, 1899), I, 46. Joseph Price describes a Quaker wedding where the men were "divideing the Bucks among the lasses" and "we hug and Kiss them agreeable to Custom till about 11 OClock then retird." See Joseph Price Diary, Sept. 21, 1796, Lower Merion Historical Society, Pa., http://www.lowermerionhistory.org/texts/price/price1796.html (accessed February 2003).

Bodily restraint and privacy were promoted under the guise of feminine modesty. As historian Laurel Thatcher Ulrich succinctly puts it in her astute analysis of the main character in Samuel Richardson's hugely popular novel, "Pamela's triumph was not in retaining her virtue but in seizing responsibility for her own behavior." Women's initial impulse in employing modesty was to limit men's physical access to female bodies and to assume the self-direction of adults. Unfortunately, by the nineteenth century modesty would sometimes metamorphose into a rigid repressiveness.[13]

A War against Women and Children

The Revolution, of course, did not operate solely on the level of high-minded, utopian abstractions or in the intended or unintended freedoms permitted by disruptions in the traditional social order. The war years brought privation and danger. Schoolmasters joined the army, and their schools closed. Household goods and foodstuffs soon became scarce, and inflation reached 2,000 percent before the end of hostilities. Neighbors turned against each other. Crops and livestock were confiscated, personal property was stolen, and buildings were torched. Some people lost everything and were "left without a shelter or the Common necessarays of Life." Soldiers vowed to wreak vengeance on their enemy's families — to eliminate them "egg and bird," that is, children and mother. Travel was risky or impossible, and yet many were driven from their homes and became refugees. Martha Lewis Grier recalled these as the "times 'which tried mens souls,'" adding, "and womens too — I think." It was not a good time to rear children.[14]

The war was dangerous for women. Women were femes covert, subsumed under the superior authority of their husbands, so that the deliberate humiliation, exposure, violation, or rape of women by the enemy, whether spontaneous or by policy, was a weapon of war designed to undermine the masculine prerogatives of their presumptive lords and masters. In 1776, drunken British soldiers offered a farmer the choice of burning down his

13. Sally Hastings, *Poems, on Different Subjects; to Which Is Added, a Descriptive Account of a Family Tour to the West; in the Year, 1800; in a Letter to a Lady* (Lancaster, Pa., 1808), 96; Laurel Thatcher Ulrich, *Good Wives: Image and Reality in the Lives of Women in Northern New England, 1650–1750* (New York, 1980), 105.

14. Anne Bezanson, *Prices and Inflation during the American Revolution: Pennsylvania, 1770–1790* (Philadelphia, 1951), 344 (weighted averages, measured against prices in 1770–1773); Eliza Chadwick Roberts Scott, "The Ocurances of Life," circa 1814, 7–8, Monmouth County Historical Association, Library and Archives, Freehold, N.J.; Orton and Slate, eds., "Journal of Martha Lewis Walton Grier Bowen," 46.

house or letting one of them kiss his youngest daughter, who was young enough to still be playing with dolls. Her father ordered her to "comply." We don't know what the daughter felt or thought of the drunken mauling or of her father's complicity in giving the soldier access to her body.[15]

Sharon Block recovered evidence of 104 rapes in the thirteen colonies in the 1740s and 1750s, nearly doubling to 203 during the two revolutionary decades after 1760. Rape was more often hushed than recorded, the subject of whispers rather than explicit news stories. An unnamed servant who expressed her support for "king and country" in the presence of American troops in Delaware was "dragged into their guard-room, where she was forcibly abused by seventeen of the villains, in the most gross, brutal, and injurious manner possible." The evidence comes only from a traveler's diary. Women's bodies were under attack.[16]

Some women's deaths were widely broadcast by partisans as indications of the barbarism of the enemy and as a warning to all women. Two of the most infamous cases were the murders of Jane M'Crea, a New York tory, and Hannah Caldwell, a New Jersey patriot. M'Crea was scalped by "Indian" allies while going to visit her fiancé in upstate New York. Caldwell was shot by a British sharpshooter while in her own house, and her corpse was stripped of clothing by soldiers looking for valuables. The fates of M'Crea and Caldwell appeared in newspapers, pamphlets, and prints. Women, as the symbolic representations and possessions of their fathers, brothers, and husbands, were targets for vengeance by the enemy.[17]

Although politically motivated violence against the enemy's masculine prerogatives as embodied in their female dependents was not new in 1775 and persists to the present day, neoclassical artistic conventions, which represented nations as females scantily dressed in draped diaphanous garb, brought the violation of women's bodies into the daily purview of the public. During the Revolution, these political cartoons represented America with

15. Lydia Minturn Post (1859 version of a 1776 diary), in Harris, ed., *American Women Writers*, 297. This account seems to have been heavily edited for Victorian sensibilities.

16. J. F. D. Smyth, *A Tour in the United States of America* . . . , 2 vols. (London, 1784), II, 302; Sharon Block, *Rape and Sexual Power in Early America* (Chapel Hill, N.C., 2006), 249. Rather than seeing change during the war, Block stresses that sexual coercion has been "profoundly transhistoric" (241).

17. James Caldwell, "Certain Facts Relating to the Tragic Death of Hannah Caldwell, Wife of Rev. James Caldwell," ed. A. L. Johnson, Union County Historical Society, *Proceedings*, II (1923–1924), 10–15; Elizabeth F. Ellet, *The Women of the American Revolution*, 3 vols. (New York, 1848–1850), II, 107–114, 221–226; Gregory Evans Dowd, "Declarations of Dependence: War and Inequality in Revolutionary New Jersey, 1776–1815," *New Jersey History*, CIII (1985), 47–67, esp. 53–55.

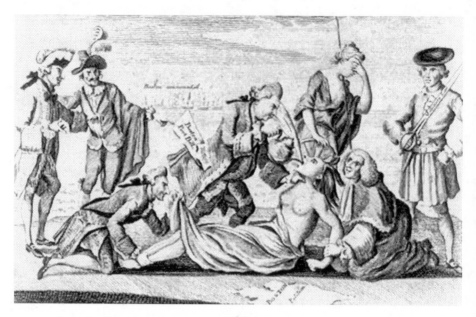

PLATE 3.

The Able Doctor; or, America Swallowing the Bitter Draught.
From *London Magazine*, May 1, 1774.

A female figure representing America is stripped, force-fed,
and sexually humiliated while a sorrowing Britain averts her eyes
from this disgraceful scene. Images of violence against
women circulated even before the war began.

stylized, symbol-laden images of women with their clothing rent from their bodies and their bare breasts exposed, women splayed like carcasses in a butcher's stall with limbs hacked off, prostrated women with men peering at their genitals (Plate 3), witchlike women with their genitals on fire, and desexed women with phallic attributes. These images of violated womanhood could be seen in the shops, taverns, and homes where these prints were displayed. Popular cartoons provided a veritable catalog of insulted and demeaned womanhood as well as a graphically precise continuation of old stereotypes of irrational, uncontrollable, passionate, and vulnerable femininity. Female bodies were under attack both in real life and in print.

One possible reaction to the politically motivated violence against women — whether imaginary or actual — would have been for women to restrict access to their persons, to gain control over their bodies. Perhaps this tendency is one reason for the widespread popularity of Mary Wollstonecraft's *Vindication of the Rights of Woman* (1792) in the United States. Wollstonecraft promoted female dignity and self-possession. She expressed a new civil category—*women's* rights—based on the sobriety and respectability of well-educated adult women. She articulated what many American women had already begun to practice: propriety and a personal reserve governed by reason that would apply equally to men as to women; at least if both boys and girls received appropriate educations.[18]

The radical implications of the *Vindication* faded from public discussion when it was revealed late in the eighteenth century that Mary Wollstonecraft had conceived two children out of wedlock. This scandalous revelation would be used for decades to denounce the proponents of women's rights as sluts. Still, some women privately persisted in their admiration. As one woman wrote to a friend, Wollstonecraft's "unfortunate deviations make one rather wish to bury all in oblivion and much as I adore her in secret, I cannot bear to hear her spoken of in company. Many an unhallowed tongue profanes her sacred name with the coarsest jests." But, despite the public ignominy, the writer promised to meet her friend and "talk over the wrongs of poor Mary," while she wrapped her copies of Wollstonecraft's books in paper so that her daughter would not be able to read them until she was old enough to distinguish virtue from disgrace. If Wollstonecraft slipped in the estimation of the reading public, then novels and later magazines continued to urge female modesty and reputation and warned of vile seducers who would play on retrograde notions of passionate, irrational femininity. Women needed to control their bodies and improve their minds.[19]

Wollstonecraft offered a fleeting, although radical in its public presentation, suggestion that women practice control over their fertility as part of the new responsibilities of sensible womanhood. Wollstonecraft urged women to breast-feed for "their own health" because then "there would be such an interval between the birth of each child that we would seldom see a houseful of babes." In addition to better health, a less crowded household would leave women time to improve their minds through the study of literature, science, and the fine arts. This message was not entirely original with

18. Mary Wollstonecraft, *A Vindication of the Rights of Woman* (1792), ed. Charles W. Hagelman, Jr. (New York, 1967), 185–198.

19. William Godwin, *Memoirs of Mary Wollstonecraft Godwin, Author of "A Vindication of the Rights of Woman,"* ed. W. Clark Durant (1799; rpt. New York, 1969); Margaret Murphey Craig (1761–1814) to Mariamne Alexander Williams (1761–1816), n.d. [circa 1798–1805], Rush Papers, Rosenbach Museum and Library, Philadelphia, II:17:12. The "wrongs of poor Mary" could either refer to Wollstonecraft herself or to her novel; see *Maria; or, The Wrongs of Woman*, ed. Moira Ferguson (New York, 1975).

Wollstonecraft—many American women had already reached similar conclusions—and these ideas did not disappear with Wollstonecraft's eclipse.
Warfare had made it clear that women had to protect themselves. At roughly
the same time, fertility rates began to decline in the United States while rates
were stagnant or rising in England.[20]

The rebelliousness of 1763–1775, the military and economic crises of the
Revolutionary War, 1775–1783, and the heated constitutional debates and
popular uprisings of the 1780s and 1790s were social as well as political upheavals that caused Americans to reassess old habits of mind and to consider
new ideas. Independence and a rejection of "slavish" behaviors challenged
and began to undermine inherited rigid social ranks and roles. The protests
and warfare that produced thirteen independent republics neither solved the
question of who would rule at home nor determined how far the guarantees
of liberty should extend. Whether Americans were wealthy or poor, free or
enslaved, radical or conservative, whether they embraced or rejected these
changes in the second half of the eighteenth century, new ideas were con-
templated, new situations were experienced.[21]

Spreading the Word

The substance of revolutionary language and of wartime experience was important in shaping women's perceptions of the rights and limitations inherent in femininity, but so was the opening of channels of communication,
both as gossip and in the proliferation of newspaper articles, pamphlets, and
broadsides. After all, few of the ideas expressed during the turmoil of the last
third of the eighteenth century were entirely new, and none was exclusively
American. The major writers of the European Enlightenment had been de-
bating natural rights to life, liberty, property, and the pursuit of happiness
long before the troubles began on the western periphery of the British Empire in America. The colonies shared in the consumer and print revolutions
that spread ideas and questioned received wisdom. Sensibility, companionate marriages, sentimentalized childhoods, and an expansive public sphere
could be found on both sides of the Atlantic. But it was the protests, parades,

20. Wollstonecraft, *Vindication*, ed. Hagelman, 282. For a long list of intrepid women, see Ellet,
The Women of the American Revolution.

21. Linda K. Kerber, *Women of the Republic: Intellect and Ideology in Revolutionary America*
(Chapel Hill, N.C., 1980); Mary Beth Norton, *Liberty's Daughters: The Revolutionary Experience of
American Women, 1750–1800* (Boston, 1980); Jay Fliegelman, *Prodigals and Pilgrims: The American
Revolution against Patriarchal Authority, 1750–1800* (New York, 1982).

battles, inflation, shortages, and sufferings that helped make the abstract tangible, that connected disparate ideas, and that triggered a more rapid and more complete overthrow of traditional habits. "The revolution interested every inhabitant of the country of both sexes, and of every rank and age ... with all the force of *novelty* upon the human mind," wrote Benjamin Rush. There was an urgency to discussions that had not existed in more peaceable times. Social barriers were breached by the crisis. One woman remembered when she and other refugees—women, children, and servants—were fleeing before British troops, looking for "a hut or barn, in any region of security," that "sometimes those who had never spoken together in the city would meet in their wanderings, and then all distinctions of rank were forgotten, and they were a band of brothers." The war temporarily opened lines of communication, so that gossip, ideas, jokes, and values spread as they would not have under peacetime conditions. Family limitation could become an aspect of public opinion through the circulation and linking of civil and political rights, individualism, restraint, birth-control methods, egalitarian marriages, limited childbearing, and expanded opportunities for children.[22]

New ideas on women's essential equality were encoded in speech and writing. The humorous adoption of the phrase "lords of creation"—used

22. Rush, "Influence of the American Revolution," in Runes, ed., *Selected Writings of Rush,* 325–333, esp. 325; H. T., "Reminiscences of Philadelphia," *Hazard's Register of Pennsylvania,* III, no. 54 (Jan. 10, 1829), 40–41. On the significance of the means of diffusion in the adoption of new ideas or patterns of behavior, see John B. Casterline, ed., *Diffusion Processes and Fertility Transition: Selected Perspectives* (Washington, D.C., 2001); Susan Cotts Watkins and Angela D. Danzi, "Women's Gossip and Social Change: Childbirth and Fertility Control among Italian and Jewish Women, 1920–1940," *Gender and Society,* IX (1995), 469–490. Diffusion should not be confused with trickle-down theories of dissemination or with gentrification, refinement, middle-class hegemony, or other monofocal conceptions of innovative behaviors. Here, innovation is seen as having multiple beginnings, purposes, and means of implementation, hence the study of visual as well as textual sources, private and public documents, legal and medical pronouncements, and statistical and individual evidence.

Some German-speaking sectarians did go against the grain, increasing fertility levels over the course of the eighteenth and early nineteenth centuries. See Rodger C. Henderson, "Eighteenth-Century Schwenkfelders: A Demographic Interpretation," in Peter C. Erb, ed., *Schwenkfelders in America: Papers Presented at the Colloquium on Schwenckfeld and the Schwenkfelders, Pennsburg, Pa., September 17–22, 1984* (Pennsburg, Pa., 1987), 25–40; Beverly Prior Smaby, *The Transformation of Moravian Bethlehem: From Communal Mission to Family Economy* (Philadelphia, 1988), 51–85. Christine Hücho has revealed the linguistic isolation of Schwenkfelder women, their heavy reliance on religious imagery, and their role in preserving a minority culture, in "Female Writers, Women's Networks, and the Preservation of Culture: The Schwenkfelder Women of Eighteenth-Century Pennsylvania" (paper presented at the Philadelphia Center for Early American Studies [currently the McNeil Center for Early American Studies], 1997). These few exceptions point to the importance both of vocabulary and of social interaction in diffusing innovative behavior.

to assail the pompous presumptuousness of the masculine sex—provides one example of a shared language of laughter, protest, and reformation. The catchphrase encapsulated the message of Genesis 1:27: "God created man in his own image, . . . male and female created he them. And God blessed them, and God said unto them, Be fruitful, and multiply, and replenish the earth, and subdue it: and have dominion over . . . every living thing." This biblical creation story presents the alternative to the Eve-as-Adam's-spare-rib myth. In this version of creation, women and men were both formed in God's image and were equally granted authority over the earth and lesser creatures. The New Testament offered additional support. In Mark 10:5–6, Jesus first overturns certain gendered inequities in Judaic marriage and divorce law and then pointedly reminds his followers that "from the beginning of creation God made them male and female." In Eden and in the Gospel, men and women were ordained by God as equals.[23]

Those who stressed an original equality believed that the egalitarian message of these biblical verses was later lost. John Milton—among many, many others—had asserted a patriarchal order from the moment of creation, so that Adam and Eve "seemed Lords of all, . . . though both Not equal as thir sex not equal seemed; . . . Hee for God only, shee for God in him." A century and more later, many literate women were beginning to reject these assumptions of "true authoritie" and "absolute rule" in men and "subjection" in women. Susanna Wright wrote circa 1778:

> Since Adam, [men], (With no superior virtue in their mind)
> Assert their right to govern womankind.
> But womankind call reason to their aid,
> And question when or where that law was made.

Increasing numbers of women decided that men's attempts to act as the "lords of creation" were blasphemous. They reverted, with laughter at the ignorant, to what they understood as the true meaning of the Bible: man and

---

23. See also Matt. 19:4 and Gal. 3:28. Jan Lewis has also noted the prevalence of references to Eve in the early Republic. Lewis's important article investigates how the biblical story of Eve's seduction by the serpent and her subsequent seduction of Adam was reworked after the Revolution into a story of Eve's positive influence in promoting male civic virtue and Edenic marriages of equals (Lewis, "The Republican Wife: Virtue and Seduction in the Early Republic," *William and Mary Quarterly*, 3d Ser., XLIV [1987], 689–721). Ana M. Acosta, *Reading Genesis in the Long Eighteenth Century: From Milton to Mary Shelley* (Burlington, Vt., 2006), discusses the ways in which enlightened exegesis reinterpreted and critiqued the book of Genesis, especially in political thought, noting that "the republican tradition of enlightenment wound up" in the Americas (7).

woman were equally in God's image and in earthly dominion. And at least one woman preferred to eliminate Adam entirely, tracing humanity back to the "daughters of Eve" and the "sons of Eve."[24]

The phrase "lords of creation" was first used sarcastically in Samuel Richardson's enormously popular novel, *Clarissa* (1748), when the character Anna Howe remarked on observing "all the noble Lords of the creation, in their peculiarities." The phrase must have struck a chord, for Richardson used it frequently in his later publications, and it appeared in other works with increasing frequency through the eighteenth and nineteenth centuries. English and some colonial sources tended to use the phrase "lords of *the* creation," that is, they referred to men's control over a static natural order. The popular educational works of Priscilla Wakefield, an English Quaker, for example, included her observation that Providence ordained that "the increase of noxious animals is generally restricted." If it were not, "this globe would be no longer habitable; we should be forced to resign our places to them, and they would become lords of the creation." According to Wakefield, humans need to outreproduce "birds and beasts of prey, and huge serpents" in order to maintain their primacy. Others, especially in America, dropped the "the" and mocked the "lords of creation," making the creation, not static and timeless, but indicative of the creative, prolific, and procreative processes that were just beginning to be called reproduction.[25]

An early use of the phrase in the colonies was by the outspoken Hannah Callender, who wrote in her diary on February 6, 1759, of "a young gentleman" who "behaved pretty tolerable, tho' plain to be seen he was not igno-

24. John Milton, *Paradise Lost; a Poem in Twelve Books* (London, 1674), book IV, lines 288–299; Pattie Cowell, "'Womankind Call Reason to Their Aid': Susanna Wright's Verse Epistle on the Status of Women in Eighteenth-Century America," *Signs*, VI (1980–1981), 799. Abigail Adams offered a variant interpretation, writing to her sister in 1799, "I will never consent to have our sex considered in an inferior point of light." She continued: "Let each planet shine in their own orbit. God and nature designed it so—if man is Lord, woman is Lordess" (quoted in Gary B. Nash, *The Unknown American Revolution: The Unruly Birth of Democracy and the Struggle to Create America* [New York, 2005], 206). See also McMahon and Schriver, eds., *To Read My Heart*, 41.

25. Samuel Richardson, *Clarissa; or, The History of a Young Lady . . .* , 7 vols. (London, 1748), I, 167–178 (Richardson used the phrase twice in the 1748 edition, added another repetition in the revision of 1751, and employed it seven times in *The History of Sir Charles Grandison; in a Series of Letters, Published from the Originals*, 3d ed., 2 vols. [London, 1754]); Priscilla Wakefield, *Mental Improvement; or, The Beauties and Wonders of Nature and Art, in a Series of Instructive Conversations*, 3d ed. (Philadelphia, 1814), 33. Mary Wollstonecraft laughed at the "faint glimmerings of mind which entitles [men] to rank as lords of creation," but, of course, did not so entitle any female, even a well-known critic and author. See Wollstonecraft, *Letters Written during a Short Residence in Sweden, Norway, and Denmark* (1795; rpt. Lincoln, Neb., 1976), 10.

rant of the title they give themselves, Lords of the Creation, but like most other potentates to be governed by their Ministers." The power of men was a self-interested delusion. Sarah Wister in 1778 stood up to some "saucy" soldiers and remarked, "I am quite a heroine, and need not be fearful of any of the lords of the creation for the future." Both women turned male dominance on its head. Already there is a suggestion that women need only assert themselves and the artifice of male dominance would collapse.[26]

Men were stubborn, however. When Philip Vickers Fithian was bested in 1773 by a young woman in a vociferous argument over the portrayal of female characters in novels, he fumed in his diary about "weak and inconsiderable Animals [women, who] tear and insult the majestic Lion [men], but the lordly Beast leaves them in their Folly, scorning to take the Advantage of so great [an] inequality!" Fithian might have triumphed on the page, but he and others were losing in the court of feminine public opinion. Indeed, in his own town a group of seven women organized "to inform each other when they heard of anything immoral or otherwise improper in the conduct of any young man." The offender would be shunned.[27]

During and after the Revolution, presumptuous lords were placed in opposition to the essential equality of peoples. "Equality is the soul of friendship," wrote Nancy Shippen in her diary, and "marriage, to give delight, must join *two minds,* not devote a slave to the will of an imperious Lord." Judith Sargent Murray published her assessment: "Yes, you lordly, you haughty sex, our souls are by nature *equal* to yours." In a similar vein, Priscilla Mason addressed a promiscuous crowd, as gatherings of men and women were called, pointing out, "Our high and mighty Lords (thanks to their arbitrary constitutions), have denied us the means of knowledge and then reproached us for the want of it. . . . Happily, a more liberal way of thinking begins to prevail." A new age was dawning. The era of corrupted biblical exegesis was being replaced by the true meaning of Genesis. Women would enjoy more scope for the exercise of their intellectual capacity through a gendered reformation that would return to the intentions of God both at the moment of creation and as reiterated by Jesus. The catchphrase soon came to encapsulate a multitude of messages concerning gendered equality, equitable marriages,

---

26. Susan E. Klepp and Karin A. Wulf, eds., *The Diary of Hannah Callender Sansom: Sense and Sensibility in a Revolutionary Age, 1758–1788* (Ithaca, N.Y., 2009), Feb. 6, 1759; Derounian, *The Journal and Occasional Writings of Sarah Wister,* 63.

27. F. Alan Palmer, ed., *The Beloved Cohansie of Philip Vickers Fithian* ([Greenwich, N.J.], 1990), 164; Mary Patterson Moore, *Grandfather's Farm: Life on the Cohansey Plantation of Squire Maskell Ewing* (1859), ed. F. Alan Palmer (Bridgeton, N.J., 1981), 13.

educational opportunities, and alternatives to domesticity. Women's declarations also paralleled one of Tom Paine's arguments against elite oppression, when he asked rhetorically, "Why are the petty Lords and Princes (as they call themselves) of Germany poor?" It was, said Paine, because they denied people their liberty. Oppression was wrong; it was impractical. Ultimately, inequality was a flimsy fiction that could easily be overthrown.[28]

Sarah Coombe Shields took the unusual step of sending an anonymous letter to a male acquaintance. She castigated the unknown recipient for "your tyranny and unkindness to your daughters." She then demanded, in the stirring language of eighteenth-century revolutions, that the man change his behavior and adopt virtue: "If tyranny is an abomination in the sight of the enlightened world; if all men who have a sense of freedom execrate the scepter'd tyrant, what must be the verdict of the humane, the benevolent and the just on a parent, who shall practice despotism upon the weak and the helpless, upon the last and the fairest of Heaven's creation?" No spare rib here. Again, the purposes of creation have been revisited and reclaimed from the weight of a tyrannical and unenlightened history.[29]

As the phrase "lords of creation" became widespread, male authors took it up. In vocalizing female opinion through fictional characters, it is interesting that men were bolder and more straightforward than women about the sexual and procreative significances of this vocabulary—indeed, they tended to be more outspoken when masquerading in feminine roles than when writing as men. According to a ragged rhyme in the *Essex Almanac* of 1771, "At length over wedlock fair liberty dawns, / And the Lords of Creation must pull in their horns." Was this awkward rhyme a lightly veiled reference to male abstinence or to male withdrawal during intercourse? Perhaps. In the 1790 play, *The Widow of Malabar*, David Humphreys has oppressed women in India cry out:

28. Ethel Armes, comp. and ed., *Nancy Shippen: Her Journal Book; The International Romance of a Young Lady of Fashion of Colonial Philadelphia with Letters to Her and about Her* (Philadelphia, 1935), 145; Judith Sargent Murray, "On the Equality of the Sexes," *Massachusetts Magazine* (March 1790), 134; Priscilla Mason, "The Salutary Oration [at the Young Ladies' Academy, 1793]," in Harris, ed., *American Women Writers*, 71; [Thomas Paine], "A Serious Address to the People of Pennsylvania, on the Present Situation of Their Affairs," *Pennsylvania Packet* (Philadelphia), Dec. 1, 1778. Shippen also writes in her journal that men who "know how to be happy, willingly give up the harsh title of master, for the more tender and endearing one of Friend" (May 15, 1783). This sentiment, from a contemporary novel, was also quoted by Abigail Adams; see Elaine Forman Crane, "Abigail Adams, Gender Politics, and *The History of Emily Montague*: A Postscript," *WMQ*, 3d Ser., LXIV (2007), 839–844, esp. 839.

29. Attributed to Sarah Coombe Shields, MS, circa 1790s, Thomas Coombe Papers, HSP.

Ah! cruel Lords of creation, see;
How weak, how full of woes, our sex is form'd;
Is it for you, . . . to add new weight
To nature's heavy yoke!

The message is clear: civilized men should refrain from multiplying women's physiological burdens, and Westerners should exhibit their superiority to supposedly primitive peoples by their better treatment of women—a justification for conquest that still has currency.[30]

Writing to a fellow doctor in 1802, Benjamin Rush proclaimed that the biblical curses inflicted on Adam and Eve had been "repealed" by "the benevolent disposition of the Creator of the world." Because many men no longer labored "by the sweat of the brow"—Adam's curse—and instead lived "in the enjoyment of all the comforts of life," women should likewise be freed of God's curse on Eve: "I will greatly multiply thy sorrow and thy conception; in sorrow thou shalt bring forth children" (Gen. 3:16). Rush proposed a number of heroic regimens designed to reduce the pain of childbirth but, as the father of thirteen children himself, did not consider reducing the number of births. Yet, the idea that an enlightened world could reinterpret the Bible in order to reduce human suffering could have far-reaching results in areas that Rush was reluctant to explore.[31]

---

30. Philo Freeman, *The Essex Almanack* . . . (Salem, Mass., 1771), 21, said to be reprinted from an unlocated English source (another version is in *Amusement; or, A New Collection of Pleasing Songs, Humorous Jests, and the Most Approved Country Dances Selected from Various Authors* [Montpelier, Vt., 1811], 53–54); David Humphreys, *The Widow of Malabar; or, The Tyranny of Custom: A Tragedy*, in *The Miscellaneous Works of Colonel Humphreys* (New York, 1790), 123.

31. Benjamin Rush, "On the Means of Lessening the Pains and Danger of Child-Bearing, and of Preventing Its Consequent Diseases," *Medical Repository of Original Essays and Intelligence*, VI, no. 1 (Jan. 1, 1803), 26–27. Still, most medical texts, whether for home use or professional training, had avoided transgressing the biblical commandment that childbirth should entail suffering. Physicians might have given birthing mothers opium in practice, but the blasphemous subject of pain relief during labor was usually avoided in the public prints. Directions for speeding up delivery were permitted, but not recipes for pain relief. See, for example, Jane Sharp, who merely explains that women who are "unruly and will not be governed . . . will suffer the greater pain in Child-birth [while] a Boy is sooner and easier brought forth than a Girle . . . for women are lustier that are with Child with Boys" (Jane Sharp, *The Midwives Book; or, The Whole Art of Midwifry Discovered* [1671], ed. Elaine Hobby [New York, 1999], 130). William Buchan, like Sharp, specifically prohibits giving alcohol or stimulants (*Domestic Medicine; or, A Treatise on the Prevention and Cure of Diseases, by Regimen and Simple Medicines* . . . , rev. ed., ed. Samuel Powel Griffitts [Philadelphia, 1795], 537–538). William Dewees provides a recipe for controlling the afterpains, but nothing else, in *A Compendious System of Midwifery* . . . (Philadelphia, 1832), 199. In central Pennsylvania in 1782, however, George Sisseholtz's wife discovered and "highly recommended" to her neighbors her own cure for "severe

Critics worried about the population implications of the phrase "lords of creation" as early as the 1780s. They accused both male and female "Lords of the creation" of putting off marriage to avoid parenthood and therefore causing "a stagnation in the rising generation." Young, unmarried women and men had become too attached to "gaiety and love of pleasure" and were excessively apprehensive about the "cares and concerns of an increasing family, or the fear of meeting with too prudent and serious companions." Traditional marriage, according to these critics, had been devalued by the corrupting messages found in novels and at the theater. Family life was seen by both men and women as a dismal prospect that offered either the worrisome financial burdens of an ever increasing family or the chilly prospect of prudent, that is, restrained, sexual relations. Neither option was enticing to the younger generation, these authors felt, and population growth was threatened.[32]

Yet the phrase continued circulating. A small-town schoolteacher published a song for her students:

The Lords of creation men we call,
And they think they rule the whole,
But they're much mistaken after all.

It was a sentiment that also linked revolutionary-era women to the women at Seneca Falls and Rochester in 1848. Maria W. Chapman concluded the world's second women's rights meeting with a similarly humorous depiction of a gendered world turned upside down, noting the "'Lords of Creation' do fear an eclipse" and that "unquestioned submission is quite out of date." The control of creation belonged to women as much as or more than it belonged to men.[33]

Women's declamations, whether humorous or serious, revealed an emerging sense that women were a social and political category whose wrongs (whether a lack of rights, of opportunity, of responsibility for self, or of sup-

pains in childbirth": aloes, myrrh, and a quart of rum; see Andrew S. Berky, trans. and ed., *The Journals and Papers of David Shultze*, 2 vols. (Pennsburg, Pa., 1953), II, 166–167.

32. "From the New-York Gazetteer," *Pennsylvania Packet, and Daily Advertiser,* June 14, 1785; "To the Young Gentlemen and Ladies of This City," *New-York Weekly Museum,* Sept. 20, 1788.

33. J. S. R., "The Lords of Creation Men We Call . . ." (Philadelphia, 1838), *Music for the Nation: American Sheet Music,* Library of Congress, http://memory.loc.gov (accessed July 2004); "Proceedings of the Woman's Rights Convention, Held at Rochester, N.Y., August 2, 1848," in *Proceedings of the Woman's Rights Conventions, Held at Seneca Falls and Rochester, N.Y., July and August 1848* (Rochester, N.Y., 1848), 12–13.

port and protection) affected all women, or perhaps only all free women. Catchphrases, humor, gossip, novels, and other forms of communication diffused recognition of the many benefits of a more autonomous femininity, bodily self-control, and, it seems, of family limitation. In all these iterations, women and many men saw themselves in a revolutionary age when the gendered inequalities imposed in previous ages were at last being overturned. God's original intention of male and female equality was being fulfilled. Birthrates wavered in the 1770s and 1780s and then began the long-term decline that persists to the present day.

A Revolution for and by Women

As revolutionary protests began, the language of women's fertility and the pregnant body started to change. Eliza Stedman, "talking Like ane american" in 1764, mocked traditional attitudes and found that, at the same time that older women were enthusiastically bearing additional children, many young women were delaying marriage and therefore not having children. She predicted that, if her satiric comments were made known, these older wives, too, "would have none." Her friend, Elizabeth Graeme, admitted, "I never was so fond of Children as Many People are." She had other interests. Other Philadelphia women were criticizing the continued emphasis on childbearing as essential to femininity. When Hannah Callender Sansom "paid a Lying in vis[it]" in 1769, she noted, "The custom of paying Vails [gifts of money] to Nurses [women who had just given birth] begins to drop." In a 1776 Quaker meeting, Suzy Lightfoot admonished "young mothers not to make such great preparations for their lying-in as they generally do, and to avoid those formal visitings upon the occasion which are too much made use of." Lightfoot worried that women appeared frivolous, and apparently many women agreed. The elaborate communal celebrations of childbearing gradually became extinct, and the quieter celebrations that continued focused on the newborn child. Women in the 1770s sewed, as gifts for the newborn, pincushions inscribed with the slogan, "Welcome, Little Stranger," the linked initials of the parents, and the date. Birthing was shifting from being woman-centered to being child-centered.[34]

34. Simon Gratz, "Some Material for a Biography of Mrs. Elizabeth Fergusson, née Graeme," *PMHB*, XXXIX (1915), 257–321 (esp. 277), 385–409 (esp. 387); Sarah Logan Fisher, "'A Diary of Trifling Occurrences': Philadelphia, 1776–1778," ed. Nicholas B. Wainwright, *PMHB*, LXXXII (1958), 418; Klepp and Wulf, eds., *Diary of Hannah Callender*, Nov. 24, 1769; Susan Burrows Swan, *Plain and Fancy: American Women and Their Needlework, 1650–1850*, rev. ed. (Austin, Tex., 1995), 128, 130.

"Teeming," "flourishing," "breeding," "fruitful," "prolific," "lusty," "big with child," "gone with child," "great with child," "big-bellied," or just plain "big" were among the exuberant, expansive adjectives that colonial American women and men had employed to refer to the pregnant body. In the last quarter of the eighteenth century, new metaphors, both sentimental and precise, replaced the language of unregulated abundance and suggest how first women and then men were reconstructing the fecund possibilities of female bodies through a vocabulary of sentiment and numeracy as they communicated these ideals orally and through poems, humor, and prose. This shift in vocabulary was begun by women, who constructed an alternative to a lifetime of childbearing, rejecting literal readings of the biblical admonitions to "be fruitful and multiply" in favor of a language of reason, foresight, constraint, and sensibility. There exists a generation and more of scholarship on the fertility transition, largely from the vantage point of nineteenth-century men's concerns over economic opportunity, the price of land, and intergenerational wealth flows. An examination of the vocabulary of pregnancy and birth allows for a woman-centered examination of the late-eighteenth-century beginning of the transition to family planning and ever lower levels of fertility.

The changed attitudes behind this vocabulary were not exactly the quiet revolution that fertility transitions have been labeled; the American Revolution provoked a widespread discussion of virtue and a critique of luxury in the context of offering women a minor place in the new Republic. In France, the only other nation to experience an early fertility transition, there was a parallel outcry against excess, irresponsibility, and luxury after the middle of the eighteenth century. The traditional language of pregnancy was no longer applicable. Men in the learned professions continued using "fertility" and "fecundity" for women, livestock, and agricultural productivity, but these were not vernacular terms. Fruitful, flourishing, teeming images were rarely invoked after the 1770s, despite their biblical origins. "Breeding" referred almost exclusively to slave women and farm animals by the 1780s, and the term was becoming a sign of contempt. The pregnant, "big-bellied" body was effaced by the beginning of the nineteenth century. The distinctive swollen breasts and abdomens of the nursing and pregnant colonial woman and the separate gatherings of women to celebrate those distinctions were disappearing behind the rational mind, tender heart, and prudent management of women citizens in the new Republic.[35]

35. John R. Gillis, Louise A. Tilly, and David Levine, *The European Experience of Declining Fertility, 1850–1970: The Quiet Revolution* (Cambridge, Mass., 1992). There is a large literature on revo-

Annis Stockton put it well around 1793:

They despise us poor females, and say that our sphere
Must move in the kitchen or heaven knows where
The nursery the pantry the dairy is made
The theatre on which our worth is display'd.

Stockton, who had previously celebrated a wealth of "prattling infants," now preferred to showcase feminine intelligence. And another poet protested against women's wit being "confined entirely by domestic arts / Producing only children and tarts." To emphasize women's minds in a revolutionary age of reason was to suppress the physical body because, as Thomas Laqueur has argued, the "body is regarded simply as the bearer of the rational subject, which itself constitutes the person." Nancy Cott has recognized that passionlessness became an ideal for women at the end of the eighteenth century. It was an attempt to emphasize women's rationality rather than their physicality and sexuality. Influential evangelicals, both women and men, preached that "Christianity had raised women from slaves in status to moral and intellectual beings" and thus "elevated women above the weakness of animal nature." But there were secular precedents for these early-nineteenth-century examples and concrete results. Academic education for women of the middle classes and basic literacy for poorer Americans, both women and men, were advocated, if not always funded, in the early national period. Revolutionary rhetoric, first in the American uprising and reinforced later in the French Revolution, at least raised the possibility of more equitable gender relations, even if the result, politically and civilly, was to revert very nearly to the prewar status quo.[36]

---

lutionary ideas and language, although not in relationship to fertility. For example, see Gordon S. Wood, *The Radicalism of the American Revolution* (New York, 1991); and Robert Darnton, *The Forbidden Bestsellers of Pre-Revolutionary France* (New York, 1995). France is usually accorded first place among nations in achieving truncated fertility; see Jean-Louis Flandrin, *Families in Former Times: Kinship, Household, and Sexuality,* trans. Richard Southern (Cambridge, 1979), 238. A simultaneous transition is suggested by the timetable in Etienne van de Walle, *The Female Population of France in the Nineteenth Century: A Reconstruction of 82 Départements* (Princeton, N.J., 1974).

36. Carla Mulford, *Only for the Eye of a Friend: The Poems of Annis Boudinot Stockton* (Charlottesville, Va., 1995), 96, 177; anonymous poet published in the *Centinel of Freedom* (Newark, N.J.), Sept. 22, 1801, quoted in Judith Apter Klinghoffer and Lois Elkis, "'The Petticoat Electors': Women's Suffrage in New Jersey, 1776–1807," *Journal of the Early Republic,* XII (1992), 181. See also Susanna Hopkins Mason, *Selections from the Letters and Manuscripts of the Late Susanna Mason; with a Brief Memoir of Her Life, by Her Daughter* (Philadelphia, 1836), 30, 277, 279; Thomas Laqueur, "Orgasm, Generation, and the Politics of Reproductive Biology," in Catherine Gallagher and Laqueur, eds., *Making of the Modern Body: Sexuality and Society in the Nineteenth Century,* special issue of *Repre-*

But, if the laws changed little, the metaphors of birth were transformed, an indication of a reconceptualization of women's relationship to fertility. After the 1760s, women no longer described themselves as fruitful or big during pregnancy; they awaited or expected the "little stranger," "the little urchin" (that is, Cupid), "the beloved object," or the "first pledge of matrimonial love." Elizabeth Seton could refer to her friend's "two precious Objects" and yet at times use less sentimental, more ominous language for her own case. She referred to her third pregnancy in financial terms—an unusually forthright admission in an increasingly sentimental age—as "expecting every day the birth of another little dependent in addition to our son and daughter." She characterized her fourth pregnancy and her subsequent newborn more ominously as "the *Shadow*," but her meaning is unclear. Did she mean the shadow of maternity, of the undeveloped character and career of a new child, of the possibility of death in childbirth, of yet another economic burden to the family, or of something else? However characterized, the focus had shifted from women's burgeoning bodies to the resulting birth. Women were, not lusty, but "in the way to become a mother" or "in the way she has *longed* for." "In the family way" appeared later. Wives did not lie in, nor were they confined to chamber, but they "gave birth." The change in definition could be sudden. Miriam Gratz felt that she had to translate her meaning when she wrote to her brother in 1769 that she and her husband were in "expectation of a new happiness (I expect a baby)." Childbearing was being reimagined.[37]

---

sentations, XIV, no. 14 (Spring 1986), 1–41, esp. 19; Nancy F. Cott, "Passionlessness: An Interpretation of Victorian Sexual Ideology, 1790–1850," *Signs*, IV (1977–1978), 219–236, esp. 227, 228. See also Kerber, *Women of the Republic*; Ruth H. Bloch, "The Gendered Meanings of Virtue in Revolutionary America," *Signs*, XIII (1987–1988), 37–58; Lewis, "The Republican Wife," *WMQ*, 3d Ser., XLIV (1987), 689–721; Carroll Smith-Rosenberg, "Domesticating Virtue: Coquettes and Revolutionaries in Young America," in Elaine Scarry, ed., *Literature and the Body: Essays on Populations and Persons*, Selected Papers from the English Institute, 1986, New Series, XII (Baltimore, 1988), 160–184; Cathy N. Davidson, *Revolution and the Word: The Rise of the Novel in America* (New York, 1986).

37. Regina Bechtle and Judith Metz, eds., *Elizabeth Bayley Seton: Collected Writings*, I, *Correspondence and Journals, 1793–1808* (Hyde Park, N.Y., 2000), 38, 47, 120, 142, 197. Perhaps she refers to the Valley of the Shadow of Death, a forewarning of possible death in childbirth, or her fear may be of multiple offspring. For a later period, see Judith Walzer Leavitt, "Under the Shadow of Maternity: American Women's Responses to Death and Debility Fears in Nineteenth-Century Childbirth," *Feminist Studies*, XII (1986), 129–154; Jacob R. Marcus, *The American Jewish Woman: A Documentary History* (New York, 1981), 10; Mrs. M[ary] Clarke, ed., *The Memoirs of the Celebrated and Beautiful Mrs. Ann Carson* (1822) (Philadelphia, 1838), 51–52; Norton, *Liberty's Daughters*, 332 n. 31; Sylvia D. Hoffert, *Private Matters: American Attitudes toward Childbearing and Infant Nurture in the Urban North, 1800–1860* (Urbana, Ill., 1989), 15, 61–70. Although most of the evidence on descriptive language comes from the well-to-do, John Fitch, poor and barely literate, wrote of

Pregnancy was becoming an obligation, a duty, that women undertook voluntarily for rational, sentimental, and instrumental purposes: to welcome a stranger and to secure a marriage by expressing romantic love. It was "expected": both planned and controlled. It was "in the way": a separate path, different from the normal course of a woman's life. The child was a gift, freely given by the woman from a selfless concern for others. There were no descriptors for the pregnant body itself. In 1803, Eliza Roberts was typical in mentioning that her "health [was] very delicate" and then that she "expected in a few weeks to become a mother." Her language circumvented any direct reference to her present state of pregnancy. The process of bearing children in which the stages of development were measured by changes in women's bodies ("going with," "big with," "great with") was eclipsed by a focus on the end result. Rarely mentioned, the pregnant body was to be hidden as ugly or shameful. No longer was the emphasis on the woman, great with child, but on externals to her physical body: her free will, her responsibilities, or the anticipated stranger as a fulfillment of the marriage vow. Childbearing had become "unnatural," exceptional, as well as all too natural, an animalistic episode in the life of an otherwise rational, civilized being. This new vocabulary of fertility was sentimental in reference to the role of women as givers of hospitality and love but also indicated that pregnancy was no longer to be the normal state of women. It is no wonder that at roughly this same time women increasingly sought professional assistance from formally educated doctors rather than from experienced midwives even in normal labors. Extraordinary events called for special measures, special training.[38]

More and more Mid-Atlantic women began defining pregnancy as an alien experience. Elizabeth Seton in New York City did confide to her best friend, "To tell the truth, I am afraid of the *Shadows* [her peculiar word for pregnancy and infants] as soon as I give up nursing." But, more commonly, women, at least in the middle states, spoke of their delicate condition and the need to exercise caution rather than defining their condition as a serious threat to health. These women were more likely to distance themselves from

friends in 1789, "The effects of Love promised further increase to their families," a circumlocution only slightly less stylized than that found among the better educated. See Frank D. Prager, ed., *The Autobiography of John Fitch* (Philadelphia, 1976), 127.

38. Scott, "Ocurances of Life," 40–41. On the rare mentions of pregnancy, see Carl N. Degler, *At Odds: Women and the Family in America from the Revolution to the Present* (New York, 1980), 59–62. For examples of unaesthetic pregnant bodies, see Virginia K. Bartlett, *Keeping House: Women's Lives in Western Pennsylvania, 1790–1850* (Pittsburgh, Pa., 1994), 144. On shame, see Richard W. Wertz and Dorothy C. Wertz, *Lying-In: A History of Childbirth in America* (New York, 1977), 77–108.

their fertility through a metaphoric language of tender pledges and little urchins than through declarations of fear or helplessness.[39]

Much of the new language of pregnancy and childbirth was popularized in the sentimental novel. The new genre of the novel allowed women to imagine a heroic, sensible, tender self. Novels held out the possibility of more egalitarian, loving marriages; they advocated the rational pleasures of reading and education for women; and they repeatedly warned of the dangers of seduction, of unrestrained passion. Novels focused on the freedom and choices of unmarried heroines and their suitors: children seldom appeared. A culture of sensibility, drawn from fiction and the psychology of contemporary medicine, engaged in a civilizing project through which women could reform men and society, fostering humanitarianism by cultivating sympathy and empathy. The liberty and autonomy that the revolutionary Republic promised men might be matched in the influence accorded to women through sensibility. Sensibility did not, however, threaten traditional feminine roles, for marriage and dependence remained at the core of women's existence, and influence over men was not power.[40]

Pamela, the heroine of Samuel Richardson's novel of the same name, refers to her firstborn as "the Pledge, the beloved Pledge of our happier Affections," in a letter to her husband, asserting her own important contribution to a marriage of social unequals. In this passage, Richardson has feminized and idealized the traditional pledge of affection or of love or the token of regard, which was a suitor's gift of a comb, carved spoon, garter, or ring to his intended spouse. These gifts had long been associated with magical binding powers and were to guarantee the man's commitment to marriage. The child was the woman's equivalent gift to her spouse, binding them together as husband and wife. But, although the novel appeared in 1740 and was immediately and enthusiastically read by the same Mid-Atlantic women who left diaries and correspondence, the sentimental language of "beloved, tender pledges" did not appear in women's writings until decades later. Then

39. Bechtle and Metz, eds., *Elizabeth Bayley Seton*, I, 193. See Jan Lewis and Kenneth A. Lockridge, "'Sally Has Been Sick': Pregnancy and Family Limitation among Virginia Gentry Women, 1780–1830," *Journal of Social History*, XXII (1988), 5–19. These authors find Virginia women describing pregnancy as a terrifying, incapacitating sickness and nonfecundity as health, reversing the polarity of colonial discourse. Few Mid-Atlantic women stressed their overwhelming fear of death or their need for their husbands to protect them from mortal danger, perhaps an indication of a developing regional difference in gender definition.

40. Davidson, *Revolution and the Word*; G. J. Barker-Benfield, *The Culture of Sensibility: Sex and Society in Eighteenth-Century Britain* (Chicago, 1992).

the phrase suddenly flourished. Anna Young Smith and her husband were refugees from British-occupied Philadelphia in early 1778. She united political liberty and marital love into a single image of domestic peace that tamed wild nature and obliterated war:

> While Love and liberty still bless'd each Shade.
> We liv'd contented in the peaceful Grove,
> With the dear pledges of Connubial Love.

Jane O'Bryan of New York City, who had been in her own words "neither opulent, nor affluent," wrote to Dolley Madison begging for her husband's release from debtor's prison on behalf of "the sweet pledges of our happy union." The dear pledges bound husband and wife together in a shared realm of marital bliss and revolutionary republicanism.[41]

The word "pledge" has several meanings. The fictional Pamela took the customary unilateral endowment of male suitors and found a female equivalent that signaled a wife's comparable initiative in cementing the marital bond. More negatively, a pledge might be a hostage designed to prevent hostilities. Ann Baker Carson enjoyed a brief respite from her husband's "caprices, jealousies, and petulancy" after their son was born in 1806, and she "fancied our mutual happiness would be secured for ever." A pledge could also refer to the security for fulfillment of a contract. Several scholars have noted the substantial changes in contractual relations that occurred during the Revolution. As Gordon Wood has argued, although not in reference to women, "colonists tried to grapple with the changes taking place in their lives almost solely in terms of their traditional personal relationships—per-

---

41. Richardson quoted in Dolores Peters, "The Pregnant Pamela: Characterization and Popular Medical Attitudes in the Eighteenth Century," *Eighteenth-Century Studies,* XIV (1981), 432–451, esp. 448; Sylvia [Mrs. (Anna Young) Smith], "Verses on Marriage," circa 1778, Thomas Coombe Papers, HSP (my thanks to Susan Stabile for the attribution); David B. Mattern and Holly C. Shulman, eds., *Selected Letters of Dolley Payne Madison* (Charlottesville, Va., 2003), 134; John R. Gillis, *For Better, for Worse: British Marriages, 1600 to the Present* (New York, 1985), 31–34.

In 1779, Captain George Bush of the Eleventh Pennsylvania Regiment recorded this song: "Kate, take my tobacco box, a soldiers all, / Lest by some d——d Hessian, I should chance to fall. / That when Tom's life is ended, you may justly prove, / You had my first, my last, my only pledge of love" (Kate Van Winkle Keller, comp. and ed., *Songs from the American Revolution* [Sandy Hook, Conn., 1992], 14). An exceptional case of mixed agricultural, religious, and sentimental imagery comes from 1755. Mary Pemberton wrote to her husband about "those tender and Pleasant Plants committed to our care, that in due time by the blessing of divine Providence they may grow up trees of Righteousness, Producing the fruits of the Spirit, thereby, be usefull Ornaments of Society, and Pledges of our mutual Love." (Judy Mann DiStefano, "A Concept of the Family in Colonial America: The Pembertons of Philadelphia" [Ph.D. diss., Ohio State University, 1970], 128).

haps most clearly revealed in the way in which they blended their enlightened paternalism into the new meaning they gave to contracts." For, instead of endorsing hierarchical relationships, revolutionary-era contracts, and we can include marriage contracts, were redefined as "positive bargains deliberately and freely entered into between two parties who were presumed to be equal and not entirely trustful of one another." The language of pledges nicely stressed the binding powers of love and disguised the force of legal inequalities while assuming a woman's right to assent to the uses of her body. Women posited an equality with men through their common share of reason and calculating prudence, or they created a symmetry by balancing women's sympathy against men's courage. Either way, there were now possibilities of self-identity beyond the cycles of fertility and nourishment.[42]

The revolutionary debate about luxury and extravagance caused women and men to emphasize prudence. The revolutionaries called on women to enforce boycotts through nonconsumption and nonimportation. Superabundance and superfluity were under attack; restraint and self-control were promoted. As early as the 1769 nonimportation movement, as J. E. Crowley has noted, "women played a key role in these expressions of industry and frugality because they were thought to have a determining influence on the fashions and therefore the luxury in American society. They would aid public virtue both by their frugality and by their example." Women had an opportunity to assert, along with men, their relative liberty, rationality, and civic virtue. They could overcome their presumed predilection for extravagance and mindlessly chasing the latest fashion by choosing to adopt simplicity, self-control, and restraint. Sumptuary women were mocked in street theater, public prints, newspapers, and magazines during the war, and their pregnancies, whether legitimate or not, were decried as evidence of sexual corruption. In 1778, one commentator burlesqued the "extraordinary natural weight which some of the ladies carry before them," referring to these women's pregnant bellies, and added, "Most of the young ladies who were in the city with the enemy, and wear the present fashionable dresses, have purchased them at the expense of their virtue." The republican wife and mother, on the other hand, would mediate between the family and the state by adopting self-control and between the present and the rising generation by replicating republican virtue.[43]

42. Clarke, ed., *Memoirs of Ann Carson*, 52–53; Wood, *Radicalism*, 162.

43. J. E. Crowley, *This Sheba, Self: The Conceptualization of Economic Life in Eighteenth-Century America* (Baltimore, 1974), 139–140; "From a Late Philadelphia Paper," *Continental Journal and Weekly Advertiser* (Boston), July, 30, 1778; Susan E. Klepp, "Rough Music on Independence Day:

And, just as the political term "virtue" came to be associated with women's sexual restraint early in the Republic, so, too, did the economic virtue of "prudence" come to be linked to women's restraint of births. The Revolution gave a national purpose to this reconfiguration of gendered expectations and held out the possibility of a more inclusive polity in which there would be a role for women. Crowley assumes a masculine subject when he writes that "liberty depended on the individual's control over the fruits of his industry," but women might find a parallel liberty in their prudent control over the fruits of their bodies.[44]

Economic ideas were changing in other ways as well. Self-interest was viewed as less of a threat to the social order under the developing market economy. Because the deliberate restriction of births had been associated with selfishness, a traditional bar to curtailed childbearing might have been lowered. However, this line of argument probably brought women too far from conventional images of selfless, charitable, and nurturing woman- hood. The postrevolutionary period saw a more powerful tendency to re- move women entirely from the economic realm, to make women's labor in- visible, and to assign all economic value to male breadwinners. Self-interest could then operate in the economic realm dominated by men, even as virtue was preserved within women's realm. Jeanne Boydston has convincingly de- scribed this process as the pastoralization of women's work: housework was natural (not skilled), effortless (not laborious), and had no monetary equiva- lent (selfless and decorative, neither acquisitive nor productive). Before the Revolution, childbearing had been considered procreation and generation. After the 1780s, childbearing was described as reproduction, a process dis- tinct from production and therefore divorced from notions of wealth. Re- production would not be of interest to the men creating the dismal science of economics, since it had no value. Birthrates became a residual function of the structures of male economic opportunity. Demographers who sought economic motives for the fertility transition could likewise focus on men, because women were not economic actors. The shift to conceptualizing childbearing as reproduction also, as Ludmilla Jordanova has argued, both "marginalizes human agency and abstracts the process [of bearing children] from the bodies and persons involved," while moving "away from associ- ating children 'naturally' with their fathers and toward associating them

---

Philadelphia, 1778," in William Pencak, Matthew Dennis, and Simon P. Newman, eds., *Riot and Revelry in Early America* (University Park, Pa., 2002), 156–176.

44. Crowley, *This Sheba, Self*, 156.

'naturally' with their mothers." The ways in which women's bodies were imagined moved both toward the world of laissez-faire economic ideas—in which women were seen as individuals who were able to control their lives through rational choices—and moved away from the values of the emerging industrial age, which emphasized men's (but not women's) productive, wealth-producing capacities.[45]

The new definitions of pregnancy that emerged during and after the Revolution were accompanied by numeracy and an emphasis on prudence in planning family size. Esther de Berdt Reed wrote to her brother in 1772: "I have fulfilled your wish of a son [her second child]. I wish I could stop with that number, but I don't expect it." She did have two more children before her early death, but a lack of success does not indicate the absence of a desire to establish a numeric limit to childbearing. Her ideal was a small family of two children. By 1778, her husband would mock his English in-laws for "going on in the old patriarchal Style begetting Sons and Daughters." Somewhat uneasily, Joseph Reed was considering restraints on his role as husband and patriarch. By 1780, as mentioned earlier, Esther Reed proposed a formal political and fiscal role for women through the appointment of "treasuresses" on the county, state, and national levels, urging women to offer "more than barren wishes for the success of so glorious a Revolution." Here, feminine barrenness was not infertility; it had become a failure to exercise political influence. Her dual aspirations for all American women and for personal, parity-specific control over reproduction link the Revolution, truncated fertility, and the expansion of women's roles. When, in 1787, Sally Redwood Fisher thought her ninth pregnancy was one too many, her husband was not convinced, remarking only that "the World would not be so well peopled as it is, if these Matters were left to the Choice of women." But his defensive recognition that women were perceiving excessive childbearing as a burden and were capable of alternate choices was in itself an indication of changing attitudes.[46]

Numbers, both ordinal and cardinal, were soon joined to sentiment and

45. Ibid., 154; Jeanne Boydston, *Home and Work: Housework, Wages, and the Ideology of Labor in the Early Republic* (New York, 1990); Ludmilla Jordanova, "Interrogating the Concept of Reproduction in the Eighteenth Century," in *Conceiving the New World Order: The Global Politics of Reproduction* (Berkeley, Calif., 1995), 369–386, esp. 372–373.

46. Reed, *The Life of Esther Reed*, 181; Paul H. Smith, ed., *Letters of Delegates to Congress, 1774–1789*, 24 vols. (Washington, D.C., 1976–), X, 102 (my thanks to Konstantine Dierks for this citation); Merrill Jensen, ed., *Documentary History of the Ratification of the Constitution* (Madison, Wis., 1976–), II, *The Ratification of the Constitution by the States: Pennsylvania*, no. 146, microfiche supplement (my thanks to Owen S. Ireland for this citation).

suggest that a prudent sensibility was tied to the calculus of women's obligations to marriage. Harriet Manigault was bemused by the 1814 visit of "Aunt Izard and her three tender pledges, as she never fails to call them." Precise numbers coexisted uneasily with the sentimental language of giving pledges, although perhaps sentiment justified actions that Abigail Adams had earlier criticized as selfish. Numbers were more commonly used for the "unselfish" purpose of calculating pity for other women through a complex factoring of age, health, number of births, and spacing of births. In 1769, Sarah Logan Fisher clucked over Peggy Howell's "6th Child before she is 29," a calculation of too many children too fast. Ann Warder was enraged in 1786 that "our worthy and much to be pitied sister Polly Emlen" had a "husband who execed the desription of my Pen for Insinsibility—Her Children are presented Yearly which, keep her in constant Ill health, this with his improper example and want of resolution render the two eldest Boyes like Tyrants." Tyranny, insensibility, a lack of self-control, and the physical damage done by annual childbearing were inseparably linked in Warder's analysis. She later added, "What a pity if girls dont know better that there Mothers should not teach them." For Warder, and for many other women, sensibility, self-control, and responsibility should be brought to bear on the timing and number of births as the duty of husbands, fathers, wives, and mothers.[47]

Elizabeth Drinker undertook that responsibility insofar as she was able, and her daughters, as shall be seen, had substantially smaller families than she did. Samples from her diary, kept from 1758 to 1807, allow the dating of one woman's shift to numeracy and sensibility. Drinker did not rank births until the late 1770s. But, starting in 1779, she began to count, and, by the early 1790s, large doses of sympathy had been added. Her worldview had been transformed during and after the Revolution.

1770	Betsy Waln brought to Bed of her Son Richard Decr. 23. 1770
1772	HS. she was brought to Bed last night or this Morning with her Daughter Jane
1774	Hannah Was brought to Bed, about 5 this Morning of her Daughter Hannah
1777	at S. Pleasants who lays in with her Daughter
1777	Catty Howell brought to Bed with her Son
1779	to Polly Mifflin who lays in with her **second Daughter**

---

47. Virginia Armentrout and James S. Armentrout, Jr., eds., *The Diary of Harriet Manigault, 1813–1816* (Rockland, Maine, 1976), 9; Sarah Logan Fisher Diary, 11 mo. [November] 1769, VIII, 93, HSP; Ann Warder Diary, 15th and 18th, 5 mo. [May] 1786, HSP.

1794   *poor Hannah Baker* brought to bed of her **sixth Child** and **first Daughter,** she lost her Husband last summer

1794   *poor Mary [Courtney]*—terrible was the succeeding hour to me, how must it have been to the poor sufferer? . . . ill la delivera d'enfant mort, the **first male child of seven,** a very fine lusty baby—**6 of the 7 dead born.** *poor Mary* appear'd very thankful that all was over

1794   S.B.—was this morning about 6 o'clock deliver'd of a daughter [no sympathy for her servant's illegitimate birth]

1794   *poor Hannah Warder,* who now lays in with twins, is *much to be pitied*

1795   Sammy Fisher . . . his wife brought to bed the day before yesterday of her **third Son.**

Drinker's mixture of precise numbers and sentiment was typical of the immediate postwar period, an indication of new conceptions of wifely duty. But, despite her new sensibilities, Drinker still felt powerless to help as she precisely calculated her daughter-in-law's burdens in 1804: "Our Son Henry at present has 6 Children, and has buried two—they have been married 9 years and 8 months, nearly—O dear!" Women had learned numeracy; teaching men sensibility was apparently more difficult.[48]

Demographers have assumed that numeracy was concerned with the number and economic costs of children. What most of these women were counting was the tax of childbearing on women's time, health, and marital commitments. They measured women's contributions to a loving marriage and indicated the point when enough was enough. No taxation without representation might well have had parallel significances for women and men, with a wife's reproductive pledge to the marriage being as finite as a husband's productive pledge. The old patriarchal model of marriage that Joseph Reed had made into a joke was being replaced by a contractual model of shared responsibilities, although it meant that childlessness was even more of a crisis for a woman, since it meant she had not lived up to her part of the marital bargain. By the nineteenth century, women hastened to produce children early in marriage as their contribution to fulfilling the marriage contract, but, after accomplishing their purpose, they curtailed childbearing when they reached their mid-thirties. If no children appeared, couples began informally adopting children—not just taking them in but also rebaptiz-

48. Elaine Forman Crane et al., eds., *The Diary of Elizabeth Drinker,* 3 vols. (Boston, 1991), III, 1761. The list is based on all births found in the index (I, 152–354, 548–637).

ing and renaming them as their own offspring. Pledges of matrimonial bliss were necessary to complete marriages, but only a few were needed. As one childless woman reportedly said in 1778, "She would be mighty glad to have only one."[49]

Free women were voicing their aspirations for a better future. Direct evidence of the thoughts and aspirations of enslaved women is lacking, but a manifest desire for freedom is apparent in their actions. African American women took the opportunity of wartime disruptions and the hesitant growth of antislavery sentiment to abscond from their masters in record numbers. The proportion of women among runaways advertised in Delaware Valley newspapers rose substantially. Women were 9 percent of Pennsylvania absconders in the colonial period, rising to 16 percent during the Revolution, and in New York and New Jersey the increase in women's stealing themselves rose from 9 to 20 percent. Put another way, only two women stole themselves in any three- or four-year period in the Mid-Atlantic colonies, while eight women are known to have sought freedom during every single year of the Revolution. The annual numbers of absconding women fell, only slightly, to six in the postwar period. The actual number was undoubtedly much higher since, as the war continued and many northern states provided for the gradual abolition of slavery, masters increasingly felt that it was a waste of time and money to attempt to regain their human property through advertisements.[50]

A good many of these absconders fled to the British army in New York City, where they could gain immediate emancipation, legal recognition of their marriages, and liberty for their children. Twenty-year-old Dinah, for example, "RAN AWAY [from Philadelphia] with the last of the British troops" when she "was big with child, and near the time of her lying in." One of the first actions of those women and men who managed to arrive safely in New York under British jurisdiction, as Debra K. Newman has discovered, was to marry, and soon a number of children were born, "listed in the records

49. Conversation recorded by Charles Willson Peale in 1778 and quoted in Charles Coleman Sellers, *The Artist of the Revolution: The Early Life of Charles Willson Peale*, 2 vols. (Hebron, Conn., 1939), I, 189; Elaine Tyler May, *Barren in the Promised Land: Childless Americans and the Pursuit of Happiness* (New York, 1995), esp. 21–40; Margaret Marsh and Wanda Ronner, *The Empty Cradle: Infertility in America from Colonial Times to the Present* (Baltimore, 1996), esp. 9–32. To trace the beginnings of formal adoptions in the 1790s, see Gloria Dei Lutheran Church, Philadelphia, Baptismal Records, Genealogical Society of Pennsylvania, Philadelphia.

50. Billy G. Smith, "Black Women Who Stole Themselves in Eighteenth-Century America," in Carla Gardina Pestana and Sharon V. Salinger, eds., *Inequality in Early America* (Hanover, N.H., 1999), 138, table 2.

as 'born free within British lines.'" Nowhere else in the former colonies was immediate freedom possible for the children of the enslaved. It is clear from their actions that the goal of self-emancipating women in running to the British was freedom for themselves and security against enslavement for their children. They were engaged in family planning based on a deep concern for the future of the children. Freedom, rather than family limitation, was the primary goal in the precisely controlled timing of these births, but they shared with other free women a concern for their own and their children's futures.[51]

Still, those African American women who left the Philadelphia region to join the British had fewer living children than their former neighbors. In this they were not unusual; the sketchy records indicate that free African Americans, like the urban poor of European descent, had smaller families than the total population. These recently emancipated women living behind British lines in 1783 had fewer children (500 children ranging from birth to age four per 1,000 women ages fifteen to forty-nine) than their former neighbors, the multiethnic, mostly free women belonging to the Swedish Lutheran Church of southeastern Pennsylvania (562 per 1,000), and many fewer than enslaved Pennsylvanians (668 per 1,000 in 1780).

The women who had left with the British certainly faced more of the hardships of war than did those left back in Pennsylvania. Infant mortality might well have been higher—there was a woman named Dinah, listed as formerly of Philadelphia and of the right age, with the British in 1783, but she did not have a child with her. If she was the same woman who had joined the British late in her pregnancy, her newborn might have died during the flight to New York City or as an infant in the refugee camps. Having fewer children might also have resulted from the reluctance of husbands and wives to start families, as it became clear that the British would lose the war and their newly won freedom was in jeopardy. And the realization that freedom did not end either prejudice or maltreatment might also have negatively affected family formation.[52]

The institutional, educational, and spiritual needs of the emerging free

51. Ann Robison, "Twenty Dollars Reward," *Pennsylvania Packet and General Advertiser,* July 16, 1778; Debra K. Newman, "They Left with the British: Black Women in the Evacuation of Philadelphia, 1778," *Pennsylvania Heritage,* IV (1977), 20–23.

52. Debra K. Newman, "Black Women in the Era of the American Revolution in Pennsylvania," *Journal of Negro History,* LXI (1976), 276–289, esp. 287; Newman, "They Left with the British," *Pennsylvania Heritage,* IV (1977), 20–23; "Census, 1783/4," in Gloria Dei Lutheran Church Records, I, MS transcription by E. D. McMahon, 1934, 755–772, HSP.

black community inspired several women to forgo marriage and parenting in the early Republic. Neither Zilpha Elaw nor Jarena Lee remarried after being widowed but devoted themselves to preaching. Each found a caretaker for her child so she could continue her religious calling. Others turned to vocations as teachers. Most, however, considered motherhood "a treasured declaration of freedom" that "allowed for a semi-autonomous role within the family, and it allowed black women to participate in the shaping of a virtuous black community," as historian Erica R. Armstrong has astutely argued for Philadelphia. Women—single and married, with or without children, most working for wages—volunteered as "mothers of the church" or in benevolent organizations to advance moral uplift and to police family life in ways that clearly distinguished a free people from the enslaved. The social, economic, and political liabilities faced by the African American community in the early nineteenth century burdened women in particular with heavy demands on their time and resources and produced both positive and negative assessments of reproduction.[53]

Most women faced fewer stark choices, and the full implications of new ideas were sometimes slow to emerge. Despite an explosion of terms to describe the outcome of pregnancy, the new metaphors still objectified and depersonalized the fetus, that future "stranger," "urchin," or "object," just as "with child" or "my flock" had formerly. The love and sentiment that accompanied the new vocabulary of birth was initially directed toward husbands and a reconfigured marital state. For Sarah Logan Fisher in 1778, as for others, children were ancillary to her love for her husband: "[We] came home in the evening and found my beloved returned, spent an Hour with our sweet Children Oh the sweet union that we feel to unite our Hearts in one—may we be sensible of the Blessing and favour of being united together and of having two such sweet pledges of our mutual Love." It would be some time before children were fully bathed in the sentimental glow of nonpatriarchal families, when vague reference to "my flock" or the newer "tender pledges" was replaced by individual recognition of sons and daughters.[54]

These new conceits of "tender pledges" required that pregnancy be the unconstrained choice of a woman who abided by the vows of love contractually and equitably expressed in the marriage ceremony. But not all preg-

53. Erica R. Armstrong, "Negro Wenches, Washer Women, and Literate Ladies: The Transforming Identities of African American Women in Philadelphia, 1780–1854" (Ph.D. diss., Columbia University, 2000), esp. 117–126 (quotations on 54, 118–119); William L. Andrews, ed., *Sisters of the Spirit: Three Black Women's Autobiographies of the Nineteenth Century* (Bloomington, Ind., 1986).

54. Sarah Logan Fisher Diary, 12 mo. [December] 1778, VI, HSP.

nancies are voluntary: some will result from seduction or force, some will be illegitimate. If women have effaced their pregnant bodies to bear "pledges" and "strangers" from love and rational choice, what happens when there is no love, no real choice? According to best-selling novelist Susanna Rowson in 1791, "Alas! when once a woman has forgot the respect due to herself, by yielding to the solicitations of illicit love, they [women] lose all their consequence." The body is gone, the woman's mind or emotions are not engaged, and only the fetus matters. Charlotte, the tragic heroine, cries to her lover, "Kill me, for pity's sake, kill me, but do not doubt my fidelity," even while she entreats him "not to forsake my poor unborn child." The "innocent witness" becomes the focus in the absence of a woman's rational decision or loving vows. The physiological irrationality of Charlotte's pleading—wishing her own death while concerned with the fate of her "unborn child"—reflects the goal of contemporary readers to separate women from the pregnant state. Both the fictive heroine and the disembodied reader were threatened with death or dissolution in the absence of rational choice, sentiment, and respectability. It was only appropriate that Charlotte died in childbirth, but her daughter lived.[55]

This transformation can also be seen in the 1822 autobiography of Ann Carson. She denounced an unnamed local doctor who had seduced his wife's cousin, Susan Elliot, and intended to abort the pregnancy. Carson reminded Elliot that "for the destroyers of innocence, perdition only is the proper punishment." Abortion had traditionally been criminal when it concealed illegal activity, so Carson condemned the doctor because he intended to remove evidence of his adultery and his corruption of a young female innocent. Elliot did not interpret this statement as a condemnation of her lover, however, but responded, "Oh! Ann, you have pronounced my condemnation." She did not see herself as the innocent victim of a seducer but interpreted the plan to abort the pregnancy as the destruction of the innocent. This moment of miscommunication captures the change in attitudes on pregnancy, fertility, and legitimacy. Pregnancy either represented a woman's choice, where choice was essential to her identity as wife and citizen, or it represented the fetus, which emerged as a being with some of the characteristics of a separate person in the absence of a woman's volition and as an innocent in the context of its criminal or immoral conception. Attitudes toward pregnancy, the fetus, and abortion were changing, and women—in their attempts to

55. Susanna Rowson, *Charlotte Temple; and, Lucy Temple* (1791), ed. Ann Douglas (New York, 1991), 62, 89, 105.

highlight their minds and hearts and to suppress differences between the sexes by hiding the distinctive pregnant body—had created a logical vacuum in which the fetus could emerge as the only significant component of pregnancy, especially when the woman's will was constrained. By the second half of the nineteenth century, churches, the medical profession, and the state would begin to intervene to protect "innocent" life from destructive "mothers," whether the pregnant woman was reputably married or not.[56]

Marriage was being transformed, and women and some men were creating an atmosphere conducive to refiguring human fertility. They expressed sympathy for women who bore what was now considered too many children too quickly. They calculated costs and consequences. They planned for the future, even if too often in vain. And we know, from a few surviving scraps of evidence, that some went beyond a verbal commitment to restricted fertility. These women provided their sisters and daughters with explicit birth-control information. In 1809, Margaret Izard Manigault was one of those who advised her daughter that it was "less fatiguing to the constitution to nurse this one, then to bring forth another." Prolonged nursing is, however, a barely adequate technique of fertility control. Other women flocked to doctors, sought out pharmacists, and bought French syringes. The Shippen sisters' confidence about their ability to stop childbearing at predetermined numbers was perhaps because they had access to one of the more reliable techniques of birth control or of abortion, although which one is unknown. "It gives me great pleasure," one sister wrote to another near the end of the century, "to hear of your prudent resolution of not increasing your family. . . . I have determined upon the same plan; and when our Sisters have had five or six, we will likewise recommend it to them." More and more women, first in the cities and then in the countryside, were stopping the cycle of reproduc-

56. Clarke, ed., *Memoirs of Ann Carson*, I, 105–107. The law was moving to restrict women's right to consent in most cases; see Holly Brewer, *By Birth or Consent: Children, Law, and the Anglo-American Revolution in Authority* (Chapel Hill, N.C., 2005), 359–365. Legal changes reflect a similar reconstruction of sexuality. In Pennsylvania until 1700, rape was considered a crime against a father or husband, who received monetary compensation for the reduced value of his property. After 1700, the fines went to the state. In 1794, however, rape became the third most harshly punished crime (after treason and first-degree murder), with sentences running twice as long as for second-degree murder. Forced pregnancy threatened women's very existence. On the later history, see Linda Gordon, *Woman's Body, Woman's Right: A Social History of Birth Control in America* (New York, 1976), 49–61; James C. Mohr, *Abortion in America: The Origins and Evolution of National Policy, 1800–1900* (New York, 1978); Angus McLaren, *Reproductive Rituals: The Perception of Fertility in England from the Sixteenth to the Nineteenth Century* (London, 1984), 113–144.

tion at predetermined numbers, freeing women from childbearing for ever larger portions of their lives.[57]

Children and the Future

The fertility transition occurred within a context of revolutionary antiauthoritarianism. The promotion of sentiment, liberality, and fairness within marriage also set in motion a reevaluation of parent-child relationships that might equalize siblings. Children's upbringing became more expensive. Sending children to sea, giving them to relatives, or handing them to the Overseers of the Poor in times of economic difficulty—all forms of postnatal family limitation—gradually became less acceptable. When Charles Willson Peale's wife died in childbirth in 1804, he vowed that their children, these "pledges of her love . . . shall not be intrusted to the care of others to rear." The familial flexibility that allowed parents to shed excess children was slowly being replaced by a sense of obligation to all offspring, not just a favored few. Still, the more immediate response to the preference for small families was to provide foundling homes and orphanages, which were filled mostly with children placed there by one or both parents. It would not be until the second half of the twentieth century that the inviolability of the parent-child bond was assumed to be the norm.[58]

Identifying favorite children or enforcing inequalities among children had become less acceptable, and a strong preference for sons alone was moderated by the postwar period. George Calvert asserted that he preferred his daughter to his newborn son: "I do not yet admire him so much as my dear little daughter. She is the sweetest little girl in the world and a blessing to her father." The editor of this letter considers Calvert's statement to be merely an affectation. Still, that Calvert thought of it at all, even if he was somewhat

57. Norton, *Liberty's Daughters*, 233; Susan E. Klepp, "Lost, Hidden, Obstructed, and Repressed: Contraceptive and Abortive Technology in the Early Delaware Valley," in Judith A. McGaw, ed., *Early American Technology: Making and Doing Things from the Colonial Era to 1850* (Chapel Hill, N.C., 1994), 68–113, esp. 88–89, 100–101; [Reed], "The Sentiments of an American Woman," *PMHB*, XVIII (1894), 361–366. The four Shippen sisters and their sister-in-law had mixed success with two, five, seven, eight, and an unknown number of children, but four bore their last child unusually early, at ages thirty-two, thirty-three, thirty-four, and thirty-six. The other was past forty-four. See Klein, *Portrait of an Early American Family*, 285 n. 105, 300; Janet Farrell Brodie, *Contraception and Abortion in Nineteenth-Century America* (Ithaca, N.Y., 1994).

58. Lillian B. Miller et al., eds., *The Selected Papers of Charles Willson Peale and His Family*, V, *The Autobiography of Charles Willson Peale* (New Haven, Conn., 2000), 324.

insincere, is one indication that parental standards were changing. William Maclay at least felt guilty about his partiality toward his son in 1790; he "wrote to every One even little Billey. I however crouded the Girls into One letter. This hardly fair. but I must be more liberal to them next time." And he was. The birth of a daughter could even be greeted with great enthusiasm. "Joy Joy," exclaimed Dolley Madison to her brother and sister-in-law in 1811: "Are you sure it is a girl? . . . I tell you plump, that I shall be sick if, in your haste to write, you have mistaken." Revolutionary antiauthoritarianism stressed the emotional bonds between parents and children, rejected any self-interested parental benefit from child labor, and enhanced the importance of daughters. Limited fertility helped make these goals possible.[59]

If, by the turn of the nineteenth century, parents began to treat all their children more equally, there were financial consequences. Girls were getting more education, although it would not be until the twentieth century that educational attainment and parental tuition outlays would be nearly equal for boys and girls. Inheritance systems and intestacy laws that provided "special treatment for eldest sons" were replaced in the early Republic by laws that "provided for the equal inheritances of children, female as well as male." Dowry systems, which had made girls such an obvious financial burden to their families and a commodity in the marriage market, were slowly disappearing.[60] In the late 1720s, Benjamin Franklin tried, unsuccessfully, to

59. Margaret Law Callcott, *Mistress of Riversdale: The Plantation Letters of Rosalie Stier Calvert, 1795-1821* (Baltimore, 1991), 36; Kenneth R. Bowling and Helen E. Veit, eds., *The Diary of William Maclay and Other Notes on Senate Debates* (Baltimore, 1988), 214, 248; Mattern and Shulman, eds., *Letters of Dolley Payne Madison*, 145. On the individualizing of children, see Susan E. Klepp, *Philadelphia in Transition: A Demographic History of the City and Its Occupational Groups, 1720-1830* (New York, 1989), 147-151.

60. Dowries were being replaced by marriage settlements that included, in rural areas, "household goods as well as garden tools for women; some household goods, farm tools and vehicles for men." Economists have attempted to link fertility with local land prices on the theory that when farmers had difficulty affording land for their sons they would be moved to reduce fertility. This theory has been used to explain why fertility levels were highest on the frontier, where there was an abundance of cheap land, and why fertility fell as population density increased. A very preliminary examination of a small number of account books shows that farmers provided movables far more often than real estate to newlyweds. The availability of affordable land may be a factor, but studies are needed of the actual cost of providing for adult children at their marriages. Curiously, no one has explored other possible explanations for higher fertility on the frontier. See the analysis of accounts in Jeannette Lasansky, *A Good Start: The Aussteier or Dowry* (Lewisburg, Pa., 1990), quotation on 72 (accounts include detailed lists of marriage portions for both English and German couples [46, 54-55, 64-69]. It seems that German fathers had, from the few accounts presented, always given goods and cash to both sexes). On land and fertility, see Yasukichi Yasuba, *Birth Rates of the White Population in the United States, 1800-1860: An Economic Study* (Baltimore, 1962); Richard A. Easterlin,

get the cash-strapped parents of one prospective bride to take out a mortgage on their home in order to fund the dowry he expected. He refused the woman when they would not do it (she apparently had no influence on the bargaining or the outcome). Hannah Callender Sansom had a large dowry as the sole surviving child of a wealthy merchant. She was married in 1762 at her father's request to a man neither she nor her mother liked. Her diary contains a detailed accounting of the commodities large and small that accompanied her into the marriage, which she later described as "a match of entire discretion, and affection to follow after." The match went ahead; the affection never developed. She made sure her only surviving daughter married for love. By the 1790s, a staple in magazines was the exotic story that linked dowry systems with primitive cultures and individual oppression. A poem in *Godeys Ladies Book* summed up these changes:

Keep, keep the maiden's dowry
And give me but my bride,
. . . For she is treasure in herself—
Worth all the world besides.

As an ideal, women were no longer to be bartered at marriage for goods and cash: they had value as rational individuals.[61]

Girls benefited from these new attitudes. As one English traveler noted with surprise in early-nineteenth-century Pennsylvania, "Females generally have a share of the patrimonial estate, and primogeniture, and the preference in favor of males, will soon be unknown." And a male orator in New Jersey proclaimed on the Fourth of July 1800: "Our daughters are the same relations to us as our sons; we owe them the same duties." Parents were obligated to their children—all of them. But the more equitable investments in the education and in the marital establishment of all children would have made

"Factors in the Decline of Farm Family Fertility in the United States: Some Preliminary Research Results," *Journal of American History,* LXIII (1976–1977), 600–614; Morton Owen Schapiro, "Land Availability and Fertility in the United States, 1760–1870," *Journal of Economic History,* XLII (1982), 599; Lee A. Craig, *To Sow One Acre More: Childbearing and Farm Productivity in the Antebellum North* (Baltimore, 1993); Barry Levy, *Quakers and the American Family: British Settlement in the Delaware Valley* (New York, 1988).

61. Kerber, *Women of the Republic;* Norton, *Liberty's Daughters;* Mary Kelley, *Learning to Stand and Speak: Women, Education, and Public Life in America's Republic* (Chapel Hill, N.C., 2006); Marylynn Salmon, *Women and the Law of Property in Early America* (Chapel Hill, N.C., 1986), 142; J. A. Leo Lemay and P. M. Zall, *eds., Benjamin Franklin's Autobiography* (New York, 1986), 55; Klepp and Wulf, eds., *Diary of Hannah Callender Sansom,* June–September 1762; Mrs. Francis Osgood, *Godeys Ladies Book,* quoted in Lasansky, *A Good Start,* 9.

childrearing increasingly expensive and could have provided a substantial motivation to limit family size.[62]

The costs of having children were, however, not just financial. By 1810, Elizabeth Fisher was asking, "Can children, be they ever so kind, repay their mother for what she has to undergo, in body and in mind, in bringing them up till they are able to do for themselves?" Her answer was forthright, "I say they cannot." Raising children could be emotionally fulfilling, but the financial and physical toll of endless childbearing was increasingly seen as excessive. Children were not sources of wealth nor were they to be comforts to their parents; rather, they were expensive investments in family formation and in the creation of an intimate domestic sphere where women could exercise self-restraint, promote bodily integrity, and assume the responsibilities that characterized adults.[63]

INTENSE CONVERSATIONS, WORRIED CORRESPONDENCE, and high hopes during a time of crisis produced and diffused new ideas about fertility and femininity. Women shared, or perhaps with appropriate education could soon share, the mental and spiritual capacities that characterized mature, virtuous humanity—traits previously considered to be purely masculine. Women need not be childish, silly, or passionate; they could be as foresighted, responsible, and thoughtful as the vagaries of life allowed. Many women, although certainly not all, embraced bodily independence and self-

---

62. *A History of North America; Comprising a Geographical and Statistical View of the United States, and of the British Canadian Possessions* . . . , 2 vols. (Leeds, 1820), II, 48; *Genius of Liberty* (Morristown, N.J.), Aug. 7, 1800, quoted in Klinhoffer and Elkins, "'The Petticoat Electors,'" *JER,* XII (1992), 179. Carole Shammas argues that the move toward equality in household governance, including inheritances, was largely window dressing and that, in Chester County, at least, sons dominated the testate provisions in their fathers' wills (Shammas, *A History of Household Government in America* [Charlottesville, Va., 2002], 56–60). But the financial obligations of parents to children included marriage gifts and education as well as the distribution of property at death. Muriel Nazzari argues that dowries, common in Europe and Latin America until the turn of the twentieth century, raised women's status in marriage, since the husband was partially dependent on his wife's financial contributions. But, since the money was never in the woman's hands, passing from her father, brother, guardian, or executor to the husband, it is difficult to see this as a source of female empowerment (Nazzari, *Disappearance of the Dowry: Women, Families, and Social Change in São Paulo, Brazil, 1600–1900* [Stanford, Calif., 1991], xv–xx). Lawrence Stone's observation that "the dowry system, and the cultural obligation to marry off the girls, meant that daughters were a serious economic drain on the family finances" seems apt (Stone, *The Family, Sex, and Marriage in England, 1500–1800* [New York, 1977], 89). This area needs further study, although finding evidence is difficult.

63. Elizabeth Munro Fisher, *Memoirs of Mrs. Elizabeth Fisher, of the City of New-York* (New York, 1810), in Sharon Halevi, ed., *The Other Daughters of the Revolution* (Albany, 2006), 102.

control. They applied numerical reasoning to their procreative physicality. They recast and reshaped their images to deemphasize bellies and to stress head and heart. They invented a selfless, domestic womanhood that limited traditional wifely obligation to a husband's lineage by elevating, through sentimentalized sensibility, the domestic circle. Childrearing was raised in social and political importance, and parents began treating all their children, whether first or last born, female or male, more equally. Families began to plan pregnancies and set goals of ideal family size and soon would contrast their restraint to the supposed practice of having children higgledy-piggledy with little thought for the long-term consequences. As one almanac put it, "Shall inferior beings [animals], merely by the power of instinct qualities, shew more care and prudence in rearing their tender offspring, than proud man, with all his lordly and boasted superiority of human reason?" The only possible answer was no. Women, by using reason and prudence, could assume the important task of guarding and rearing the next generation—but only if they had fewer children.[64]

64. Tom Tattle [pseud.], *The Pennsylvania, New-Jersey, Delaware, Maryland, and Virginia Almanac for the Year of Our Lord, 1800* (Philadelphia, 1799), entry for April.

—— 4 ——

Beauty and the Bestial

IMAGES OF WOMEN

Poor Richard recycled a timeworn sentiment when he wrote: "A Ship under sail and a big-bellied Woman, / Are the handsomest two things that can be seen common." The proverb makes for an awkward rhyme, but the linked images of ships and pregnancy had been harbingers of good fortune since classical Greco-Roman times. The graceful curves of a merchant ship's billowing sails and of a woman's body big with child promised men the wealth that came from both commercial success and productive children. Images of the Roman goddess Fortuna commonly portrayed her bearing a cornucopia spilling an abundance of fruit as she steadied a ship's rudder or a ship's wheel: these attributes symbolized fertility and good fortune for Fortuna's devotees. These aesthetically pleasing images represented one view of women and their bodies. But darker implications were never far from the surface in either trade or women. Ships might sink, women might miscarry, children could be born deformed or grow disobedient, and the seemingly certain promise of wealth would evaporate in a flash. Men could as easily be "oppress'd by Dame Fortune" as rewarded. Fate was fickle. Fortuna's bright promises could suddenly and inexplicably shift into blind malevolence. The ocean was dangerous and so were women.[1]

1. Benjamin Franklin, *Poor Richard: The Almanacks for the Years 1733–1758* (New York, 1964), 29; Susan E. Klepp and Billy G. Smith, eds., *The Infortunate: The Voyage and Adventures of William Moraley, an Indentured Servant* (University Park, Pa., 2005), 14.

These positive and negative linkages were not simply fossilized artistic remnants of an antique past but remained current into the seventeenth and eighteenth centuries. The midwife Jane Sharp rehearsed another hoary version of both the beauty and the horror of womanhood by citing, "Menstrua: quasi Monstrua," a common, if confused, Latin tag that held that a menstruating woman was "a Monstrous thing," unlike any other creature, yet Sharp added that menstruation was "named Flowers because Fruit follows." Colonial women's physicality had both idealized human features and less than human connotations. It was at once ugly and beautiful.[2]

In the American colonies, it was not just the Bible's repeated command to increase and multiply that sustained the old regime of high fertility, nor did economic, demographic, and patrilineal considerations alone dictate pregnancies every two years of a woman's married life. There was an aesthetic of high fertility and the pregnant body that communicated social and cultural values of fecund femininity. The colonial iconography of fruitful, flowering women would be replaced by a different set of symbolic meanings around the time of the American Revolution. The diffusion of novel ideas about childbearing and women was not simply textual, oral, and aural; it was visual as well.

I would not have thought to include visual representations of women in a study of family planning and the fertility transition except for a chance remark made some years ago by Carroll Smith-Rosenberg at the American Philosophical Society while she was showing slides to illustrate female representations of citizenship and the nation. When flashing the illustration *Columbia Trading with All the World* (not included here) on the screen, she quipped, "This was not how my mother taught me to sit." Just so. This image of a respectable woman in neoclassical mode, rather demure in countenance, head modestly and submissively bowed, represents the bounty of the New World in her full, lightly veiled breasts. Columbia plucks fruit from a cornucopia held by Minerva, the goddess of war, wisdom, and the arts, while a native American in feathered headdress looks on. Columbia turns away from a giant, phallic horn held by a dark-skinned male in an elephant mask, perhaps representing Africa or the East Indies, who is linked with a stern mariner, perhaps a pirate. Columbia sits squarely, facing the viewer, with her knees splayed, her body and unguarded genitals open to the public gaze in a pose that might even now be thought to verge on the obscene. When

2. Jane Sharp, *The Midwives Book; or, The Whole Art of Midwifry Discovered* (1671), ed. Elaine Hobby (New York, 1999), 215.

and why did women's bodies become more private, more sheltered and constrained, less overtly sexualized, more individualized? These reconfigurations will help to provide a basis for acquiring control over fertility.[3]

Emblems of fertility were rare in eighteenth-century English portraits, although the motifs and postures that many colonials came to prefer could occasionally have been found in the seventeenth century and the first decades of the eighteenth century. The prevalence of these emblems was quite different in the colonies. Fruits and flowers became increasingly common in American women's portraiture through the first three-quarters of the eighteenth century as birthrates, already high, soared to their peaks in the cities in the 1760s and in the countryside in the 1770s. Yet negative connotations of "the Sex" often underlay the portrait artist's depictions of these prosperous, fecund colonial women. During and after the American Revolution, however, the visual iconography of pregnancy, fertility, and the female body shifted dramatically. New messages of maturity, regulation, rationality, and domesticity were embraced by those who commissioned, purchased, or simply viewed paintings in private homes or only saw mezzotint copies in books, magazines, and shop windows. Childrearing, rather than the promise of fecund abundance, became the dominant theme, and some of the negative references were assigned to children rather than to adult women. At the time of the American Revolution, a new aesthetic of the female body began that would help communicate ideas of virtuous womanhood, bodily self-control, and limited, even disavowed, fecundity.

By twenty-first-century standards, colonists lived in a visually impoverished representational world. Painted pictures, prints, and illustrations were rare. There were few painters in the colonies, and such as there were worked in the least prestigious branch of the trade, producing portraits and miniatures on order for paying customers. Ambitious artists had to travel to England to partake in a more sophisticated world of instruction, specialization, public exhibition, and patronage. There were even fewer colonial artisans or artists capable of making prints, engravings, or woodcuts. Most such items and illustrations were imported until the upheavals of the 1760s, when po-

3. Published as Carroll Smith-Rosenberg, "Dis-Covering the Subject of the 'Great Constitutional Discussion,' 1786–1789," *Journal of American History*, LXXIX (1992–1993), 841–873. This chapter draws heavily on David Steinberg, "The Characters of Charles Willson Peale: Portraiture and Social Identity, 1769–1776" (Ph.D. diss., University of Pennsylvania, 1993), particularly his analysis of posture in the portrait of John Beale Bordley in chap. 3. Ellen G. Miles generously provided comments on an earlier draft of this chapter as well as a crash course in art history as social history. Anne Verplanck's wide learning made her supportive comments particularly valuable. None of these experts, however, are responsible for what follows.

litical debate fueled a demand for political cartoons, and the 1780s, when illustrations for American books and magazines began to be included in publishing projects.

Still, imported prints were posted in taverns and were cheap enough to be purchased even by people of fairly modest means. Mezzotints generally cost between one shilling and a crown (two and a half shillings). They had become an important export item; in 1778, England exported prints worth two hundred thousand pounds, many to the former colonies. These prints often appeared in the New World remarkably quickly after their creation. For example, Pennsylvania-born artist Benjamin West painted a portrait of his wife and son in London sometime in 1768. Philadelphians were able to view a print of this portrait of their former neighbors by the end of February 1770. The sophisticated print culture of London could not be replicated in the colonies, and American-produced prints were both rare and primitive. Crude woodcuts of generic ships, horses, or runaway servants and slaves appeared in newspaper advertisements, and more elaborate designs sometimes graced the mastheads of these weekly publications. An almanac would usually have one or two woodcuts, commonly an illustration of astrological signs and their locations on the human (male) body and less often a fanciful cover image of the local town or countryside. A few crude political cartoons were published in the colonies by the 1760s commenting on local events; these had become far more common by the 1770s. It was only after the Revolution that books printed in America began to carry frontispieces or that American magazines and almanacs sported more sophisticated illustrations.[4]

For the average colonist, imported satiric prints were the most likely source of visual representation of women. Although no prints portraying pregnancy by eighteenth-century American graphic artists—who were few in number and generally amateurs—have been found, British prints circulated widely in American cities and could be seen in taverns, booksellers' shop windows, and general merchandise stores even by those who would not or could not purchase one. These English productions provided the only direct portrayals of pregnant bodies and suggest some of the reasons for the absence of formal portrayals of actual pregnancy in women's portraits. Pregnancy could be positively valued as beautiful in its promise of future

4. Desmond Shawe-Taylor, *The Georgians: Eighteenth-Century Portraiture and Society* (London, 1990), 26; Susan E. Klepp and Karin A. Wulf, eds., *The Diary of Hannah Callender: Sense and Sensibility in a Revolutionary Age, 1758–1788* (Ithaca, N.Y., 2009), February 1770, 50. One shilling would be roughly thirty dollars in 2008; see Samuel H. Williamson, ed., *How Much Is That?* http://eh.net/hmit (accessed April 2009).

wealth and male heirs, but it also had strongly negative connotations that demeaned, not so much pregnancy, but women's physicality, the bestial side of their natures.

The most popular of eighteenth-century printmakers was the ingenious William Hogarth. Hogarth, like another arbiter of taste, Josiah Wedgwood, saw the enormous economic potential of marketing moderately priced goods to the growing number of middle-class consumers. His complex and multilay-ered prints made the content of his far more expensive paintings widely avail-able to the public. The symbols in his prints appealed to the values of the rising middling sort by promoting a strong work ethic, moral reform, companionate marriages, patriotism, moderation, restraint, anticruelty, and sincerity. His works condemned (while sensationally depicting) aristocratic excess, sexual immorality, mercenary marriages, social climbing, laziness, drunkenness, po-litical corruption, gambling, criminality, superstition, and more. It must have been comforting to the middling sort to know that vice was located primarily among the elite and the poor and virtue was cultivated by folks like them-selves, that is, if they continued to carefully guard their behavior.[5]

It was through this combination of sensationalism and moral up-lift that Hogarth pictured the pregnant body. He twice used the image of Mrs. Tofts—who from 1724 to 1726 had actually confounded prominent doc-tors by convincing them that she had given birth to rabbits—as a symbol of unreasonable, devious femininity. His 1762 print *Credulity, Superstition, and Fanaticism* (not included here) shows the ungainly Mrs. Tofts writhing on the floor while rabbits stream from underneath her skirts. She still has her appetites, despite her feigned pain, and cranes to drink a dose of medi-cine, probably an anodyne or narcotic. A foolish boy is nearby with a large bottle of liquor. Hogarth had earlier used a similar image of Tofts to satirize the ignorance and credulity of the male medical profession, who knew so little about female physiology that an ignorant woman could deceive them. Gullible men and irrational females, both governed by ambition and weak minds, were the targets.[6]

In his 1738 series on the four times of the day and the four seasons of the year, Hogarth emphasized the fecundity of afternoon / fall harvest season by placing a tall, heavyset, and very pregnant woman at the center of the pic-ture. This big-bellied woman is not beneficent, but signals the large uncon-trolled appetites of a fat female (Plate 4). She is the one who dominates and

5. Jenny Uglow, *Hogarth: A Life and a World* (New York, 1997), esp. 217–276.
6. Sean Shesgreen, *Engravings by Hogarth: 101 Prints* (New York, 1973), print 95.

unmans her pathetic, cuckolded husband—he is shorter than she, carries a child (children were supposed to be the woman's responsibility) and, thanks to a well-placed cow, sports the horns that signal his humiliation and lack of mastery. Even the woman's son and dog are oppressed, emasculated by this powerful, but stupid, amorous, and bovine female figure—again the cow comes in handy in illustrating her mixed human and bestial traits. Pregnancy is a graphic sign of women's irrationality, fickleness, and corruption. It is a visually acceptable signal of the illicit sexual acts that led to this autumnal afternoon's walk in the bountiful, but disordered, countryside.

In 1750/1, the artist used a pregnant woman as the ultimate victim of a boy's education in cruelty—the dead woman is lovely and helpless not only because of her age and sex but also because she is pregnant (Plate 5). She might have commanded masculine protectiveness had she been respectably married or if she had maintained her sexual innocence; instead, she is the victim of violence. The rendering of the dead woman is somewhat sympathetic, even though she had participated in the crimes and illicit lusts that had so inflamed her heartless lover and murderer. She is, however, sympathetic only in death. Like the trepanned heroines of contemporary novels who conveniently die of grief and shame at the end of the story, this fallen woman, had she lived, would simply have been another common wench lost in the city's criminal underground.

More positive portrayals of the pregnant body occur in Hogarth's prints but far more rarely than negative images. Hogarth uses a young, pregnant woman to represent England in the 1750/1 satire on the British army, *The March to Finchley* (Plate 6). She is at the center of the picture, pleading with the guilt-stricken officer not to go and fight in a distant war. She begs him not to abandon her even as a superstitious hag attempts to distract him from his duty. The pregnant woman is moderately well dressed, but her skirt hem is in tatters. The message seems to be that England is dependent, helpless, and impoverished. The woman's hemline illustrates one of the cruder, cant phrases for pregnancy, "the rising of the apron," a phrase often applied to unmarried serving women who tried to hide their pregnancies but were betrayed by their skirts. She and England need the domestic support of an undistracted (male) army. In this midcentury image and in later satiric prints, pregnancy has become associated with poverty, not wealth. In this case, visual messages were in advance of most published writings.[7]

7. Ibid., print 74. A Revolutionary War–era British cartoon protesting the low wages of British soldiers uses an even more ragged woman—barefoot and pregnant—along with her three nearly

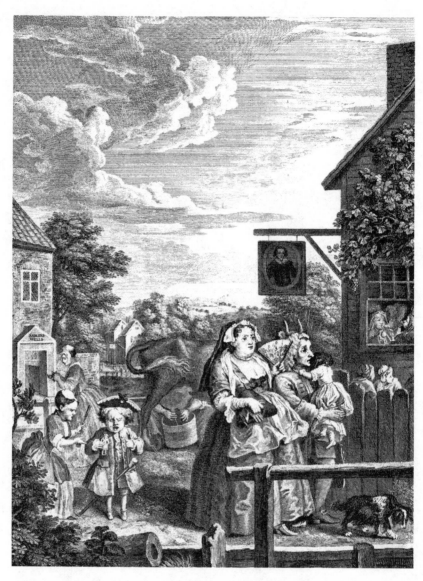

PLATE 4.

Evening, plate III of *The Four Times of the Day.* By William Hogarth, 1738.

In an autumn evening, a London family walks in the countryside. This is no companionate marriage of loving equals: the gross, pregnant wife has cuckolded her pathetic husband. He wears, symbolically, the horns of the cow. She seems to have two bodies: one human and pregnant, the other bovine.

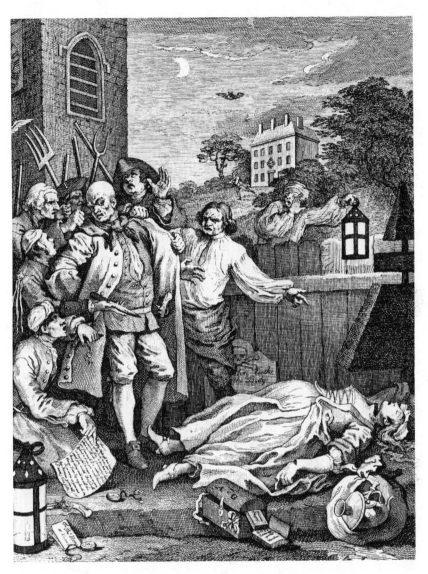

PLATE 5.

Detail of *Cruelty in Perfection*, plate IV of *The Four Times of the Day*.
By William Hogarth, 1750–1751.

A young and pregnant woman was involved in a criminal
gang and has been murdered. The pregnancy is evidence of the
unrestrained appetites that led to this violent end.

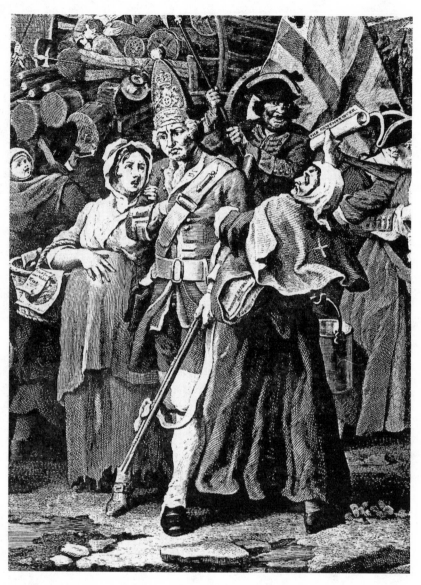

Detail of *The March to Finchley*. By William Hogarth, 1750–1751.

A respectable and very pregnant woman pleads for protection and
support from a British army officer about to deploy to a distant location.

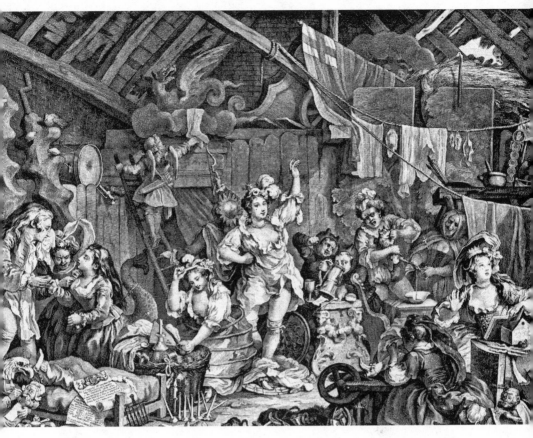

PLATE 7.

Strolling Actresses in a Barn. By William Hogarth, 1738.

The many passions and failings of
unrestrained women appear in this scene.

Irrationality, passion, deviousness, and seductiveness were among the
negative valuations of womanhood in the eighteenth century. Hogarth's decidedly unsympathetic depiction of actresses dressing for a performance
provides a veritable catalog of women's failings (Plate 7). Starting from the
left of the image, there is a venal mother who is prostituting her daughter to a
lovesick man who has already lost his breeches. A predatory (and unnatural)

---

naked children to point to the impoverished, helpless state of soldiers' wives. The woman is mocked
by a mischievous street urchin, who points to her swollen belly and her skirts, which, like those of
the woman in Hogarth's *March to Finchley,* illustrate "the rising of the apron." These prints anticipate Malthus's assumption that excess births would inevitably produce a rise in poverty.

woman in an eagle costume feeds her puking infant pap instead of nursing it as the laws of nature demand. Moving to the right, there is a vain woman in dishabille combing her hair and peering admiringly at her own reflection in a mirror while a bold and seductive woman, also in a very loose gown, hikes up her skirts—a false Cupid behind these two women will no doubt pierce the heart of some hapless man, but the Medusa at the women's feet signals the ugliness within. Two devilish brats and their angry, coarse mother loudly quarrel; women's unruly tongues, like those of their infants, are a source of social disorder. A witchlike woman embodies the superstitious, credulous aspects of womanhood as well as the ugliness of elderly women who have outlived their useful, productive, and procreative years. A patently hypocritical woman appeals to the heavens but seems more concerned with the appearance of prayer and how it shows her bosom to advantage than with real piety. A devious woman turns her back on the viewer—is she sewing or thieving? Both of the latter women exhibit the easy sinfulness and deviousness of the female sex. Venality, vanity, delusion, uncontrolled passions, dishonesty, stupidity, insincerity: these are among the many shortcomings of the female sex.

These latent feminine traits can be made manifest in the pregnant body— for a pregnancy bears public witness to the lusts of its origin. Never included among Hogarth's negative or positive images of pregnant women was the physical toll of nearly continual childbearing on women. That was simply woman's lot. The pregnant body was not only handsome, as celebrated by Poor Richard and others, but it was also immodest and shameful. Even in respectably married women, pregnancy signaled the physical passion that initiated pregnancy. There are, not surprisingly therefore, no painted portraits of individual elite women big with child. Nothing—not respectability, handsomeness, youth, or modesty—could override the implications of base desire in a pregnant woman. What might be limned in comic prints could never be shown in an image of an actual woman, even if she in fact spent much of her life pregnant. What can be learned about fertility or family limitation from the surviving portraits of individuals?

Portraits were not common objects in the eighteenth century; they were expensive, and the custom of purchasing and displaying paintings was confined to the households of the wealthiest inhabitants. Most Quakers, even if wealthy, condemned portraiture as vane and worldly, so not even all of the elite would have commissioned portraits of family members. How much influence could these representations have had when present only in the houses of a portion of the elite? Perhaps not much. Still, respectable strangers did call unannounced at these grand houses, expecting—and often receiving—guided tours of private collections. In addition, these big houses saw a succession of servants, seamstresses, tailoresses, whitewashers, day laborers, wet nurses, artisans, neighbors, employees, tenants, and others who might pass through day after day. Charles Willson Peale advised those forced to "wait at a gentlimans House" to use the time to study "any amusing coll[e]ction of Paintings or even good prints." The impact of the portraits might have been more wide-reaching than later scholars usually imagine. What we do not know is what these interlopers, artisans, and servants thought of these images. Even though these portraits were hung only in private households, they drew on widespread beliefs about women's place in the family and in the Empire.[8]

The few portraits of colonial women from the seventeenth century tended to be dominated by religious symbolism; cherries for Christ's love, symbols of fidelity like dogs, and hymnals or testaments (usually closed) were among the commonplace icons of feminine piety. By the eighteenth century, the religious imagery had faded as the messages signaled by portraits became more secular.

There was often little that was original about eighteenth-century colonial portraits. The settings, clothing, and attributes of wealthy colonial women were frequently direct quotations from engraved prints of fashionable British aristocrats as painted by the most fashionable studios in London. Most colonial portrait painters owned a collection of such prints from which customers could choose. In the resulting portrait it was often only the face and hands that were colonial; the hairstyle, dress, architecture, postures, and settings might well be meticulously copied from London sources. Although these portraits reveal much about patriotic British loyalties, shared aesthetic values among the Empire's gentry, and provincial aspirations for recognition by the imperial center, they are less forthcoming about the values of colonial women. Even when there is no obvious print source for an American portrait, the better established painters owned clothing, chairs, vases, pillars, and draperies that sitters might adopt. The dress, jewelry, and the setting might simply be an indication of a particular painter's stock in trade. Clothing, as Margaretta Lovell has shown by tracing the appearance and multiple reappearances of a single blue gown, could be borrowed from kin

8. Lillian B. Miller et al., eds., *The Selected Papers of Charles Willson Peale and His Family*, V, *The Autobiography of Charles Willson Peale* (New Haven, Conn., 2000), 229. Hannah Callender describes making several such visits in the 1760s; see Klepp and Wulf, eds., *Diary of Hannah Callender*, Sept. 9, 1758, for one example.

and friends. These portraits are not candid photographs. A painting was supposed to produce a "likeness" that was less a photographic image than a representation of the client's idealized self-aspirations. Images of women represent carefully plotted emblems of femininity, and they carry both the positive and the negative gendered stereotypes of the times. Colonial portraits of women reveal certain social attitudes, but they do not easily yield insights into women's perceptions.[9]

A number of questions emerge from women's portraits. Whose ideals are being represented in the picture? Who decides whether to copy an English print or to add a column, some drapery, a pet squirrel, a pile of books, or other commonplace symbols that might represent antiquity, wealth, authority, learning, virtue, fidelity, taste, or any number of other values—was it the client or purchaser? In portraits of married women, the client, the one who hired the painter and eventually paid the bill, would normally have been the husband; for single women, it would have been the father. Men controlled the family's purse strings, and arranging a commission would, presumably, have been a man's decision. But there are other possibilities. In the lengthy face-to-face sittings that portraiture required, the sitter might have been able to influence both posture and props. Or, the artist, as a master of his craft, might have insisted on his own interpretation. It could be that there was a shared, even unspoken, perception by customer, sitter, and artist of the latest fashion. The resulting picture might have entailed a negotiation between the various parties. It is usually not at all clear whose values are being represented on the canvas.

Some of the forces at play during a sitting for a portrait are satirized in the 1825 painting by Charles Bird King of an itinerant portrait painter at work (Plate 8). The sitter is a farmwife who has donned finery that was probably borrowed—her workaday apron and gown are visible underneath the elegant outer apparel. The illusion of serene elegance on the canvas is at odds with the surrounding dirt and disorder of a farm kitchen. Hams hang from smoke-darkened rafters, and clutter spills from the mantelpiece. The marital bed beckons in the background but is off-limits. Meanwhile, a number of children, a young African American servant, a slovenly boy, and a dog sprawl on the none-too-tidy floor, and a fussy infant reaches from the cradle for a teething ring. The artistic vision of the professional painter is sharply

9. Margaretta M. Lovell, *Art in a Season of Revolution: Painters, Artisans, and Patrons in Early America* (Philadelphia, 2005), chap. 3; T. H. Breen, "The Meaning of 'Likeness': American Portrait Painting in an Eighteenth-Century Consumer Society," *Word and Image*, VI (1990), 325–350.

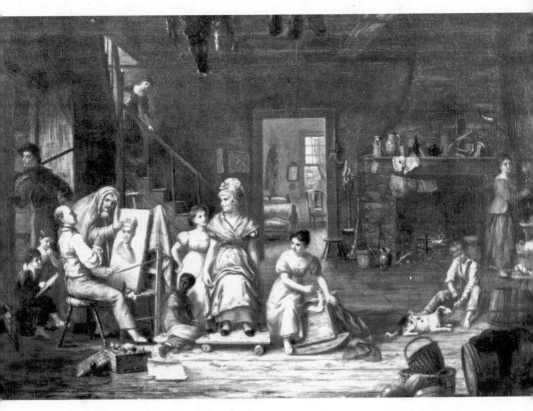

PLATE 8.

The Itinerant Artist. By Charles Bird King, circa 1825–1830.
Permission, Fenimore Art Museum, Cooperstown, New York.

This comic painting depicts the struggles faced by a beleaguered American portrait painter.

criticized by an elderly woman, perhaps the sitter's mother, and the artist draws back, affronted. As an additional insult, two children hang at his elbow as if being an artist was child's play. A younger, lovelier woman looks down on the squalid scene like some angel from above, but she is not his subject. The artist cannot follow his muse but must truckle to his customer. The men in the picture are beleaguered—the only other adult male, the husband, escapes the overly feminized domestic confusion with his hunting rifle in hand. Portrait painting was not a simple business.

There were multiple influences present when portraits were being planned and painted. Emulation of metropolitan styles was certainly a sincere and common form of flattery and self-identity in the early colonies. But, beginning in the 1720s, many colonial paintings of women, created in different locales by different artists, began to deviate from European models. These innovative portraits with their unusual iconographic symbols were produced by most of the portrait artists operating in America: Gerardus Duyckinck, John Hesselius, Charles Willson Peale, Benjamin West, John Singleton Copley, John Smibert, John Wollaston, and others. A colonial celebration of fecundity and abundance came to be highlighted through rounded baskets of fruits and flowers placed in the center of the canvas on the laps of young marriageable women, recently married women, or postmenopausal women who were seeking a youthful image. Such references were not entirely new. Women's portraits in the early colonial period often did contain a single small flower or a wreath, but these props pale by comparison to the showy fruit and flowers included in the portraits of the late-colonial era. Certainly, conventions of the baroque period influenced painters. Bright colors, complex curved lines, and ostentatious or pastoral settings were part of the vocabulary of contemporary aesthetics. But very few English portraits contained the images of bountiful fecundity that began to appear in paintings across the Atlantic. It was in colonial portraits, painted far from the centers of taste and fashion, that these fruits and flowers were most elaborate.[10]

One other common colonial motif can be found in the poses of women. The postures of colonial women changed from the standing positions usual in English aristocratic models to seated poses. Provincial commoners, even wealthy ones, were portrayed as lower, more docile than the assertive, dominant women of England's hereditary elite. In addition, art historian Deborah I. Prosser points out that the frontal poses of colonial women "suggest openness, an invitation to the viewer to visually engage the sitter." This openness is made more pronounced by the parted legs of the female subjects. Men, on the other hand, are positioned "with hand on hips or jutting elbows,

10. A sampling of similar motifs in the portraits of colonial American women are: [Gerardus Duyckinck, attributed], *Phila Franks*, circa 1735, in Richard Brilliant, *Facing the New World: Jewish Portraits in Colonial and Federal America* (New York, 1997), 33; [John Wollaston, attributed], *Margaret Oswald*, circa 1758, in Roger W. Moss, *Historic Houses of Philadelphia: A Tour of the Region's Museum Homes* (Philadelphia, 1998), 119; John Smibert, *Mrs. David Miln*, 1723, in Richard H. Saunders, *John Smibert: Colonial America's First Portrait Painter* (New Haven, Conn., 1995), 41; Unknown artist (possibly John Hesselius), *Mary Sorber, Mrs. John Redman*, circa 1749, in Nicholas B. Wainwright, comp., *Paintings and Miniatures at the Historical Society of Pennsylvania* (Philadelphia, 1974), 36; William Johnston, *Mrs. Thomas Mumford*, 1763, in Michael Quick, *American Portraiture in the Grand Manner, 1720-1920* (Los Angeles, Calif., 1981), 99; John Singleton Copley, *Jeremiah Lee and Mrs. Jeremiah Lee*, 1769, ibid., 104-105; Robert Feke, *Susannah Faneuil Boutineau*, 1748, in Richard H. Saunders and Ellen G. Miles, *American Colonial Portraits, 1700-1776* (Washington, D.C., 1987), 109; Robert Feke, *Mrs. James Bowdoin II*, 1748, in Ellen G. Miles, ed., *The Portrait in Eighteenth-Century America* (Newark, Del., 1993), 78.

[to] connote greater authority and physical distance" from the viewer. In the very few family groups painted in the eighteenth century as well as in paired portraits of husband and wife, men stand, but their wives sit docilely beneath their husbands' towering figures. Men were more likely to look directly at the viewer; women focused on the dominant male. Men in paired portraits were pictured in more cultivated, usually indoor, built environments; they were in standing positions, surrounded by emblems of the classical past, by their houses and farms, busy at their desks, or engaged with the tools of their trades. They were civilized; women were natural. Women's arms were placed to hint at (but never actually portray) rotund bellies, and those rounded baskets of colorful fruit or flowers were held at the lower torso or thighs, knees spread apart so that it appeared as if these female bodies were pouring forth nature's bounty in fecund abundance. Outdoor settings—either wild or cultivated—also bespoke the productivity of American females. Colonial women were presented as sexual beings, as cornucopias pouring out symbolic babies and future wealth from their bodies. The fruits and flowers of their bodies were pregnant with meaning. By the middle of the eighteenth century, then, many colonial women's portraits deviated from the English mezzotints that frequently determined content, particularly in posture and props. There are few English examples so blatant in their celebration of procreation. A showy visual vocabulary of abundance was largely colonial.[11]

A young woman's portrait was often taken on the occasion of her marriage and reflected, as Margaretta Lovell has noted, "her transition to a sexually active and sexually available state." These depictions were, on the surface, celebrations of a woman's potential procreative abundance as well as her husband's pleasure in her sexual availability. They could also be somewhat titillating. An anonymous poet wrote under one woman's portrait, "Where the pleas'd Eye darts forth a Vestals Fire / And undesiring kindles up Desire." Women's portraits had an erotic element. The painter Charles Willson Peale described at some length the flirtatious quality of a series of sittings with twenty-year-old Susannah Caldwell, "in the prime of [her] youth." He instructed her to "look at him as if she wis[h]ed to [cap]tivate—the idea was put into p[rac]tice, and the result had nearly b[een] effected into a reality." The artist, he continued, "if he cannot fall in love with his copy . . . is in danger from the original, whose native charms he endeavors to develope." Part

11. Deborah I. Prosser, "'The Rising Prospect or the Lovely Face': Conventions of Gender in Colonial American Portraiture," in Peter Benes et al., eds., *Painting and Portrait Making in the American Northeast*, The Dublin Seminar for New England Folk Life, *Annual Proceedings*, XIX (Boston, 1994), 183.

of the artist's job was to make his female subjects as enticing as possible. The prevalence of these fertile and sexualized images in the colonies followed the rising birthrates in the Middle Colonies, and, like statistical and linguistic evidence of celebrated fertility, they peaked in the 1760s and 1770s.[12]

An early example of an American emphasis on fecundity is the portrait of Phila Franks, attributed to Gerardus Duyckinck I, circa 1740, which quotes in many of its details a mezzotint of the Duchess of Bolton from 1703 (not included here). The English duchess stands, spilling a basket of fruit and flowers as an offering to the monarch whose crown is visible on the massive pedestal or alter at her side. The basket of flowers is held away from her body. In the colonial version, the carved pedestal with its royalist imagery has disappeared, allowing the flowers a more prominent position in Franks's portrait. Franks more closely clings to the basket, and she holds it next to her body. Franks does not stand but is seated on a bench. Rather than emphasize her belly through props and posture, as other portraitists would soon do, Duyckinck shows Franck, like other of his female sitters, largely covered by a cloak. Soon colonial portraits would be more explicit.[13]

John Wollaston's 1750 portrait of Experience Johnson provides a rich example of a mid-eighteenth-century American image of female fertility (not included here, but see the similar poses in Plates 10 and 19, below). It borrows

12. Lovell, *Art in a Season of Revolution*, 73; "The Following Lines Were Wrote under H. Paytons Picture," in Catherine La Courreye Blecki and Karin A. Wulf, eds., *Milcah Martha Moore's Book: A Commonplace Book from Revolutionary America* (University Park, Pa., 1997), 188; Miller et al., eds., *Selected Papers of Peale and His Family*, V, *Autobiography of Peale*, 155. Although a number of art historians have noted that fruit and flowers were associated with women in colonial portraits, none have probed the deeper meanings and temporal distribution of these emblems. Useful as background here are Margaretta M. Lovell, "Reading Eighteenth-Century American Family Portraits: Social Images and Self-Images," *Winterthur Portfolio*, XXII (1987), 243–264; Karin Calvert, "Children in American Family Portraiture, 1670–1810," *William and Mary Quarterly*, 3d Ser., XXXIX (1982), 87–113; Breen, "The Meaning of 'Likeness,'" *Word and Image*, VI (1990), 325–350; Steinberg, "The Characters of Charles Willson Peale"; Wayne Craven, *Colonial American Portraiture: The Economic, Religious, Social, Cultural, Philosophical, Scientific, and Aesthetic Foundations* (Cambridge, 1986), esp. 329; Deborah I. Prosser, "In Their Faces: Eighteenth-Century American Portraits and English Mezzotint Prints as Historical Evidence" (paper presented at the Philadelphia Center for Early American Studies [currently the McNeil Center for Early American Studies], Apr. 2, 1993); Prosser, "'The Rising Prospect or the Lovely Face,'" in Benes et al., eds., *Painting and Portrait Making*, Dublin Seminar for New England Folklife, *Annual Procs.*, XIX (1994), 181–200; Roland E. Fleischer, "Emblems and Colonial American Painting," *American Art Journal*, XX, no. 3 (1988), esp. 34 n. 9. Even in European art criticism, "the fruit basket as a symbol of fertility has been sadly neglected"; see Jan Baptist Bedaux, "Fruit and Fertility: Fruit Symbolism in Netherlandish Portraiture of the Sixteenth and Seventeenth Centuries," *Simiolus*, XVII, nos. 2–3 (1987), 150–168, esp. 150.

13. Reproduced in Waldron Phoenix Belknap, Jr., *American Colonial Painting: Materials for a History* (Cambridge, Mass., 1959), XXX, after 292.

important elements from a late-seventeenth-century source, Pierre Mignard's portrait of Louise Renee de Kéroualle (often anglicized to Carwell) (Plate 9). It is a surprising choice for colonial imitation. Kéroualle was Charles II's mistress and a Roman Catholic to boot, but the sexual implications of a royal mistress and the productive and possessive implications of the portrait, so rare in English portraits, might have appealed to the purchaser, whomever he or perhaps she was. The two subjects have similar poses, hairstyles, and necklines. Kéroualle's arm, however, embraces a slave boy, who holds a shell filled with pearls at her lap. Prosperity emerges from England's commerce in African laborers and East Asian rarities like pearls. Imperial ambitions, personified in the king, can conquer and appropriate this French mistress as well as the commercial products of Africa and the South Sea islands. The colonial interpretation differs in important details and symbolism from this model. Experience Johnson holds a basket filled with brightly colored flowers at her lower belly—there are no exotic pearls, no enslaved lackey. Is her fecundity an offering to the Empire by a patriotic colonial, herself or her husband? Poor Richard, that same year, argued: "People increase faster by Generation in these Colonies, where . . . there is Room and Business for Millions yet unborn. [In] England for Instance, as soon as the Number of People is as great as can be supported . . . the Overplus must quit the Country, or they will perish by Poverty, Diseases, and want of Necessaries." The growth and prosperity of the British Empire depends entirely on the generative powers exhibited by colonials. Expansion is embodied in Johnson's person, not in imperial booty.[14]

The details of the portrait further suggest productivity. Experience Johnson's left arm assists in swelling the curvature of her profile in imitation of the pregnant state. The viewer's eye is torn between the face and the colorful, fruitful basket at the lower abdomen. Her legs are parted, as are Kéroualle's, but the fabric of Johnson's dress assumes folds between her legs that flow from her torso as if an infant (male?) were emerging, legs first, arms above the head. She is seated outdoors, in nature—the raw physicality of womanhood dominates the portrayal. The emphasis on nature might also have had positive, early Romantic connotations of dramatic beauty in the gaudy sunrise or sunset, but the darkening skies certainly indicate a less sunny side as well.

Experience Johnson's portrait and others of similar posturing and attributes are quite different from the usual presentations of English nobility or

14. *Poor Richard Improved for 1750*, in Leonard W. Labaree et al., eds., *The Papers of Benjamin Franklin* (New Haven, Conn., 1959–), III, 438–439.

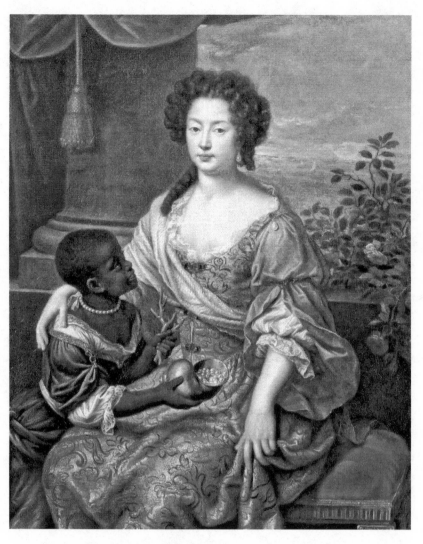

PLATE 9.

Louise Renee de Kéroualle, Duchess of Portsmouth. By Pierre Mignard, 1682.
Permission, National Portrait Gallery, London.

This portrait of a mistress of Charles II presents the subject in a
seated pose and with iconographic props suggesting fecund wealth. A seashell
serves as a cornucopia spilling pearls. Wealth seems to flow from Kéroualle's body,
assisted by an enslaved lackey. Both the pose and the props were uncommon in
England and confined largely to the seventeenth century, but quite similar images
became commonplace in the mid-eighteenth-century British colonies.

of colonial men. Men are engaged in the rational pursuits of the man-made world of civilized society. They are active in commerce, in government, in reading, and in other intellectual pursuits. Situating women outdoors emphasizes both the strength of their physical drives and the weakness of their minds. The 1751 portrait of Elizabeth Waldron (not included here) borrows heavily from the 1723 mezzotint of Bessey, countess of Rochford, but, where the countess holds a crown in her lap, her colonial counterpart holds several apples. Jane Clark, painted by John Smibert in 1732, sits on a grassy embankment as she plucks a ripe peach from a basket, seemingly about to offer this delicacy to the viewer (Plate 10). Just as Eve tempted Adam with forbidden fruit, so does Clark tempt her audience, especially the owner of the painting. The basket rests on her inner thigh, between her splayed legs, as if emerging from her body. The landscape is wild and uncultivated. It is a pastoral vision of an available Eden.[15]

Fruits and flowers pour from colonial women's open bodies. Botanic symbols of fecundity in overflowing round baskets are usually placed below the sitter's waist between outspread legs. Women are subservient and sit in these portraits just as birthing women in the eighteenth century sat propped up in bed or in a special chair. These are elaborate representations of colonial women's sexualized productivity and are examples of an artistic convention that saw women more "as incubators than as persons with intellect, character, and an individual perspective on life." Men are reasonable, civilized, and self-assured.[16]

In New England, John Singleton Copley used even more blatantly fecund images in the 1750s and 1760s. He painted Martha Swett Lee (not included here) with an apron filled with brightly colored fruit, while her right arm furthers the image of a rounded belly. She appears to be rather old for such fertile images—could Copley have been hinting that she was "mutton dressed as lamb," to use the vulgar phrase for women who attempted to hold on to their youth? Her husband, according to art historian Jules David Prown, "is presented as a man of affairs, standing at a table holding a letter, hand on hip, in complete control of the situation," and towering over, we might add, the naked woman's head and torso carved amid flourishing branches and leaves in the table leg. In his portrait (also not included here), "numerous

15. The portrait of Elizabeth Waldron is reproduced in Prosser, "'The Rising Prospect or the Lovely Face,'" in Benes et al., eds., *Painting and Portrait Making*, Dublin Seminar for New England Folklife, *Annual Procs.*, XIX (1994), 188.

16. Saunders, *John Smibert*, 76.

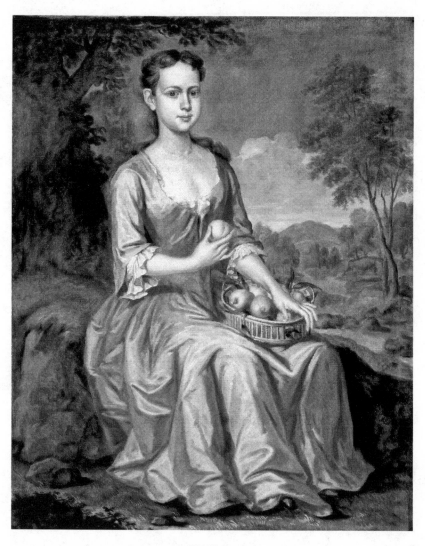

PLATE 10.

Jane Clark. By John Smibert, 1732.
Courtesy of the Massachusetts Historical Society.

Jane Clark was seventeen when her portrait was
painted. Her basket is filled with oranges and peaches that
mirror the sheen of her peach-colored silk or satin dress. She
seems to offer a piece of fruit to the viewer, and perhaps she
herself is ripening fruit waiting to be plucked.
She would be married by 1735.

lines, from the quill pen to the great embroidered banding on his waistcoat, converge on the head"; the same artistic centering is absent from his wife's portrait, although Prown fails to comment on it. The husband is indoors in a room filled with richly figured textiles and with a well-tended farm as a backdrop, whereas his wife is placed outdoors and linked with a spare temple in an uncultivated forest.[17]

The portrait of Mrs. Ezekiel Goldthwait, an accomplished gardener and mother of fourteen children, shows her, in Prown's astute analysis, reaching for "a barely disguised symbol of fecundity, and her extended hand emphasizes her identification with it. . . . The picture bulges with rounded forms [that] echo the plump figure of Mrs. Goldthwait herself and emphasize the sense of amplitude and plenty" (Plate 11). But in comparison with a later French caricature, Copley seems to be coming close to evoking negative intimations of grasping, barely controlled female appetites as well as more benevolent celebrations of plenty through female and horticultural fecundity. Goldthwait's gesture carries suggestions not only of plenty but of unrestrained hunger. The mixed nature of femininity contrasts to the more focused iconography of men's portrayals.[18]

The well-known 1769 portrait of Elizabeth Storer Smith has usually been analyzed in terms of its rich fabrics (Plate 12). Margaretta Lovell adds a perceptive reading of "the limp, muscleless grasp with which she supports (or rather, fails to support) a heavy bunch of grapes." And she finds the "very real gender-specific social conventions [that] differentiate between the kinds of objects (man-made or natural) and the type of appropriation (firm, possessive grasp or limp gesture) that link individuals to the outside world and to outside experience." Here, however, it appears that the symbolism is more concrete. The grapes spill from between Storer Smith's legs like a newborn child, while she sits as in a birthing chair. Her lower body is placed in line with the fields seen through the window, where the harvested hay has already been raked into lines. The portrait links the fruitful productivity of femininity and farms, but the expression on Smith's face is not happy.[19]

When colonial portrait painters deviated from slavish copies of English mezzotints, women's bodies were depicted as hollow, open vessels emblematic of superabundance and growth. Women were made into living cornu-

---

17. Jules David Prown, *John Singleton Copley, 1738–1815* (Washington, D.C., 1965), 60–61.

18. Ibid., 61.

19. Lovell, "Reading Eighteenth-Century American Family Portraits," *Winterthur Portfolio,* XXII (1987), 247.

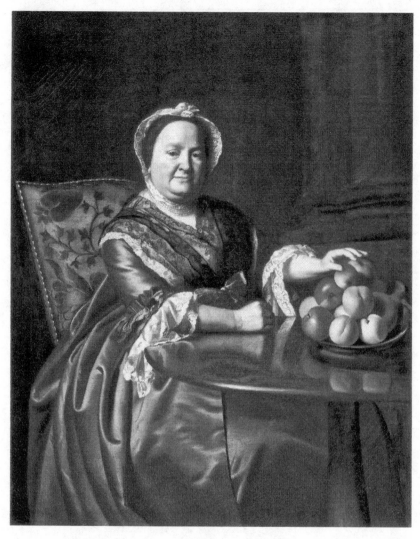

PLATE 11.

Mrs. Ezekiel Goldthwait (Elizabeth Lewis). By John Singleton Copley, 1771.
Oil on canvas, 127.32 x 101.92 cm. (50 ⅛ x 40 ⅛ in.). Museum of Fine Arts,
Boston. Bequest of John T. Bowen in memory of Eliza M. Bowen, 41.84.
Photograph © Museum of Fine Arts, Boston.

Elizabeth Goldthwait is about to eat one of the apples from her garden.
She was as prolific of children as she was of fruit.

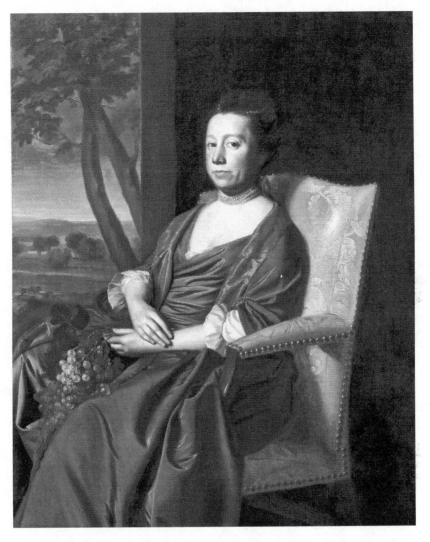

PLATE 12.

Mrs. Isaac Smith (Elizabeth Storer). By John Singleton Copley, 1762. Yale University
Art Gallery, New Haven. Gift of Maitland F. Griggs, B.A., 1896.

The autumnal colors suggest the harvest season. A large bunch of grapes seems
to pour from the body of Elizabeth Smith, who was pregnant at the time this portrait
was painted. The procreative powers of field and female promise wealth.

copias through postures symbolic of the pregnant body. These are all positive values, and yet the more negative referents to irrationality, physicality, and ungovernable appetite are never far from the vocabulary of the visual text.

Did women approve of their portrayals? Probably they did; colonial-era women gloried in their large families, as has been seen, but, for the most part, they left no direct comment on their visual representations. Only a few widows ordered portraits, and preliminary research indicates these women chose more modest and more serious dresses, poses, and props for their depictions than are shown in the portraits of married women, where presumably the husband hired the painter and had considerable influence on the presentation. Was the more somber portrayal of widows seen as an age- or status-appropriate presentation, as a symbol of mourning for a dear departed spouse, or as a declaration of a feminine aesthetic emerging because there was no husband to pay for the picture and determine its content?[20]

A few, rare exceptions to the lack of commentary by women on their portraits come from chance remarks by William Logan. In a letter to his brother-in-law in 1758, Logan proposed to send along his sister's portrait because John Smith, as her husband, "hast the Original and most right to it." Hannah Logan Smith wanted nothing to do with this painting, however, for she said she "intends when she Gets possession of it, to destroy it," according to her brother. Why she wanted it destroyed is unknown. It could have been unflattering, it might have been demeaning (especially if sexualized), and it was certainly frowned upon as vain among fellow Quakers. This last point might well have been the important issue for Hannah Logan Smith, for she was a prominent Quaker minister and therefore likely to be held to an even more austere standard than other Quakers. In the end, she might have gotten her wish — the painting has apparently not survived. Much later, in 1773, there was an even more pointed protest, this time by Logan's wife, Hannah Emlen Logan. "Nothing on earth," he wrote to a family member, "could prevail with my spouse to sitt at al[l] [for portrait painter John Hesselius], or to have hers taken by any man." Logan thought his wife's stubbornness was due to female vanity, since Hesselius, an old man by the time, apparently had a reputation as being less than successful in his portraits of women. Hannah Logan's comment, however, suggests that her objection was, not about the artist's purported inability to produce a flattering feminine likeness, but about the impropriety of posing for any man, whether that man was Hesselius or not.

20. Prosser, "'The Rising Prospect or the Lovely Face,'" in Benes et al., eds., *Painting and Portrait Making*, Dublin Seminar for New England Folklife, *Annual Procs.*, XIX (1994), 181–200.

Peale's musings on the erotic tensions between his female subject and himself suggests that she might have had a point. Hannah Logan's comment suggests that on the eve of Revolution the sexualized, fecund images of the American female body were being rejected as inappropriate and immodest.[21]

As Revolution spread and birthrates began to drop, the late colonial iconography of femininity was abandoned. Colonial trappings were replaced by other symbolic devices. The visual representation of flourishing, teeming procreation diminished partly in response to the debate over luxury. There were pointed comments about women's irrationality that accused women of admiring "'shadowy Ornaments' rather than those 'Qualifications which are substantial and really useful.'" In a time of crisis, such frivolity could not be tolerated. From France, where fertility rates were already in slow decline, Montesquieu observed: "In a popular state public incontinencey [by women] may be considered as the last of miseries, and as a certain forerunner of a change in the constitution. . . . In Republics women are free by the laws and restrained by manners; luxury is banished thence, and with it corruption and vice." Luxury could be seen as both gendered and sexualized but could also be rejected. A revolutionary republic required hardworking, committed citizens in order to overcome its vice-ridden oppressors. The nonimportation movement and the privations of war offered American women an opportunity to influence politics as engaged citizens. New understandings of liberty, rationality, and civic virtue could be achieved by rejecting abundance and luxury in favor of simplicity, self-control, and restraint. Americans would not be slaves. Virtue, prudence, and self-control were new goals for women (and for many men). Contractual equity within marriage, sensibility, and numeracy were also important. The old luxury of excess was replaced by the refined luxuries resulting from self-control. Childbearing was to be planned and purposeful. It was a selfless sacrifice for the sake of the children's future. Bernard Ulrich Dahlgren and Martha Rowan Dahlgren "lived in conjugal affection and felicity," according to their minister. "They had five children, of whom a male died aged 1 year, the other 3 sons and a daughter are living, healthy and well-educated." Status, wealth, and success could be measured, not by sheer abundance of resources, but by their quality. A loving, egalitarian family, health, and education could be accomplished with a limited

21. William Logan to John Smith, Nov. 17, 1758, John Smith Letterbook, Historical Society of Pennsylvania, Philadelphia. See also Dianne C. Johnson, "Living in the Light: Quakerism and Colonial Portraiture," in Emma Jones Lapsansky and Anne A. Verplanck, eds., *Quaker Aesthetics: Reflections on a Quaker Ethic in American Design and Consumption* (Philadelphia, 2003), 136.

number of children. Women, in particular, were increasingly celebrated as the proper rearers of children (because they were moral and pious) rather than as passive bearers of men's children (or preeminently sexual beings).[22]

The emergence of American-themed political satires during the Revolution might have assisted in the transformation of feminine images. In the viciously partisan political prints of the 1760s, 1770s, and 1780s, the allegorical figures of lightly clad, round-bellied, splay-legged women who embodied nations, colonies, or the Empire—like that of *The Able Doctor; or, America Swallowing the Bitter Draught*—become vulnerable to attack. The war produced an atmosphere of particularly hostile misogyny. In the political cartoons emanating from all sides during the revolutionary conflict, females are pictured as mutilated, sodomized, tortured, subjected to voyeurism, and resexed through phallic imagery as coarse males or hermaphrodites. The graphic revolutionary-era political allegories of exposed, mutilated, and disgraced female bodies, not to mention the very real rapes and murders of female noncombatants during the wide-ranging war, might have prompted the seemingly safer self-disciplining of the female body, particularly the genitals. New standards of proper feminine posture indicate that the openness of the female body, the splayed legs and the attention paid to the genitals, so apparent in the portraits of earlier decades, was being replaced by a carefully regulated, self-guarded bodily privacy. The openness of the colonial female body had become dangerous by the Revolution. Neoclassical conventions of virtue and reason, Renaissance images of the Virgin and child, stress on a separate, protected female sphere, and a heightened emphasis on childrear-

22. J. E. Crowley, *This Sheba, Self: The Conceptualization of Economic Life in Eighteenth-Century America* (Baltimore, 1974), 139–140; Charles de Secondat, baron de Montesquieu, *The Spirit of the Laws* (1748), 2 vols., trans. Thomas Nugent (New York, 1949), 101–102; [Esther de Berdt Reed], "Sentiments of an American Woman," *Pennsylvania Magazine of History and Biography*, XVIII (1894), 363; William B. Reed, ed., *The Life of Esther de Berdt, Afterwards Esther Reed, of Pennsylvania* (Philadelphia, 1853), 181; Sarah Logan Fisher, "'A Diary of Trifling Occurrences': Philadelphia, 1776–1778," ed. Nicholas B. Wainwright, *PMHB*, LXXXII (1958), 418; Nancy F. Cott, "Passionlessness: An Interpretation of Victorian Sexual Ideology, 1790–1850," *Signs*, IV (1978), 219–236; Linda K. Kerber, *Women of the Republic: Intellect and Ideology in Revolutionary America* (Chapel Hill, N.C., 1980); Ruth H. Bloch, "The Gendered Meanings of Virtue in Revolutionary America," *Signs*, I (1987), 37–58; Jan Lewis, "The Republican Wife: Virtue and Seduction in the Early Republic," *WMQ*, 3d Ser., XLIV (1987), 689–721; Carroll Smith-Rosenberg, "Domesticating Virtue: Coquettes and Revolutionaries in Young America," in Elaine Scarry, ed., *Literature and the Body: Essays on Populations and Persons* (Baltimore, 1988), 160–184; Cathy N. Davidson, *Revolution and the Word: The Rise of the Novel in America* (New York, 1986); Theodore G. Tappert and John W. Doberstein, trans. and eds., *The Notebook of a Colonial Clergyman: Condensed from the Journals of Henry Melchoir Muhlenberg* (Philadelphia, 1975), 211. Quotations from Gloria Dei Lutheran Church, Philadelphia, Burial Records, July 20, 1824, Genealogical Society of Pennsylvania, Philadelphia.

ing rather than childbearing began to characterize women's portraits in the early Republic.

A determined woman could subvert the irrational message of the old fecund emblems. Nineteen-year-old Judith Sargent (later Murray) stands with elbow jutting assertively and looks directly at the viewer, circa 1770–1772 (Plate 13). She has shifted the typical prop of a basket of flowers from her belly to her hip, where it is partly hidden by her arm and is firmly in her grasp. The basket is too decentered to suggest a gravid silhouette. Copley has made a valiant effort to recapture the fecund symbolism of the flowers by having some leaves and buds fall (upward!) from the basket and cast their shadows on her abdomen and genitals. Most pointedly, the artist has made the fecund imagery survive Sargent's unconventional stance by having a rounded curtain act as the shadow of a grossly pregnant woman in the background. Yet, despite Stuart's various connivances, the portrait fails to represent a female self embodied fully in fecund physicality. Certainly, hers is no "limp, muscleless grasp." She is in control. Sargent Murray would later become a leading advocate of women's rights, female rationality, and domesticated equality through her "Gleaner Essays," 1792–1794. This portrait seems to be a transitional piece, an early hint that the iconography of fertility is about to lose its centrality in women's likenesses.

Another transitional piece is Charles Willson Peale's 1772–1775 portrait of Ann Baldwin (Mrs. Samuel) Chase of Maryland and her two daughters (not included here). The infant is seated on Chase's lap, positioned to swell her profile, but most of her lower body is covered by the child's clothes. The fertility that had been symbolized by fruit is made manifest in the living child. Women's importance lies, not in the fecund possibilities of their bodies, but in their roles as republican wives and mothers. Her older daughter holds an apron filled with fruit, and the infant daughter has just begun to grasp an orange in anticipation of her future career as a childbearer. The physicality of childbearing and the hungry grasping of fruit are childish and unworthy of virtuous womanhood. Peale's 1771 portrait of Mrs. and Mr. Edward Lloyd (not included here) includes no fruit, although the lute the wife holds retains the rounded silhouette and openness of earlier representations. A flower is in her hair, not at her belly or breast. A child stands between her husband and herself, linking the two adults as predicted by the language of a "pledge of matrimonial love and felicity" that kindled "that flame which the altar of Hymen had sanctioned" and produced "days of domestic felicity." The child is associated with the mother's head, not her belly, but her husband remains superior. By 1774, Peale's depiction of the Elie Valette family (not

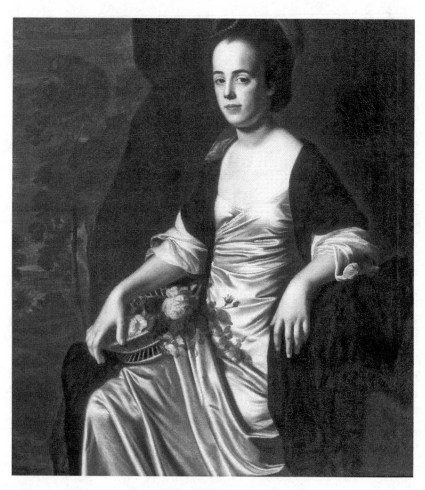

Judith Sargent Murray strikes a more assertive pose
than was usual in women's portraits.

included here) has the husband and wife on the same plane, connected by two children.[23]

Also from Peale is the portrait of Mrs. John Dickinson and her daughter, Sally, painted in 1772 (not included here). The production of this particular portrait had been delayed until after Dickinson had given birth. It is the child who holds a rounded lapful of lilacs, not the adult. The heads of mother and child dominate the picture. The mother stands, leaning slightly toward the child, and her right arm hides her abdomen. She steadies her daughter with both hands. Both figures are placed next to a sun-dappled staircase, and the steps lead upward. The concerned mother will guide her daughter into a promising future. Tranquillity and progress are implied. In Peale's female portraits of this period, women embody kindness and the beauty that comes from virtue. This was a form of authority; a bride could have "a refining effect on her new husband as well as on all that transpired in her new home." Women had a sphere of their own, a domestic realm.[24]

American artists avoided quoting luxury-loving British aristocrats in the last third of the eighteenth century and instead borrowed Renaissance images of the Madonna and child for their portrayals of republican women. Women in these paintings are virginal, pure, self-controlled. A fully developed example is the portrait of Elizabeth Wurtz Elder and her children, painted by Jacob Eichholtz in 1825 (Plate 14). Elder's white dress and that of her infant connote purity. The grapes do not spill from her body—she does not even touch them—but are clutched tightly by her older daughter while the younger daughter, just a toddler, lunges greedily after them. Unrestrained passions are infantile. The mother and son are restrained, upright. Virtuous women are above lowly appetites, and, like the Renaissance presentations of the Virgin Mary and infant Jesus, they have lost the obvious sexuality of colonial portrayals. Adult women are rational. Only young children and servile people have too little self-command and reason to resist impulsive behaviors. Children, especially, need careful training and supervision if they are to be virtuous citizens, and this is the important role of women.

23. Mary Clarke, ed., *The Memoirs of the Celebrated and Beautiful Mrs. Ann Carson* (Philadelphia, 1838), 52–54 (see also Chapter 3, above); Charles Willson Peale, *Edward Lloyd Family*, 1771, *Mrs. Samuel Chase and Her Daughters Matilda Chase and Anne Chase*, 1772–1775, in Edgar P. Richardson, Brooke Hindle, and Lillian B. Miller, *Charles Willson Peale and His World* (New York, 1983), 44, 206; Charles Willson Peale, *The Family of Elie Valette*, 1774, in Sidney Hart, "Charles Willson Peale and the Theory and Practice of the Eighteenth-Century Family," in Lillian B. Miller, ed., *The Peale Family: Creation of a Legacy, 1770–1870* (New York, 1996), 109.

24. Hart, "Charles Willson Peale," and David Steinberg, "Charles Willson Peale Portrays the Body Politic," both in Miller, ed., *The Peale Family*, 114, 129.

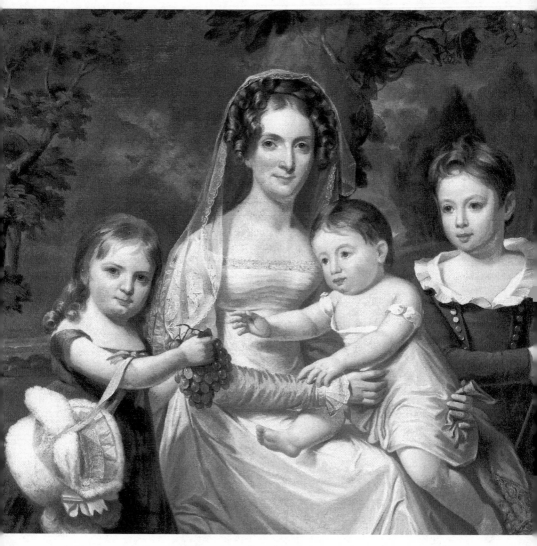

PLATE 14.

Mrs. Elizabeth Wurtz Elder and Her Three Children.
By Jacob Eichholtz, 1825. Oil on canvas, 41 ½ x 47 ½ in. (108.0 x 120.7 cm.),
1923.12. Courtesy of the Pennsylvania Academy of the Fine Arts,
Philadelphia. Bequest of Mrs. Blanche Elder Howell.

Elizabeth Elder is the embodiment of virginal purity, posed as a Madonna
and dressed entirely in white. Only the infant reaches greedily for the fruit held
by the second youngest child. Adult women control their appetites.

Nancy Shippen Livingston enthusiastically embraced the symbolism of her now lost 1783 portrait by Joseph Wright. Her daughter Peggy was "dress'd in White and has a peach in her dear hand—sweet innocent!" she recorded in her diary. Nancy herself was painted in an imaginary silken dress the color of lilacs, with pearls in her flowing hair, but "what adorns me most is my Angel Child sitting in my lap and one of my arms encircling her dear waist." Purity, innocence, and sentimentality infuse the picture, so similar in Livingston's description to other pictures of the time. Like a Renaissance Madonna and child, the republican mother is honored for her sexual virtue, not her sexual availability; for guiding the next generation, rather than producing it; and for sentimental and moral associations, not the production of wealth. The anonymous poet quoted previously added a critique of earlier portrayals of women: "The wanton Glance, may short-liv'd Passion move / But awful Virtue fixes solid Love." There was a republican aesthetic that rejected the obvious sexuality and procreative proficiency of colonial women.[25]

These new conventions lead toward Copley's famous 1773 double portrait of the Mifflins—where husband and wife are on one plane, and both engage in rational entertainments (not included here). The few, small flowers have migrated to her heart, the shadow of the table hides her lower extremities, and her husband adores her, fondly gazing at her head while she directly engages the viewer with her measured gaze. The lines in the painting, including Mifflin's husband's arm and the open book, the highlighted lines in the dress, and the components of the ribbon-making machine (a politically charged activity during a period of nonimportation) all point to her head. Behind her a classical column towers above mere nature.[26]

The painting of the Samels family also shows husband and wife on the same plane (Plate 15). Mrs. Samels focuses on her tea table, and the children are independent of the parents. The oldest girl has an open book in her lap. No longer do women sit with their legs splayed; they now keep their ankles crossed or their knees held decorously together. Their lower bodies are regulated, constrained, and covered by the position of the arms, by books, or by tables. They sit or stand more or less at an angle; they have adopted the posture that was specific to men in the colonial period. In addition, the heads and arms are dominant and freer. The same enclosure of the legs and

25. Ethel Armes, ed., *Nancy Shippen: Her Journal Book* (Philadelphia, 1935), 154; "The Following Lines Were Wrote Under H. Paytons Picture," Blecki and Wulf, eds., *Milcah Martha Moore's Book*, 188.

26. John Singleton Copley, *Mr. and Mrs. Thomas Mifflin (Sarah Morris)*, 1773, in Carrie Rebora et al., *John Singleton Copley in America* (New York, 1995), 319.

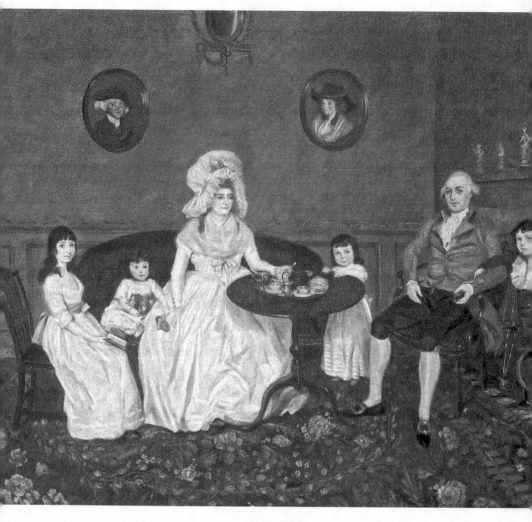

PLATE 15.

Samels Family. By Johann Eckstein, 1788. Oil on canvas, 64.77 x 76.2 cm.
(25 ½ x 30 in.). Museum of Fine Arts, Boston. Ellen Kelleran Gardner Fund, 59.194.
Photograph © Museum of Fine Arts, Boston.

In late-eighteenth-century American family portraits, women often moved to
the center; they dominate the domestic realm. The eldest daughter has adopted
her mother's bodily restraint. Men and boys are on the periphery distant
from the tea service and are less concerned with posture.

pubic area does not, however, apply to men. They can sprawl if they wish. Their rationality need not be proven: it is not in conflict with their sexuality. Women are portrayed as rational; they are no longer simply fertile icons passively perpetuating their husbands' lineages, but they remain different. In the picture of the Samels family, for example, males and females occupy separate spaces. But, as women move into the center of domestic spaces, men move to the margins. The "concurrent retreat of the husband from centrality in the domestic sphere is nowhere as emphatic in the documents [of the time] as it is in these paintings," as Lovell points out. The home was women's domestic sphere; men were public actors, engaged in politics, business, and the professions. Women's purity is fragile and needs careful guarding in a secure domestic setting. Men have more liberty in posture and in life.[27]

Also segregated by gender is the well-known portrait of the Washington family painted by Edward Savage in 1789–1790 (not included here). Martha Washington points to the proposed District of Columbia on a map. Her granddaughter, too, seems engaged in a serious conversation, while George and her grandson think serious thoughts but seem to pay little attention to the women's contributions. Instead, the males stare into the middle distance. The worlds of men and women are clearly separated by the table. Scott Casper notes that the women are linked to George Washington's favorite slave, who is standing in the shade behind the women. Females and slaves are still the property of the paterfamilias, and the icons of power and authority—globe, spurs, sword—are associated with the males. The persistence of slavery and of other hierarchies undoubtedly informed the choice of symbols in this painting and suggest a regional difference between slaveholding states and nominally free states.[28]

Another new convention separates infants from older children and adults. There are several paintings from the 1820s in which babies are distanced from their mothers and held by African American servants. The family portrait from York, Pennsylvania, in the late 1820s is an example (Plate 16). Infants, merely physical beings without reflection or sensibility, are placed in the company of African Americans and separated from the more mature,

27. Lovell, "Reading Eighteenth-Century American Family Portraits," *Winterthur Portfolio,* XXII (1987), 257.

28. Edward Savage, *The Washington Family,* circa 1789–1790, in Edgar P. Richardson, *American Paintings and Related Pictures in the Henry Francis du Pont Winterthur Museum* (Charlottesville, Va., 1986), 77; Scott E. Casper, "The Washington Family in American Culture: Imagining the National Family" (paper presented at the symposium, "George Washington and the American Nation," David Library of the American Revolution, Dec. 4, 1999). Many of the slaves working at Mount Vernon were Martha Washington's property, not her husband's.

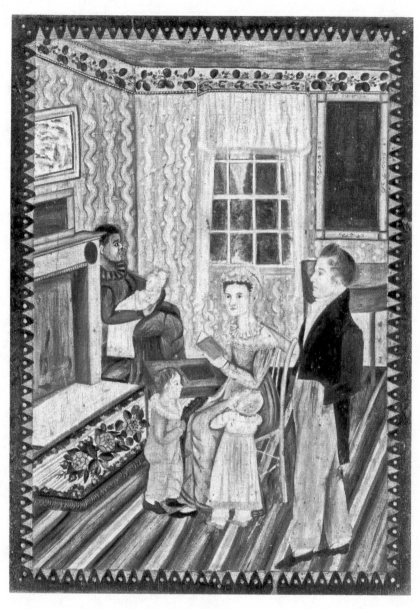

PLATE 16.

York, Pennsylvania, Family with Negro Servant. Unknown artist, circa 1828.
Courtesy, Saint Louis Art Museum, Bequest of Edgar William
and Bernice Chrysler Garbisch.

A republican wife and mother instructs her children. The presumptively less
rational members of the household are tucked away in a corner, separated from the rest,
yet both adult women have adopted the more restrained posture of the period.

thinking members of the family. This grouping of an infant and an African American nurse comes at a time when the stereotypical figure of the African American woman as "Jezebel" was being developed by whites—sexualized, passionate, irrational, and deceptive. Or she might be considered a mammy, instinctively maternal. Again, as was seen elsewhere, African American women come to embody older, usually negative stereotypes once applied to all women.[29]

In the rejection of high fertility in life and in individual portraits, there might be a similar rejection of children. The decidedly odd picture of Anne Bingham painted by Gilbert Stuart shows her turning away from the child, as if she had found something else of greater interest (Plate 17). Certainly, young children are not endlessly entertaining, but to memorialize such a diversion on canvas is quite contrary to social norms. Yet a few contemporary women did express some disenchantment with young children. Hannah Pemberton wrote, "I am not so doatingly fond of very young Infants, as some are, I have no Idea, of kissing every little dirty mouth, that is held up for notice." She then added, "But when the dawn of Reason begins to make its beautiful appearance, and they can take notice; I think them the most engaging little creatures in the world." Reason brings beauty; without it there can be no aesthetic pleasure.[30]

Far more typical are the values presented in the group portrait of the Peale family, painted by James Peale in 1795 (Plate 18). The adults stand side by side, and, as this is a domestic scene, the wife and mother is in the foreground. The mother seems to offer good advice to the oldest daughter, who has already separated herself from the younger children and entered women's sphere. The father points authoritatively to the little ones. One young girl reaches out, again greedily, to grab the fruit offered by her brother. Fruit has continued to provide important visual cues in portraits, but only in portraits of very young girls. For the most part, fruit and the grasping appetite for sweet oranges, apples, peaches, and pears have become infantile and unworthy of respectable married women, the republican wives and mothers of a sovereign nation.[31]

29. Deborah Gray White, *Ar'n't I a Woman? Female Slaves in the Plantation South* (New York, 1985).

30. Hannah Pemberton to Thomas Parke, Aug. 29, 1780, quoted in Judy Mann DiStefano, "A Concept of the Family in Colonial America: The Pembertons of Philadelphia" (Ph.D. diss., Ohio State University, 1970), 95.

31. Philippe Aries noted in *Centuries of Childhood: A Social History of Family Life*, trans. Robert Baldick (New York, 1962), 57–61, that the fashions of earlier generations become children's clothing as a way of emphasizing the separateness of childhood and the inferiority of children to adults. This

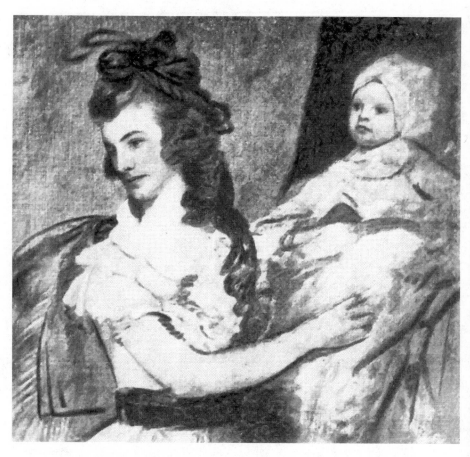

PLATE 17.

Mrs. William Bingham (Anne Willing). By Gilbert Stuart.
Private collection, reproduced in Anne Hollingsworth Wharton,
Salons Colonial and Republican . . . (Philadelphia, 1900), opposite 140.

A highly unusual portrayal of a distracted mother.

The extent of the transformation in values and iconography can be seen
by comparing two paired sets of superficially similar portraits, one in each
set painted before the Revolution, one after. The 1751 portrait of Elizabeth
Peel by Benjamin West is an early example from the then very young artist
(Plate 19). Peel is posed with a basket of flowers held before her stomach,
swelling her silhouette as if pregnant and placed conspicuously between her

---

generational shift in the emblems of inferiority applies not only to children but to African Americans as well.

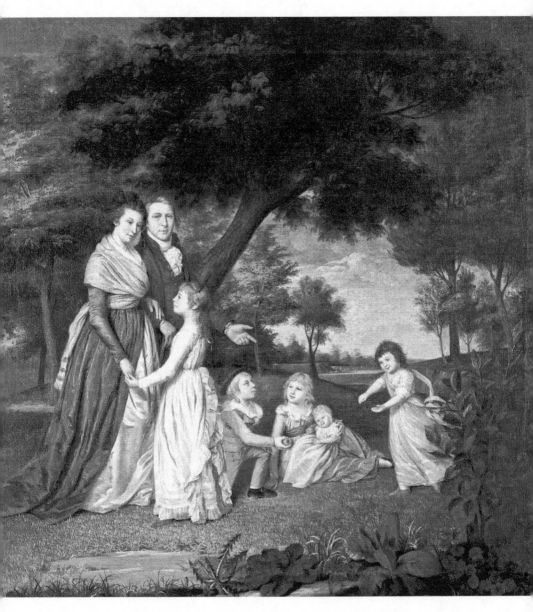

PLATE 18.

The Artist and His Family. By James Peale, 1795. Oil on canvas, 31 ¼ x 32 ¾ in.
(79.4 x 83.2 cm.), 1922.1.1. Courtesy of the Pennsylvania Academy of the
Fine Arts, Philadelphia. Gift of John Frederick Lewis.

James Peale has placed his wife in the foreground, and his pointing finger
distinguishes the irrationality of the littlest children who are fighting over an
apple from the calm rationality of the adults and their older daughter.

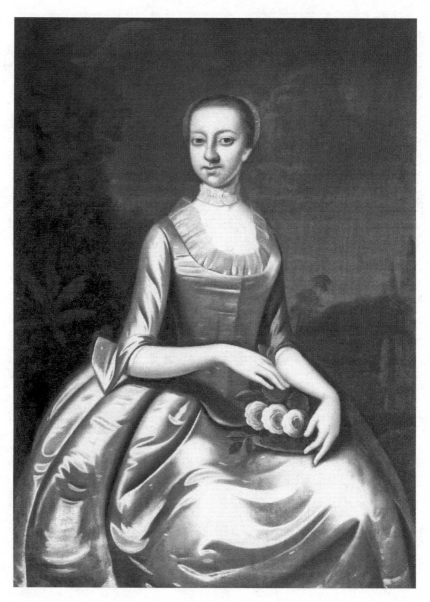

PLATE 19.

Elizabeth Peel. By Benjamin West, circa 1757. Oil on canvas, 47 ⅛ x 34 ⅜ in. (119.7 x 87.3 cm.), 1923.8.13. Courtesy of the Pennsylvania Academy of the Fine Arts, Philadelphia. Gift of John Frederick Lewis.

Elizabeth Peel adopts a common colonial pose. Her small head is dwarfed by her voluminous skirts; her right hand and arm suggest roundness, as does the basket of full-blown flowers held between her parted legs.

outstretched legs as if spilling from the female body in luxuriant abundance. The position of her hands and arms furthers the suggestion of a rounded belly. The brightly colored flowers serve to distract the viewer's attention from the face. Peel sits facing the viewer with her legs splayed, a leaf points to her crotch. Flowers signal that women are physical creatures, producers of wealth. They are divided between head and reproductive organs, obviously less rational and more animalistic than men. Peel sits outdoors in an untamed natural setting rather than in the built environment of civilized society. The features present in this portrait were commonplace in the middle decades of the eighteenth century.

The 1790 portrait of Hannah Maley Cuyler, by an unknown artist, provides a contrast on several levels (Plate 20). Cuyler serves as a model of the new ideals of femininity. Her hands and arms hide her abdomen. Her knees are held closely together, and her body is self-contained, no longer open to the public gaze. She is holding a dark-colored, open book as if she were momentarily interrupted when reading. She has intellectual interests. On the dressing table are a fan, which suggests sociability, a pin cushion for her artistic, decorative skills, and a pocketbook—she has control of at least some money. Her watch and keys at her waist suggest her domestic responsibilities. A miniature portrait of her husband connects to her heart. She is in an indoor setting, unlike the otherwise similarly posed pictures of Experience Johnson or Elizabeth Peel painted thirty and forty years earlier. The domestic realm, not an untamed wilderness, is her domain. She is rational, competent, and adult.

In John Hesselius's 1763 double portrait of Rebecca Young and her granddaughter, the youthful Rebecca Woodward cradles a heap of strawberries by pulling up her apron in prediction of a fecund future, while the older (and probably postmenopausal) grandmother holds a single small, bright red strawberry at her lower abdomen (Plate 21). The real fruit of her loins, the granddaughter, is likewise placed between her outspread legs. The granddaughter comfortingly pats her grandmother's inner thigh. Descendants dutifully care for their predecessors. The two are outdoors in what may be an Italian garden; the sun appears to be setting behind the grandmother, but she has left a legacy in her offspring.

In Charles Willson Peale's double portrait, circa 1777–1780, of Rebecca Edghill Mifflin and her granddaughter, Rebecca Francis, the grandmother instructs her granddaughter, holding a book of emblems on her lap, while the child points to a page illustrating the emblems for conjugal concord, filial love, virtue, and duty (Plate 22). The imagery is moral, intellectual, and sen-

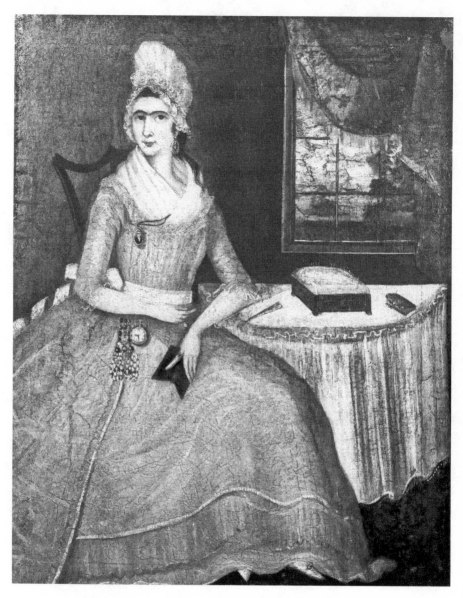

PLATE 20.

Mrs. Johannes Cornelius Cuyler (Hannah Maley Cuyler). Anonymous, circa 1790.
Courtesy, Albany Institute of History and Art.

Compared to colonial women's portraits, Hannah Cuyler exhibits
her many interests and responsibilities. The position of her arms hides her
belly rather than highlighting it as was typical in colonial portraits.

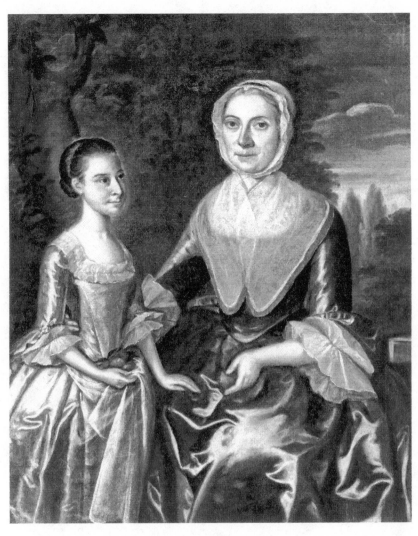

PLATE 21.

Rebecca Holdsworth Young and Granddaughter Rebecca Woodward.
By John Hesselius, 1763. Courtesy, Winterthur Museum.

Succulent strawberries are gathered in the granddaughter's apron, a symbol
of a fecund future. Even the grandmother holds a single berry. The granddaughter
dutifully comforts her forebear by patting her thigh.

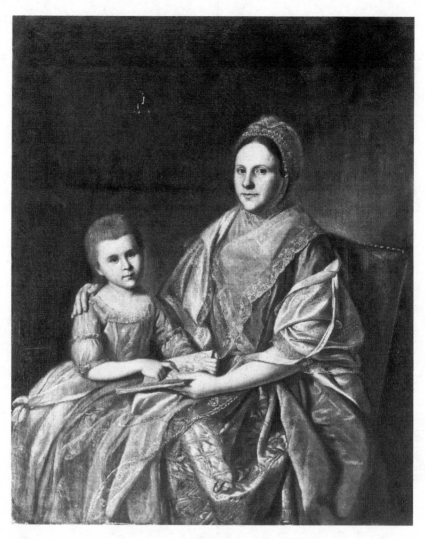

PLATE 22.

Mrs. Samuel Mifflin (Rebecca Edghill Mifflin) and Granddaughter
Rebecca Mifflin Francis. By Charles Willson Peale, circa 1777–1780.
Metropolitan Museum of Art, Egleston Fund, 1922 (22.153.2).

Books have replaced fruit.
The grandmother protects the child.

sible rather than fertile. The women are located in the domestic realm rather than out in nature. The book and the older woman's arms cover the older woman's abdomen; her legs are placed together. The young girl leans on the grandmother but is outside her body. The child imitates her grandmother's posture by having her arm cover her abdomen. Unlike the double portrait of grandmother and granddaughter by Hesselius, it is the grandmother who virtuously and selflessly comforts and protects the child by wrapping her arm around the granddaughter's shoulder. Children are a responsibility, not a source of future economic benefit. These two women of the early Republic— Cuyler and Mifflin—are not represented as cornucopias, as empty vessels pouring forth abundant wealth. They are responsible adults at least within the realm of childrearing and domesticity.

The emblems associated with women changed during and after the Revolution; the books, tea tables, embroidery projects, musical instruments, and maps that appeared with increasing frequency during and after the Revolution suggested the range of their activities and interests. Perhaps as important as the kind of props was their muted coloring, which no longer distracts the viewer from the character of the face. Indeed, props, tables, and women's arms were so arranged that women's abdomens and lower limbs were partially or fully hidden. The body language of restraint and control had replaced the outspread knees of earlier decades. Even though most of the evidence concerning these new standards of comportment comes from the images generated by the upper classes, an 1810 portrait sketch by Baroness Hyde de Neuville suggests a more widespread disciplining of the female body as an African American servant sits in a chair with her limbs tucked close to her body (not included here). The posture of the nursemaid from York, Pennsylvania, does not differ from her employers' (see Plate 16).[32]

Hints of the old fecund emblems survived very occasionally in the portraits of childless women. In the double portrait of the childless Benjamin and Eleanor Ridgely Laming, painted by Peale in 1788 (not included here) and analyzed by Ellen G. Miles and Leslie Reinhardt, phallic symbolism is as

---

32. Baroness Hyde de Neuville, *The Scrubwoman*, undated, in Jadviga M. da Costa Nunes and Ferris Olin, *Baroness Hyde de Neuville: Sketches of America, 1807–1822* (New Brunswick, N.J., 1984), 20. See also Gwendolyn DuBois Shaw, *Portraits of a People: Picturing African Americans in the Nineteenth Century* (Andover, Mass., 2006). In New England, there are portraits of women with a book as a prop even in the seventeenth century. There was never more than one book, however, indicating that it was the Bible. The book was closed, and it was held at the lower torso. It was a religious talisman rather than a symbol of intellectual pursuits. At the end of the eighteenth century, there were more books, many small octavo volumes (probably novels), and the books were likely to be open and associated with the head. Women were engaged in reading.

prominent as fruitful symbolism. The garden is meant to represent a place where, according to the Italian poet Torquato Tasso, "All seem impregnate with the seeds of love." The phallic symbolism is blatant, yet the fruitful imagery is restrained in comparison to the large baskets and filled aprons of fruit so common in the prewar period. These dual icons are perhaps an indication that there could be anxiety about the man's physicality as well as the woman's, and in fact the Lamings' only child had recently died. The fertile imagery attempts to compensate for difficulties in conceiving but is an unusual deployment of icons, redolent of a previous generation. The images of symbolic fertility persist for another generation or two in the South and West, in some rural areas and among German speakers—all regions and groups that were slower to embrace lower fertility. Even in these groups, the fruitful, flowering images disappeared by about the 1830s.[33]

Again the question is about the sources of these changes in iconography: Who was in charge, patrons, painters, or sitters? Something is known of the production of two portraits, both from 1795. Robert Morris paid sixty guineas to have Gilbert Stuart paint a dual portrait of his daughters (Plate 23). The painting shows the two women seated behind a table playing chess, looking boldly at the viewer. Morris criticized the painting; the grounds of his disapproval are unknown, and Stuart slashed the canvas. After her marriage, Hetty Morris Marshall had her husband negotiate for the painting. He paid Stuart the full price and had it restored. These women appreciated, and perhaps dictated, their portrayal as rational, confident, and independent individuals.[34]

The portrait of Angelica Peale Robinson and her husband, Alexander Robinson, was painted by Angelica's father, Charles Willson Peale (not included here). He wrote in his diary that the portrait had to be carried out with "dispatch, as the situation of Angelica required that no time should be lost, as it was daily expected that she would be in the straw," that is, she was in the ninth month of pregnancy and about to give birth. A few years later, a Pennsylvania farmer, who was not otherwise noted for his savoir faire, commented that a neighbor's wife was "in Straw as the Vulgar Say." Peale's vulgarity might have reflected his dislike of his son-in-law and hence of the marriage. His daughter's portrait gives no sign, however, that these barnyard

33. Torquato Tasso, quoted in Ellen G. Miles and Leslie Reinhardt, "'Art Conceal'd': Peale's Double Portrait of Benjamin and Eleanor Ridgely Laming," *Art Bulletin*, LXXVIII, no. 1 (1996), 56–74, esp. 67.

34. Anne Hollingsworth Wharton, *Salons Colonial and Republican* . . . (Philadelphia, 1900), xii, 97.

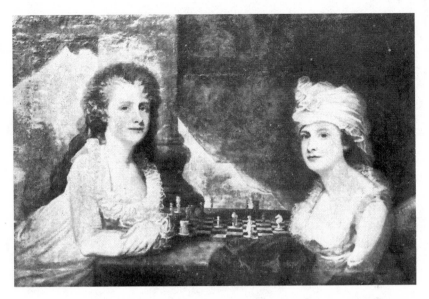

PLATE 23.

Maria Morris Nixon and Hetty Morris Marshall. By Gilbert Stuart.
Private collection, reproduced in Anne Hollingsworth Wharton,
Salons Colonial and Republican . . . (Philadelphia, 1900), opposite 96.

Two sisters play chess and look confidently at the
viewer in this repaired painting.

functions were about to occur. Angelica Robinson's head is dominant; her belly, insofar as it can be seen, is flat. But symbolism may be at work here as well, if two 1824 letters from Sevin Bell to Madelaine LeMoyne are accurate codebooks for this earlier period. The suggestion of a shawl is the clue. Judge Bell wrote to his married niece: "Mrs. Claypoole has been wearing *the shawl* for some time. . . . Our Parson's Lady will certainly increase the number of our congregation as soon as law and decency will permit, but she is so far from wearing a shawl that she appears to make a boast of it." Women had to hide their gravid bodies, just as the euphemism "wearing the shawl" veiled these comments on pregnancy. The parson's lady's obvious pride in her non-pregnancy was despite community expectations of her early impregnation. Bell continued, "We have scarcely a wife in town who is not either minding an infant or waddling about with the rotundity of a beer barrel." The aesthetics of the gravid female body had been reversed since Poor Richard's time — no longer evoking a handsome, billowing sail in the wind, the pregnant woman had all the grace of a wooden barrel. By the nineteenth century, the pregnant body was ugly, humiliating, redolent of poverty, and best hidden from sight.[35]

The state took over the productive role previously assigned to women. When the Second Continental Congress in 1776 drew up its list of the king's "repeated injuries and usurpations," the seventh was that he "endeavored to prevent of population of these states" by discouraging immigration. State policy, not women's bodies, was the source of growth. Americans celebrated the rapid growth of their population in the early national period. William Barton patriotically applauded America's "inherent, radical and lasting source of national vigor and greatness;—For, it will be found, that, in no other part of the world . . . is the progress of population so rapid, as in these states." Politics, not procreation, was key: "The benign influence of our government produces early marriages," he noted, as did the healthfulness of the climate (low mortality), simple manners, and the attractions of the western country to immigrants. It was the state and its fiscal policies rather than the labor of individual married women that produced wealth—women reproduced, merely replicating the previous generation. They no longer procreated or generated babies and wealth. Men took more pride in being "free, white, and twenty-one" and had somewhat less interest in their private family lives. Men were citizens in a democratizing polity. Virtuous women were at home—at least in theory.[36]

Fertile images were banished from individual women's portraits, but neoclassical symbolism dominated symbolic images of the newly independent states. A few examples will suffice. In W. D. Cooper's 1789 frontispiece *America Trampling on Oppression,* the new United States is the slightly pregnant Minerva, goddess of war and wisdom (Plate 24). She mediates between Benjamin Franklin, representing healing, the arts, and science, and George Washington, representing the martial arts and patriotism. At her feet are a

35. Charles Willson Peale, *Alexander Robinson and His Wife, Angelica Peale,* 1795, in Richardson, Hindle, and Miller, *Charles Willson Peale,* 217; Peale, quoted in Charles Coleman Sellers, *Portraits and Miniatures by Charles Willson Peale,* American Philosophical Society, *Transactions,* XLII (Philadelphia, 1952), 183; Joseph Price Diary, Apr. 16, 1804, Lower Merion Historical Society, Pa., http://www.lowermerionhistory.org/texts/price/price1804.html (accessed March 2003); Sevin Bell, quoted in Virginia K. Bartlett, *Keeping House: Women's Lives in Western Pennsylvania, 1790–1850* (Pittsburgh, 1994), 144. For another example, with my thanks to Anne Verplanck, see the analysis of the portrait of Sarah Walsh Varick wearing a large shawl in Tammis K. Groft and Mary Alice Mackay, eds., *The Albany Institute of History and Art: Two Hundred Years of Collecting* (New York, 1998), 150–151. This portrait might have been painted posthumously; Varick died in childbirth.

36. William Barton, *Observations on the Progress of Population, and the Probabilities of the Duration of Human Life, in the United States of America* . . . (Philadelphia, 1791), 2.

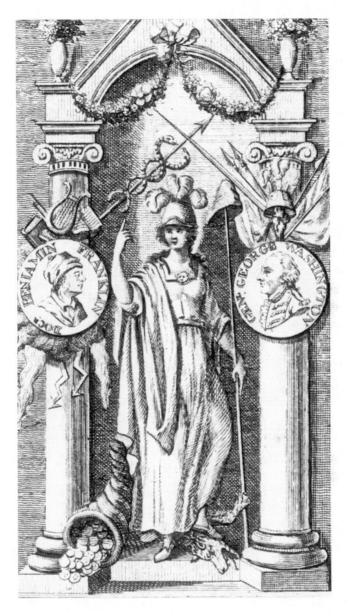

PLATE 24.

America Trampling on Oppression. By W. D. Cooper. Frontispiece
to E. Newberry, *History of North America* (London, 1789).

A slightly pregnant America tramples on the wolf of oppression.
A cornucopia pours out hard cash, not fruit. The images of Benjamin Franklin
and George Washington represent peace and war. Growth and prosperity are
guaranteed by the feminized pregnant state, not by fecundity of real-life women.

cornucopia filled to overflowing with coins and the trampled wolf of oppression of the title. Prosperity and victory are assured for the future. America is not the fickle Fortuna. In *America Guided by Wisdom,* George Washington is only a frozen statue in shadows, while America, again slightly pregnant, with her cornucopia overflowing with local produce, her constitutional shield, and flag of the United States, is advised by Athena (not included here). The two female goddesses watch over commercial ships guided by the speed and communicative powers of Mercury. On land is a beehive of industry and a sheaf of wheat guarded by Ceres, the goddess of agriculture and fertility. In the far background, a woman spins. Robert Edge Pine's 1778 allegory adopts similar themes (not included here). He portrays a group of feminized virtues who are "expressive of *Population.*" These are Peace, Virtue, Liberty, Concord, Industry, and Plenty, and they will repair the damages done in America by a lengthy, destructive war. Growth comes from virtuous, republican government.[37]

These images became official. The coats of arms of the city of Philadelphia and the state of New Jersey, among many other cities and states, featured the sailing ships and the burgeoning female bellies reminiscent of Franklin's tag (not included here). These themes were also adopted for coins, medallions, and other bric-a-brac of sovereign nations. To these ships and bulging bellies were added cornucopias, plows, liberty caps, the scales of justice, and maps or charters. Again, it is government as embodied in iconic females, not individual women, that will bring wealth, progress, and prosperity to the country. Unlike Fortune, they are not fickle; they are not dangerous or arbitrary. The most demeaning characteristics associated with women had been suppressed. These are virtuous creatures in the images of the gods, and they are the ones supporting the growth of a new republic. Their symbolic pregnancies free real women from the debilitating tasks of generating large populations, providing an expanding labor force and consumer markets, and furnishing a powerful military with soldiers and sailors. Smaller numbers of

37. *America Guided by Virtue* and several other examples of the new Republic as a slightly pregnant goddess can be found in Alfred F. Young and Terry J. Fife, *We the People: Voices and Images of the New Nation* (Philadelphia, 1993), 197–199. The best source for Robert Edge Pine's allegory is http://www.nps.gov/history/history/online_books/inde/anderson/chap5c.htm. An unusual use of neoclassical images is a deck of playing cards with Thomas Jefferson as the King of Clubs, the goddess Ceres with her cornucopia as the Queen, and Joseph Brant, a prominent Iroquois, as the Jack. See Sara Day, "'With Peace and Freedom Blest!' Woman as Symbol in America, 1590–1800," Library of Congress, http://lcweb2.loc.gov/ammem/awhhtml/awo5e/awo5e.html; and Caroline Winterer, "From Royal to Republican: The Classical Image in Early America," *JAH*, XCI (2005), 1264–1290.

well-educated children, happy marriages, and options for women could now be safely promoted.[38]

PORTRAITS IN THE late eighteenth century, just as women's writings, experimented with new definitions of a rational, prudent, sentimental feminine self. Pregnancy and fertility were distanced. Childrearing, education, and companionate marriages emerged as alternative sources of personal, familial, and public identity. These visual and aesthetic changes were perhaps limited to the elite who could afford to have their portraits painted. But early in the new nation many of the middling sort could afford to commission miniatures, and, by the 1790s, cut silhouettes captured the individualized profiles of far less wealthy Americans. All these artistic forms—portraits, miniatures, and silhouettes—indicate an emphasis on women's heads, rather than on their torso or genitals; women's bodies had become privatized. They were less like animals and more thoughtful, virtuous, and mature adults. These changes occurred as women began planning and counting the number of children they would bear, marrying later, concentrating childbearing into the early years of marriage, and ceasing childbearing earlier, freeing up their lives for other activities and interests.[39]

The revolutionary debates on luxury and wartime attacks on women and children prompted a rejection of the superabundant, flourishing, flowering images associated with the feminine body and expressed through high birthrates. The Revolution also brought prints in which the publicly accessible female body was tortured and dismembered—the home became both a refuge and a source of authority. Some of these changes are articulated in the writings of the period, but some appear most clearly through the body language of sitters for portraits; women's extremities become enclosed, regulated, concealed, domesticated, and privatized. Emblems, too, shift from a vocabulary of fruits and flowers to books, music, maps, artistry, and other rational engagements.

Colonial women's portraits often announced their sexual availability and hinted at the lusts that would produce those flourishing fruits and flowers

38. Thomas Sully's *Coat of Arms for Philadelphia*, 1789, is in Randall M. Miller and William Pencak, *Pennsylvania: A History of the Commonwealth* (University Park, Pa., 2002), 132. State and local coats of arms can be found at http://www.ngw.nl/int/usa/states.htm.

39. Robin Jaffee Frank, *Love and Loss: American Portrait and Mourning Miniatures* (New Haven, Conn., 2000); Charles Coleman Sellers, "Joseph Sansom, Philadelphia Silhouettist," *PMHB*, LXXXVIII (1964), 395–438.

pouring from women's bodies. The potentially fecund female body embodied beauty in the rounded forms of baskets and arms, certainly, but also carried hints of the fickleness and greed of the lusty female. After the Revolution, a new aesthetic in portraits celebrated married women's virginal virtue and their steadying maternal and domestic roles. Abundance and fecundity continued only in the symbolic representations of the Republic, of liberty, or of agriculture. Children moved away from their mothers' laps and toward women's heads and hearts, but children, especially daughters, also tended to move away from their fathers. Yet, for all these changes, women continued to be femes covert; they belonged to their husbands and reflected their husbands' status. Their freedom from fertility and their rationality, especially as expressed within the domestic realm, came at the price of bodily constraints that did not apply to men. There were spatial limitations, too, that confined women to the domestic sphere. Public spaces were inherently dangerous. Women's bodies were still redolent of the symbolic meanings of wealth, power, and status placed on them by the larger society. Women were indeed self-defined in human and humane ways that their mothers and grandmothers might not have been, as the distinctly gendered roles of motherhood, restrained virtue, and domesticity replaced the overt sexuality and animal appetites of colonial images.

5

Potions, Pills, and Jumping Ropes

THE TECHNOLOGY

OF

BIRTH CONTROL

In 1766, a printer in Germantown, Pennsylvania, advised his readers that the common herb "tansy is of a warm and dry nature, and possesses the fine virtue of loosening all thick humors of the body, here and there, but particularly in the matrix [womb]; of dispelling . . . mother fits [hysterics, convulsions, eclampsia, or other conditions], of killing and expelling worms; of warming a cold matrix and bringing a lot more into good order" (Plate 25). This now odd-seeming collection of varied conditions and their single remedy brings us into a medical world almost totally foreign in its assumptions and practices. It does suggest the resources eighteenth-century women had when they were concerned about their physical state or the size of their families. In this particular case, tansy could, it was claimed, restore menstruation (a thick humor), bring regularity of menstruation (good order), and promote pregnancy and male offspring (heating a cold womb) and healthy obstetrics (dispelling mother fits). Not incidentally, internal parasites could be expelled with the same medicine. There were many such cures, ancient

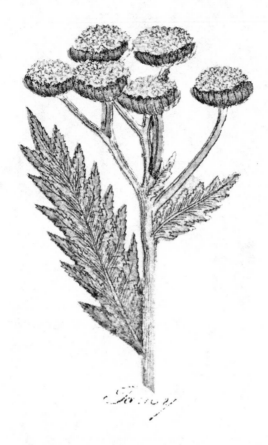

PLATE 25.

Tansy. From Nicholas Culpeper, *Culpeper's Complete Herbal and English Physician* . . . (1826; rpt. Manchester 1981), after 198.

Tansy was one of many medicinal herbs used in the eighteenth century.

and new, available to housewives, midwives, pharmacists, and doctors in the eighteenth and nineteenth centuries.[1]

The medical advice directed at women of the time offers little that looks familiar to twenty-first-century eyes. There are few references to the use of barrier methods of contraception before the late eighteenth or early nineteenth centuries. References to coitus interruptus (male withdrawal before ejaculation) as a method of preventing conception often occur in the context of illicit sexual encounters, leading scholars to conclude that contraceptive practices were unthinkable for the majority of married couples. There is little evidence that sexual abstinence was ever widely practiced by married couples or that there was any comprehension of an infertile period during the menstrual cycle for most of the eighteenth century. Demographers have stressed either the late average ages at marriage as a device for limiting family size

1. William Woys Weaver, trans. and ed., *Sauer's Herbal Cures: America's First Book of Botanic Healing, 1762–1778* (New York, 2001), 319.

or prolonged lactation by married women as somewhat effective and commonplace methods of postponing or spacing births before the nineteenth century. But even the use of lengthy breast-feeding was, according to some historians and demographers, a matter of local custom and was not used by individual women to restrict fertility. Most American historians have argued from "the few public accounts of abortion, infanticide, and contraceptive practice" that "control of birth was not significant in colonial America."[2]

But not everyone agrees with this negative assessment. Contraception is assumed in several studies. Robert Wells found evidence of "deliberate family limitation" among Quaker families living in Pennsylvania, New York, and New Jersey. These women steadily reduced fertility levels and family size from the middle of the eighteenth century. Beverly Smaby suggested "direct birth control" explained both the reduced fertility of the Moravians of Bethlehem, Pennsylvania, during the Revolutionary War and a subsequent period of crisis in their religious community as well as the higher fertility levels when times were more propitious. Other studies, detailed in Chapter 1, above, show falling birthrates, child-woman ratios, and age-specific marital fertility rates. How can these cases of restricted fertility be reconciled with the presumed absence of contraceptive and abortive technology?[3]

The Regulation of Fertility: Eighteenth-Century Definitions

Colonial women did not envisage an ideal number of children, so they did not try to stop childbearing after achieving some intended family size.

2. Norman E. Himes, *Medical History of Contraception* (1936; rpt. New York, 1970), ix, 209–238; Angus McLaren, *A History of Contraception: From Antiquity to the Present Day* (Oxford, 1990); John M. Riddle, *Contraception and Abortion from the Ancient World to the Renaissance* (Cambridge, Mass., 1992); Catherine M. Scholten, *Childbearing in American Society, 1650–1850* (New York, 1985), 13–14. Most demographers and economists have argued that before the nineteenth century a system of "natural fertility" prevailed. According to this view, the only certain control over fertility in preindustrial Europe was age at marriage and celibacy rates, but, once marriage occurred, biology, not human volition, governed fertility. Etienne van de Walle, "De la nature a la fecondite naturelle," *Annales de démographie historique, 1988* (Paris, 1989), 13–17, summarized this argument; see also his "Fertility Transition, Conscious Choice, and Numeracy," *Demography*, XXIX (1992), 487–502. A provocative view of American and French fertility declines is in Rudolph Binion, "Marianne au foyer, Révolution politique et transition démographique en France et aux États-Unis," *Population*, LV (2000), 81–104, and Jean-Pierre Bardet et Etienne van de Walle, "À propos de l'article de Rudolph Binion," and Rudolph Binion, "Réponse," both ibid., 387–396.

3. Robert V. Wells, "Family Size and Fertility Control in Eighteenth-Century America: A Study of Quaker Families," *Population Studies*, XXV (1971), 80–81; Beverly Prior Smaby, *The Transformation of Moravian Bethlehem: From Communal Mission to Family Economy* (Philadelphia, 1988), 75.

Women rarely, if ever, spoke about restricting fertility in the first seventy years of the century, but they did regulate their health and well-being by employing medicines and procedures known as emmenagogues, which, as defined by Dr. Joseph Carson, "provoke and maintain the periodical occurrence of the menstrual secretion." Rather than planning the future size of their families or curtailing the span of their childbearing years, women focused on their present circumstances, especially their current physical and emotional health, as apparent in the regularity of their menstrual cycles.[4]

Pregnancy was difficult to determine before the twentieth century, and most women would have agreed with Dr. Samuel K. Jennings: "An entire suppression of the menses attends almost every case of pregnancy. But as suppressions may be brought on by other causes this cannot be an infallible mark." The absence of menstruation could be equally a sign of pregnancy or a sign of illness. So, in 1778, Sally Logan Fisher of Philadelphia was "much dissapointed" with the onset of menstruation, since she had just miscarried and longed for another child. In 1805, Lydia Tallender of the same city defined her amenorrhea as a sign of illness, not pregnancy. According to her husband, she "had not had the female customs for 2 mos, and been unwell; . . . pills given for the effecting the return of the aforementioned caused puking and purgation, which after a while was checked." The lack of a necessary connection between amenorrhea and pregnancy allowed both women and doctors to view a missed menstrual period as a question of health before quickening. Although by the middle of the eighteenth century few women or doctors believed in the old idea that quickening was the mystical moment when the fetus was endowed with a soul, quickening remained important as the first certain sign of a viable pregnancy. Before that point, amenorrhea (called lost, hidden, obstructed, or suppressed menses) might be diagnosed. Elizabeth Bayley Seton's pointed comment in 1800, "Emma had *lost*, and has found *again*," makes no sense today, but it signaled to her closest friend that their acquaintance was no longer afraid of a possible pregnancy or illness. Women watched their bodies for signs. If a woman saw her amenorrhea as pathological, then pregnancy was excluded as a possible underlying cause. A woman was either gravid or obstructed, and the two conditions bore no necessary relationship to one another.[5]

4. Joseph Carson, *Synopsis of the Course of Lectures on Materia Medica and Pharmacy Delivered in the University of Pennsylvania* (Philadelphia, 1867), 82–84.

5. Samuel K. Jennings, *The Married Lady's Companion; or, Poor Man's Friend* (1808; rpt. New York, 1972), 75; Mary Beth Norton, *Liberty's Daughters: The Revolutionary Experience of American Women, 1750–1800* (Boston, 1980), 80; "Strangers' Burials," Sept. 3, 1805, Gloria Dei Lutheran

Some women who knew that they were pregnant might, of course, have lied about their condition. When Winifred Carter miscarried in Virginia in 1771, her curmudgeon of a father-in-law, Landon Carter, "suspected her being with child some months ago," but she did not admit to pregnancy. Her behavior caused him to think that "there must have been some intention to forward the abortio[n]." Three years later, she again miscarried, reputedly saying that "she had not felt her child these 2 months, a thing she had never spoak of to one soul." Landon Carter added, when Winifred "told me she was not with child . . . [this] was intended to discover [tell others] the Child was dead within her." Her statements seem both unconvincing and self-serving, at least as reported by her suspicious and unsympathetic father-in-law. More typically, however, a woman's word on her condition was not challenged, especially if she was respectably married.[6]

The two symptoms that distinguished the pathological condition of obstructed menses from pregnancy were, according to one doctor, "mental despondency" and hysteria. The emotional state of the woman was the primary clue to her physical condition. "Grief and distress" were considered the predominant symptoms in cases of amenorrhea and could be accompanied by stomach pains, headaches, and melancholy. Hysteria was, in the eighteenth century, a disease with both mental and physical symptoms. Despondency and physical symptoms resembling early pregnancy were thought to define hysteria. The most popular home guide to health stated, "A sudden suppression of the menses often gives rise to hysteric fits," beginning with fatigue, "lowness of spirits, oppression and anxiety." Additionally, hysteria was indicated if the woman felt "as if there were a ball at the lower part of the belly, which gradually rises towards the stomach, where it occasions inflation, sickness, and sometimes vomiting." Another medical source added a curious collection of symptoms: "an unusual gurgling of the bowels, as if some little

---

Church, Philadelphia, Burial Records, Genealogical Society of Pennsylvania, Philadelphia (Tallender died, not from the emmenagogues, but from yellow fever); Regina Bechtle and Judith Metz, eds., *Elizabeth Bayley Seton: Collected Writings*, I, *Correspondence and Journals, 1793–1808* (Hyde Park, N.Y., 2000), 121. Dr. George DeBenneville wrote angrily, "Some woman are so Ignorant, They do not know whin she are Conceived with Child, and others so easy, They will nott Confess when they do know it," but he did not include amenorrhea as one of the signs of pregnancy. Rather, he listed some very dubious symptoms such as "coldness of the outward parts," the "belly waxeth very flat," "the Veins of the eyes are clearly seen," or the appearance of a "small living creature" in the woman's urine after thirteen days of storage (George DeBenneville, "Medicina Pensylvania; or, The Pensylvania Physician," circa 1760–1779, 124, microfilm, American Philosophical Society, Philadelphia). He passed on this information to his married daughter, Harriet DeBenneville Klein.

6. Jack P. Greene, ed., *The Diary of Colonel Landon Carter of Sabine Hall, 1752–1778*, 2 vols. (Charlottesville, Va., 1965), II, 620, 859, 861.

animal were there in actual motion, with wandering pains, constituting colic of a peculiar kind." Anxiety, low spirits, and a feeling of oppression could, of course, have been caused by fears of an unwanted pregnancy. The physical signs thought to be specific to the disease of hysteria—an inflated belly, perceived motion, vomiting, and colic—mirror some of the early symptoms of pregnancy.[7]

In popular discourse, a missed menstrual period was called "taking the cold." This term was a survival of the Galenic system of medicine in which a balance of the four humors—black bile, yellow bile, blood, and phlegm— determined health. Since menstrual blood was a "hot" humor, its absence must signify the dominance of a cold humor. Dr. William Buchan's *Domestic Medicine* warned, "More of the sex [women] date their disorders [amenorrhea] from colds, caught while they are out of order [expecting menstruation], than from all other causes." This merging of two physical conditions— the common cold and pregnancy—can be seen both in medical tracts and in women's recipe books. Rheumatism and pleurisy, thought to be caused by colds, were linked to obstructed menstruation through the "stoppage of customary discharges." All these conditions were conflated and the treatments merged so that emmenagogic medicines were considered cures for rheumatism. Riding on horseback was also recommended for rheumatism, presumably because it would dislodge any obstructed customary discharges. Consumption, another obstructive disease, was also a possibility. Rosalie Calvert told her brother in 1802 that her "doctors thought I was going into consumption, but the outcome is that you will have another nephew or niece in several months." Although these doctors' wildly inaccurate diagnoses seem ludicrous in the twenty-first century—how could anyone confuse pulmonary tuberculosis with pregnancy, we might ask—traditional humoral assumptions about suppressed fluids made the confusion logical. In the empirical and eclectic medical practice of the eighteenth century, few strictly followed any one system of medicine, but the humoral categories persisted well into the nineteenth century. Catching a cold had layers of meaning for women in the colonies and in the new nation.[8]

7. Andrew S. Berky, *Practitioner in Physick: A Biography of Abraham Wagner, 1717–1763* (Pennsburg, Pa., 1954), 112; William P. C. Barton, *Outlines of Lectures on Materia Medica and Botany, Delivered in Jefferson Medical College, Philadelphia*, 2 vols. (Philadelphia, 1827–1828), I, 104; William Buchan, *Domestic Medicine; or, A Treatise on the Prevention and Cure of Diseases . . .* , ed. Samuel Powel Griffitts (Philadelphia, 1795), 455–456; Jennings, *Married Lady's Companion*, 54.

8. James C. Mohr, *Abortion in America: The Origins and Evolution of National Policy, 1800–1900* (New York, 1978), 7; Buchan, *Domestic Medicine*, 395–396, 529; Margaret Law Callcott, ed., *Mistress of Riversdale: The Plantation Letters of Rosalie Stier Calvert, 1795–1821* (Baltimore, 1991), 34.

The emotional and physical state of the woman determined whether she would view her "suppressed menstruation" as a sign of pregnancy or as a sign of illness. The illness might be labeled obstructed menstruation, which was considered a separate disease, or the obstructed menstruation could be interpreted as one symptom of despondency, hysteria, colds, pleurisy, or rheumatism. There were additional possibilities. Intestinal parasites might be diagnosed. The hard, bulging bellies of the worm-infested, the inflated abdomens of the hysteric, and the swollen bodies of the dropsical could look much the same. Since small animals might seem to rumble through one's innards causing colic and hysteria, and since intestinal worms could cause similar internal sensations, then the conditions must therefore be related. Even though amenorrhea was not involved in cases of worms, emmenagogic medicines could be given, an indication that a concern with external appearance was often paramount in women's perceptions of disease treatments. Yet, in this application of emmenagogic medicines, eighteenth-century medicine came close to erasing the distinction between emmenagogues and abortifacients, for, if foreign creatures might be expelled by emmenagogues in cases of worms, these medicines might also be understood to work to expel the fetus before quickening. Signs of obstructed fluids, amenorrhea, colds, abdominal swelling, discomfort, parasites, and anxiety united these "diseases" into overlapping categories and provided medical diagnoses that could be quite distinct from pregnancy.

Therapeutics as well as diagnostics linked these disease classifications. Emmenagogic medicines were often used in cases diagnosed as dropsy, intestinal worms, rheumatism, pleurisy, and other diseases, since in all cases the expulsion of foreign or dangerous fluids, the destruction of little animals, and the reduction of abdominal swelling were the goals. Women did not need to stress their amenorrhea when employing emmenagogic drugs or procedures, since amenorrhea might be only one among many pathological indicators of an illness. Botanist C. S. Rafinesque provides one example. Juniper's properties, he noted, "increase all the secretions, but may produce hemorrhagy and abortion, acting chiefly on the uterus. Pregnant women ought never to use them; but they are very useful in dropsical complaints, menstrual suppressions, also in rheumatism, gout, worms, etc." A line was drawn between the symptoms of pregnancy and of disease that is by no means clear today, and disease categories and treatments overlapped in a seemingly imprecise fashion that is quite at odds with twenty-first-century nosology. The illogic is only retrospective. Women in the eighteenth century read their mental and physical signs to distinguish between sickness and pregnancy, and, if ill health was determined, then the opinions of others—friends, kin, neighbors, pharmacists, doctors, midwives—might help sort through both reported and visible symptoms to try to pinpoint the cause. Emmenagogic medicines were universally applicable in cases of congestion, swelling, infestation, and anxiety no matter what the underlying disease might be determined to be. Definitions of disease provided women with a vehicle for dealing with unwelcome pregnancies. There are few references to the deliberate prevention of conception or to induced abortion in the eighteenth and nineteenth centuries but many to the regulation of the menstrual cycle through the treatment of one or more of these diseases.[9]

English-language health manuals, diaries, and letters did not discuss the fertility effects of these emmenagogic practices and medicines, because the focus was entirely on the woman's health. But about one-third of Pennsylvania women were German, not English. In the German-language health guides published in eighteenth-century Pennsylvania, most recipes concerned the finding of "hidden or lost menses" and the subsequent restoration of menstruation and health, just as in the English guides. However, German women could also suffer from carrying "dead fruit." Christopher Sauer's *Small Herbal of Little Cost,* printed in Germantown from 1762 to 1778, gave women recipes designed "to expel the dead fruit." Later in the century, midwifery manuals published at Ephrata, Pennsylvania, recorded the same cures as effective in expelling the fetus, "be it dead or alive." No such explicit reference to abortion appears in English printed material.[10]

Even among the English it must have been known, if little recorded for posterity, that restoring menstruation could abort a pregnancy. In the eighteenth century and well into the nineteenth century, descriptions of violent exercise or the ingestion of various herbs and minerals could be found in books of household medicine both under sections describing behaviors to avoid in pregnancy and in sections dealing with cures for the disease of "obstructed menses." The strong association of emmenagogues with the destruction of "little animals" and their simultaneous use as insecticides and vermifuges indicate a conceptual linkage with contraceptive and abortive functions. Women usually made only oblique references to their use of these

9. C. S. Rafinesque, *Medical Flora; or, Manual of the Medical Botany of the United States of North America . . . ,* 2 vols. (Philadelphia, 1828, 1830), II, 16.

10. Christa M. Wilmanns Wells, "A Small Herbal of Little Cost, 1762–1778: A Case Study of a Colonial Herbal as a Social and Cultural Document" (Ph.D. diss., University of Pennsylvania, 1980), 464, 470–471. See also James Woycke, *Birth Control in Germany, 1871–1933* (London, 1988), 16–19.

medicines and practices. Two months after weaning her son in 1757, Esther Edwards Burr was bedridden for two days and then rode from Princeton to Brunswick: "Found the Ride of service," she wrote to a friend. One month later, she was "poorly." She did not remark that these illnesses came in monthly cycles, nor did she discuss the possible consequences of these ailments. Margaret Hill Morris included no emmenagogues in her collection of cures. Yet her recipe for rheumatism encompassed ingredients and dosages that were usually used to restore menstruation. Euphemisms and now quite foreign perceptions of disease can obscure the intentions of eighteenth-century women.[11]

Also blurring the intentions of women was that these same remedies were used as prophylactics. One preventive method was to employ an emmenagogue just before the menstrual period was due in order to ensure its arrival. A second prophylactic technique was that "after birth, nursing mothers took it [a tea of the herb savin] to hold off renewed menses," since renewed menses would have signaled a resumption of fertility. Here savin is primarily an antifertility agent, not an emmenagogue. Because, according to one visitor, "in Philadelphia a husband resumes conjugal relations with his nursing wife a month after the birth" instead of following the tradition of sexual abstinence as long as the child was nursing, medications might have been necessary to protect both mother and child against another pregnancy. Definitions of disease—obstructed menses, colds, rheumatism, even worms or internal parasites—along with a reticence in speaking or writing about private female topics have hidden the contraceptive and abortive technologies available to women in the eighteenth and nineteenth centuries.[12]

11. For examples, see John Wesley, *Primitive Remedies* (Santa Barbara, Calif., 1975) (orig. pub. as *Primitive Physick; or, An Easy and Natural Method of Curing Most Diseases*, 5th ed. [Bristol, 1755]), 23, 89–90; Jennings, *Married Lady's Companion*, 43–49, 77–80; Carol F. Karlsen and Laurie Crumpacker, eds., *The Journal of Esther Edwards Burr, 1754-1757* (New Haven, Conn., 1984), 267, 270 (see also 211). "For the Rheumatism—half an ounce of gum guiacum in fine powdr; ¼ os [ounce] Valerian root in powder[,] 1 Dram of Camphor, mix them well together in a morter and with a little syrup make a mass for pills. Take 4, night and morning" (Margaret Hill Morris [1736-1816], "Receipe Book," 4, photocopy, Quaker Collection, Haverford College, Haverford, Pa.). On insect metaphors used for describing first trimester fetuses, see Chapter 6, below.

12. Bradford Angier, *Field Guide to Medicinal Wild Plants* (Harrisburg, Pa., 1978), 155; Kenneth Roberts and Anna M. Roberts, eds. and trans., *Moreau de St. Méry's American Journey (1793-1798)* (Garden City, N.Y., 1947), 289. Many, but not all, books of domestic medicine advised against the resumption of sexual relations while nursing; see Paula A. Treckel, "Breastfeeding and Maternal Sexuality in Colonial America," *Journal of Interdisciplinary History*, XX (1989-1990), 25–51.

The Regulation of Fertility: Techniques

There were a large number of cures for the disease of obstructed menses, and women combined herbal decoctions, bleeding, vigorous exercise, and "baths" to treat their amenorrhea. In 1828, Dr. W. P. C. Barton provided his medical students with an unusually inclusive list of emmenagogic medicines and procedures. He described thirteen classes of medical treatments. There were forty medicinal herbs and minerals designed to be swallowed in liquid form or as pills. He also advocated bloodletting, vigorous exercise such as dancing and horseback riding, and application of pressure to the abdomen with brushes and "frictions" (a forcible rubbing of the lower torso). He recommended baths of various sorts. The methods described by Barton would today be considered attempts to abort, and some, like jumping rope, are still practiced popularly in efforts to terminate pregnancy. The use of footbaths and bathing would seem especially ineffectual, but among the Pennsylvania Germans a footbath was a euphemism for a vaginal douche. It was defined in German medical texts as "bathing inside from below upward." No such definition has been found in English, although perhaps this usage was understood both by physicians and lay practitioners. Similarly, the German health guides can explicitly describe contraceptive and abortive tampons, yet at times they employ the circumlocution of medicines "laid upon the thighs" instead of referring directly to tampons. When Barton recommended fomentations and cloths laid upon the pubic region, these might well have connoted douches and tampons to his readers. The veiled language of the day makes it difficult to recover the full range of contemporary American practice. Unstated assumptions almost certainly contributed to wide variation in individual women's abilities to achieve their goals.[13]

The emmenagogic, contraceptive, or abortive practices of the eighteenth century were not associated with the act of sexual intercourse, but, as befits a technology largely controlled by women, focused on menstruation and women's perception of a possible pregnancy or disruption of health. Medications might sometimes be prescribed or prepared by men, but they were administered by women. The treatments were taken orally or anally or applied externally. There are explicit references to vaginal intrusion in Ger-

13. Barton, *Outlines of Lectures*, I, 105–107; Johannes Adam Lorinzer, a sixteenth-century German botanist and physician, quoted in Wells, "Small Herbal," 467. For a discussion of the distinctive childbearing patterns in particular families based on an analysis of birth intervals, see Stephanie Grauman Wolf, *Urban Village: Population, Community, and Family Structure in Germantown, Pennsylvania, 1683–1800* (Princeton, N.J., 1976), 271–273.

man; none in English. There are no references to uterine intrusion. Vomiting, purging, and sweating were the expected results of all these treatments. The emmenagogic practices of the eighteenth century seem harsh two hundred years later, as does much of eighteenth-century medical practice. But the intrusive methods of later contraceptive practice initially struck most Philadelphians as "hideous."[14]

It may be that physical remedies for obstructed menses like jumping rope, horseback riding, or carriage rides were the most commonly employed. They would have been readily available to women. Landon Carter suspected his daughter-in-law of such activity. After one stillbirth, he wrote: This "is her own fault, a woman that hardly moves when not with child, always is Jolting in a Chariot when with Child. This is the 3d destroyed this way." It is possible that oral communication informed many women of tampons and douching techniques. It is, however, the herbal remedies designed to be swallowed as liquids or pills that prevail in the historical record, not these other practices. Some herbs dominate the literature, recurring frequently in popular and professional medical books, in the advertisements of druggists, and in the writings of women. Savin (*Juniperus sabina* L.), juniper or red cedar (*Juniperus virginiana* L.), rue (*Ruta graveolens*), aloes (*Aloe barbadensis*), pennyroyal (*Hedeoma pulegiodes*), madder (*Rubia tinctorum*), and seneca snakeroot (*Polygala senega*) were the most common drugs used, both among the English and Germans. These substances were employed to ensure the onset of the menstrual cycle, to bring a return of menstruation, or to prolong amenorrhea during lactation.[15]

The plant most commonly mentioned in the restoration of menstruation was European savin or the related, chemically identical American species of juniper or red cedar. As early as the seventeenth century, savin, a plant native to the Mediterranean and a known abortive agent since Roman times, was being grown in Pennsylvania. A 1702 description of the colony included notice of "a little tree, which looks like Juniper, and is called the Savan; it has the property of making a mare barren, or bring out her foal before the time. For that purpose you need only give her a handful of it." By 1750, both natu-

---

14. Roberts and Roberts, eds. and trans., *American Journey of Moreau de St. Méry*, 314–315. On women's concern with menstruation, see, in particular, Etienne van de Walle and Elisha P. Renne, eds., *Regulating Menstruation: Beliefs, Practices, Interpretations* (Chicago, 2001); Lucile F. Newman, ed., *Women's Medicine: A Cross-Cultural Study of Indigenous Fertility Regulation* (New Brunswick, N.J., 1985); Mary Chamberlain, *Old Wives' Tales: Their History, Remedies, and Spells* (London, 1981).

15. Greene, ed., *Diary of Colonel Landon Carter*, II, 859, 861.

ralized European savin and the native red cedar were growing in abundance along the banks of the Delaware River and its tributaries. The uses of these related plant species were widely known. Frederika von Riedesel had been in the United States for less than two months in 1777 when she heard something of the abortifacient properties of American cedar. Juniper was sold in various forms at the Philadelphia market at midcentury, and imported and native preparations of juniper—both savin and red cedar—were staples in drugstores and other shops. By the early nineteenth century, savin "was the single most commonly employed folk abortifacient in the United States." Drunk as a tea made from the berries or tips of the stems, it was used to restore menstruation and to prevent impregnation during lactation.[16]

Druggists and physicians sold pills of imported aloes mixed with other ingredients as a treatment for amenorrhea. As a medical student in 1759, William Shippen successfully treated a case of "obstructed menses" with three pills containing aloes, myrrh, sulfate of iron, valeriana, rue, dittany, asafetida, and other items. In the early nineteenth century, the Dispensatory of the United States of America noted of aloes, "It is perhaps more frequently employed than any other remedy, entering into almost all the numerous empirical preparations habitually resorted to by females in that complaint [amenorrhea] and enjoying a no less favorable reputation in regular practice." Barbados aloes were always specified and were available from pharmacists in the form of Hooper's Female Pills, a popular proprietary medicine combining Barbados aloes with iron sulfate, hellebore, and myrrh as the major ingredients and widely advertised in Philadelphia newspapers from the middle of the eighteenth century.[17]

16. Thomas Campanius Holm, *A Short Description of the Province of New Sweden, Now Called, by the English, Pennsylvania, in America*, trans. Peter S. DuPonceau, Historical Society of Pennsylvania, *Memoirs*, III, part 2 (Philadelphia, 1834), 163; Adolph B. Benson, ed., *Peter Kalm's Travels in North America: The English Version of 1770*, 2 vols. (1937; rpt. New York, 1964), II, 635; William P. C. Barton, *Compendium Florae Philadelphicae* . . . (Philadelphia, 1818), 200; Marvin L. Brown, Jr., ed. and trans., *Baroness von Riedesel and the American Revolution: Journal and Correspondence of a Tour of Duty, 1776–1783* (Chapel Hill, N.C., 1965), 49; Gottlieb Mittelberger, *Journey to Pennsylvania*, ed. and trans. Oscar Handlin and John Clive (Cambridge, Mass., 1960), 55; Joseph W. England, ed., *The First Century of the Philadelphia College of Pharmacy, 1821–1921* (Philadelphia, 1922), 110–112; Barton, *Outlines of Lectures*, II, 196; Mohr, *Abortion in America*, 9.

17. Betsy Copping Corner, *William Shippen, Jr.: Pioneer in American Medical Education* (Philadelphia, 1951), 14, 37–38; George B. Wood and Franklin Bache, *The Dispensatory of the United States of America*, 2d ed. (Philadelphia, 1834), 68. See, for example, the advertisement of chemist Christopher Marshall in the *Pennsylvania Gazette* (Philadelphia), Jan. 2, 1749/50. The ingredients in Hooper's Female Pills are four hundred parts Barbados aloes, two hundred parts desiccated iron sulfate, one hundred parts dark hellebore, one hundred parts myrrh, one hundred parts soap, fifty

For women with kitchen gardens, rue, another plant native to the Mediterranean but naturalized first in England and then in North America, and the native American pennyroyal were favored remedies. Rue was used primarily as an emmenagogue and abortifacient, although it was considered an important remedy in rheumatism as well. Francis Daniel Pastorius grew it in his garden in Germantown early in the century and associated it with mothers, time, and age for its ability to regulate the periodicities of life. It was one of the "common herbs for domestic remedies" by midcentury. Among the Pennsylvania Germans it had the additional reputation of being able to "prevent impregnation," a rare reference to contraceptive intent.[18]

The other common garden drug, pennyroyal, was "a popular remedy throughout the country for female complaints. . . . It is chiefly beneficial in obstructed catamenia, and recent cases of suppressions, given as a sweetened tea." According to the United States Dispensatory, pennyroyal is capable of "exciting the menstrual flux when the system is predisposed to the effort. Hence it is much used as an emmenagogue in popular practice and frequently with success." The native American pennyroyal, also called squaw mint both to distinguish it from the unrelated European plant and to indicate its function and origin, was domesticated in gardens and grew wild throughout the region, especially on newly cleared land and at the side of roads.[19]

Seneca snakeroot, or rattlesnake root, was another native American species but was not domesticated. It became a commodity, however, and was gathered in the South and shipped to Philadelphia vendors from the early decades of the eighteenth century. Benjamin Franklin, or, more likely, Deborah Franklin and her mother, sold the newly discovered seneca root from the Philadelphia post office in 1740. It was valued for various medicinal purposes but became closely associated with emmenagogic functions. By the late eighteenth century, consumers were spared the trouble of steeping their own roots when it was sold as Snakeroot Cordial at local pharmacies. Snake-

parts white cinnamon, and fifty parts ground ginger; see Roslyn Stone Wolman, "Some Aspects of Community Health in Colonial Philadelphia" (Ph.D. diss., University of Pennsylvania, 1974), 360.

18. Francis Daniel Pastorius, *Deliciae Hortenses; or, Garden-Recreations and Volumptates Apianae* (1705–1711), ed. Christoph E. Schweitzer (Columbia, S.C., 1982), 16, 28; Israel Acrelius, *A History of New Sweden . . .* (1874), trans. William M. Reynolds, HSP, *Memoirs*, XI (Philadelphia, 1876), 151; David E. Lick and Thomas R. Brendle, "Plant Names and Plant Lore among the Pennsylvania Germans," Pennsylvania-German Society, *Proceedings and Addresses*, XXXIII, part 3 (1923), 62.

19. Rafinesque, *Medical Flora*, I, 233. The author adds that pennyroyal's usefulness in restoring menstruation "is proved by daily experience." See also Wood and Bache, *Dispensatory of the United States*, 365; Benson, ed., *Peter Kalm's Travels*, I, 103, II, 632.

root became an important export item as it entered into foreign pharmaco-poeias. It continued to be considered an important emmenagogue through the first three-quarters of the nineteenth century.[20]

Other emmenagogic medicines appear in the written records. Gum guaia-cum was imported from the Caribbean, madder from Holland. Black helle-bore was "very highly esteemed by some practitioners." There were some ethnic and regional differences in medical practice. Two important plant groups used by the Germans in Pennsylvania were smalledge (wild parsley or wild celery, *Apium graveolens* L.) and various species of the Artemisia family. German women also ingested ragwort (*Seneca aureus*) and called it the life herb for its ability to "correct female irregularities." The Shakers of New Lebanon employed scaly dragon claw (*Pterospora andromedea*) as an emmenagogue. In rural areas, American dittany (*Cunila mariana*), moun-tain tea (*Gautiera ripens*), or winter witch hazel (*Hamamelis virginica*) were among the drugs used. One of the few plants listed solely as a contraceptive was wild ginger (*Asarum canadense*). It was used "by the Indian females to prevent impregnation." Some in the German community thought that wild ginger was not only a contraceptive but also an aphrodisiac. This dan-gerous combination of attributes earned it the name "thing of evil" in rural Schwenksville, Pennsylvania. This list of plants thought to have emmena-gogic properties is not exhaustive but gives some indication of the range of plants in use. There was no shortage of drugs designed to restore menstrua-tion.[21]

The herbal remedies that dominated the emmenagogic and abortive lit-

20. Snakeroot "is highly extolled by many practitioners in the treatment of amenorrhoea" (John B. Biddle, *Materia Medica, for the Use of Students,* 4th ed. [Philadelphia, 1871], 257). In 1740, snakeroot was sold from the post office "with Directions how to use it in the Pleurisy, etc." The "etc." could cover the indelicate topic of emmenagogues and was a euphemism for menses in German. By 1789, no directions were needed for the cordial. See *Pa. Gaz.,* June 12, 1740, Feb. 1, 1789 (adver-tisement of Seth and Isaac Willis); Wells, "Small Herbal," 468; England, *College of Pharmacy,* 110. In 1791–1792, fifty-three hundred pounds of snakeroot were exported from Philadelphia, 40 percent of the country's annual exports of this product; see Tench Coxe, *A View of the United States of America . . .* (Philadelphia, 1794), 414.

21. Wood and Bache, *Dispensatory of the United States,* 345; Wells, "Small Herbal," 461–469; Lick and Brendle, "Plants and Plant Lore," Pa.-German Soc., Procs., XXXIII, part 3 (1923), 62, 157. Ragwort is also called the life root, the female regulator, or squaw-weed. See Joseph E. Meyer, *The Herbalist,* ed. Clarence Meyer and David C. Meyer (Glenwood, Ill., 1981), 119; Rafinesque, *Medical Flora,* I, 139, 165, 204, 230, II, 69; Frederick Pursh, *Flora Americae septentrionalis . . . ,* ed. Joseph Ewan (1814; rpt. Hirschberg, Germany, 1979), 596; Liese M. Perrin, "Resisting Reproduction: Recon-sidering Slave Contraception in the Old South," *Journal of American Studies,* XXXV, no. 2 (2001), 255–274.

erature are often portrayed as part of a traditional and largely static body of knowledge rooted in folklore and in medical authorities that dated back to the classical Greeks. Even if it is true that these treatments had changed little in Europe, the attempt to transport European medical practices to America brought change and encouraged experimentation. Some established remedies were carried over from the Old World: rosemary, rue, and savin, among others. The European plants most successfully naturalized and domesticated in British North America were plants that had first been naturalized in England and Germany, often from the Mediterranean region. Women also duplicated Old World remedies by seeking closely related American species that they called by familiar names: dittany, madder, and savin. African women labeled several species of plants as snakeroot and were familiar with cotton-root. The botanists of the late eighteenth century and early nineteenth century got much of their information on local flora from women who had explored, identified, and experimented with a wide variety of plant species.[22]

There seems to have been some selectivity in the transit of herbal medicine, since not all common English remedies were transported to the New World. Ergot of rye, for example, seems not to have been adopted as a drug in Pennsylvania. English pennyroyal failed to find advocates, since American pennyroyal, a plant with somewhat similar "shape, smell and properties" was found to be "more efficient" as an emmenagogue. On the other hand, imported savin was preferred over locally available savin or juniper, in part because it was "scarce, and dear," but largely because it was believed to be a stronger medicine.[23]

Cross-cultural borrowing can be seen in the interest in native American emmenagogues and related plants. Squawbush (*Vibirnum opulus*, also known as cramp bark), squaw mint (*Hedeoma pulegioides*, also known as pennyroyal), squawroot (*Cimicifuga racemosa* or *Caulophyllum thalictroides*), squaw vine (*Michella repens*, a native relative of madder), and squaw-weed (*Erigon philadelphicum*, also known as fleabane) were among the plants

22. "African Slaves in the United States and Birth Control," in Vern L. Bullough, ed., *Encyclopedia of Birth Control* (Santa Barbara, Calif., 2001), 11–12; Martia Graham Goodson, "Medical-Botanical Contributions of African Slave Women to American Medicine," in Darlene Clark Hine, ed., *Black Women in American History: From Colonial Times through the Nineteenth Century* (New York, 1990), 473–484; William J. Simon, "A Luso-African Formulary of the Late Eighteenth Century," *Pharmacy in History*, XVIII (1976), 114; George Way Harley, *Native African Medicine: With Special Reference to Its Practice in the Mano Tribe of Liberia* (London, 1970), 61–62, 215–216, 224.

23. Rafinesque, *Medical Flora*, I, 232; Barton, *Outlines of Lectures*, II, 196.

borrowed from or attributed to the medical knowledge of native American women. One native plant—pennyroyal—was domesticated in the eighteenth century, and both black and seneca snakeroot were prepared commercially. The process of investigation and experimentation was not one-sided. European plants, including rosemary and rue, were adopted by some American and African American women. Turpentine, chemically similar to some preparations of savin, was common in African American communities in the nineteenth and twentieth centuries.[24]

Investigation of new sources was encouraged because there were as yet no distinct lines between folk and professional medical practices. Women's medicinal recipes for household use were as likely to be copied from medical books as they were to be handed down orally. Oral tradition did not necessarily differ from professional medical advice. Neither women nor doctors were strongly bound by traditions in this period. Elizabeth Coates Paschall, a Philadelphia shopkeeper, proudly recorded many medical recipes as "my own Invention" and discussed the efficacy and safety of drugs with a wide range of people, including doctors, botanists, apothecaries, midwives, relatives, friends, servants, and customers, in her effort to discover the best cures. Doctors and medical botanists asked questions of women practitioners and sometimes adopted their advice. Although emmenagogic usage contained some traditional aspects in the New World, contact with native American and African medicine, a changed environment, and a fascination with new remedies encouraged experimentation.[25]

24. Meyer, *The Herbalist*, ed. Meyer and Meyer, 18, 21, 33, 92, 119; Rafinesque, *Medical Flora*, I, 88, 99, 162–165, 234; Perrin, "Resisting Reproduction," *Journal of American Studies*, XXXV, no. 2 (2001), 260. Squaw-weed and squawroot were adopted in England by the mid-nineteenth century, at a time when herbal abortifacients or emmenagogues are usually considered to have been abandoned. See Malcolm Stuart, ed., *The Encyclopedia of Herbs and Herbalism* (London, 1979), 262, 274; Virgil J. Vogel, *American Indian Medicine* (Norman, Okla., 1970), 243–244; Gladys Tantaquidgeon, *A Study of Delaware Indian Medicine Practice and Folk Belief* (Harrisburg, Pa., 1942); William N. Fenton, "Contacts between Iroquois Herbalism and Colonial Medicine," in Smithsonian Institution, *Annual Report of the Board of Regents, 1941* (Washington, D.C., 1942), 503–527; Goodson, "Medical Botanical Contributions," in Hine, ed., *Black Women*, 473–484.

25. Elizabeth Coates (Mrs. Joseph) Paschall, Receipt Book, circa 1749–1766, photocopy, College of Physicians of Philadelphia; Ellen G. Gartrell, "Women Healers and Domestic Remedies in Eighteenth-Century America: The Recipe Book of Elizabeth Coates Paschall," *New York Journal of Medicine*, LXXXI, no. 1 (January 1987), 23–29. Oral tradition was not confined to women's chatting over the garden gate. After abortion was made illegal in Pennsylvania, Dr. Joseph Carson's printed lecture outline on the drug savin warned of its "criminal use." One student's notes, scribbled into his textbook, reveal, however, that it was "one of the most powerful agents of abortion" and then proceeded to record other specific abortion techniques. What was said in class could obviously not be published. See Joseph Carson, *Synopsis of the Course of Lectures on Materia Medica and*

Experimentation did not diffuse all forms of medicine equally. English and urban practices came to dominate over German and rural medicine. With only a few exceptions, the experiments of rural women were not incorporated into urban pharmacologies as they were codified in the early decades of the nineteenth century. Neither the explicit language nor the drugs specific to German practice seem to have had any direct effect on English writings. African and native American remedies were generally secondary to other drugs. After the turn of the nineteenth century, few new plant species were added to the lists of accepted drugs. The period of experimentation had come to an end.[26]

Starting in the middle of the eighteenth century, domestic emmenagogues based on herbs gathered from gardens and fields were gradually supplanted by commercial preparations. These were imported from England or made by local pharmacists and physicians. Emmenagogic drugs were an important part of a flourishing international pharmaceutical industry. Proprietary medicines and standardized preparations like Hooper's Female Pills, Hungary Water (an infusion of rosemary), and Dr Ryan's Worm-destroying Sugar Plumbs ("highly serviceable to the Female Sex") were advertised in local newspapers. Bulk drugs, including savin, madder, guaiacum, and other emmenagogues, were imported from various parts of the globe. Preparations of herbs—gums, infusions, essences, tonics, waters, cordials—could be purchased from pharmacists, physicians, or druggists. Medical chests containing an assortment of simple herbs, patent medicines, and prepared drugs were regularly advertised for sale by doctors and pharmacists for rural families with no access to apothecaries. These chests included emmenagogues. Commercialization began standardizing and publicizing prepared emmenagogic medicines even in remote rural areas by the turn of the nineteenth century.[27]

Pharmacy . . . , 3d ed. (Philadelphia, 1863), 181 (copy at Van Pelt Library, University of Pennsylvania, Philadelphia).

26. Renate Wilson argues for a "specifically German medical culture and market in eighteenth-century North America," albeit one that "drew on and perpetuated similar traditions of knowledge" that were familiar to English practice. See Renate Wilson, *Pious Traders in Medicine: A German Pharmaceutical Network in Eighteenth-Century North America* (University Park, Pa., 2000), 6–7.

27. An error-ridden compilation of the ingredients in commercial emmenagogic medicines can be found in "A Collection of Medicinal Preparations by Saml Fahnestock M D; Together with the Virtues and Dosis, York Town, Pennsylvania, June 22d 1798," College of Physicians of Philadelphia. Fahnestock was almost exclusively interested in emmenagogic drugs. Suppressed menses was the most common complaint of Chester County women seeking professional medical advice in the early nineteenth century. See Joan M. Jensen, *Loosening the Bonds: Mid-Atlantic Farm Women, 1750–1850* (New Haven, Conn., 1986), 33; S. Stander, "Transatlantic Trade in Pharmaceuticals during

The Regulation of Fertility: Results

The herbal remedies most commonly mentioned in eighteenth-century sources are still classified as emmenagogues, contraceptives, and abortifacients in some national dispensatories, particularly in Asia and Africa. Even in the United States, many of these drugs continued to be listed into the 1950s, albeit as "no longer official" or "abandoned," having been dismissed by the medical profession as either ineffectual or dangerously toxic. Laboratory tests, however, have shown that, for example, aloes, mints, and rue produce antifertility effects in rats and mice by acting on the smooth muscles of the uterus or by disrupting ovulation. Although hellebore is a dangerously toxic substance, most herbs are not. Yet the effects of fresh or dried herbs cannot be uniform. The active ingredients can vary based on the size or freshness of the plant, growing conditions, or methods of preparation. So it was that herbal remedies were rarely simple, and lay and professional practitioners often combined multiple ingredients and added vigorous exercise, "baths," and other techniques to their cures.[28]

The success of aggressive medical treatment can be seen in Elizabeth Coates Paschall's recollection, in about 1750, of an event that must have taken place in the 1720s or 1730s—a very rare firsthand account of an induced abortion. "I once was verry Bad with a violent pain in my Back and Bowells and three months Gone with Child," she wrote in her book of medical recipes. Three months gestation was before quickening. She decided that the pregnancy was the cause of her colic, as she called her condition, but on her own efforts she "Could not be Delivered." She then sought professional advice: "It was Judged Both By the Doctor and midwife that if I was not Speedily Delivered I Should Dye." The male doctor confirmed her diagnosis but played no other role. "The midwife tried to Deliver me butt found it Impossible." With the failure of professional help, Paschall turned to another

---

the Industrial Revolution," *Bulletin of the History of Medicine*, XLIII (1969), 326–343; Harold B. Gill, Jr., *The Apothecary in Colonial Virginia* (Charlottesville, Va., 1972). Quaker influence in the trade is noted in Roy Porter and Dorothy Porter, "The Rise of the English Drug Industry: The Role of Thomas Corbyn," *Medical History*, XXXIII (1989), 277–295; see also Robert A. Buerki, "Caleb Taylor, Philadelphia Druggist, 1812–1820," *Pharmacy in History*, XXX (1988), 81–88; advertisement of Nicholas Brooks in *Pa. Gaz.*, May 24, 1780 (quotation).

28. Arthur Osol et al., *Dispensatory of the United States of America*, 25th ed. (Philadelphia, 1955), seems to have been the last year when these herbs were listed. See James A. Duke, *Handbook of Medicinal Herbs* (Boca Raton, Fla., 1985), 517–522; Norman S. Farnsworth et al., "Potential Value of Plants as Sources of New Antifertility Agents," *Journal of Pharmaceutical Sciences*, LXIV (1975), 535–598.

source of expertise: the authority of an aged woman. "An Elderly woman proposed Giving me a Glister [enema]" containing chamomile (an emmenagogue) and other ingredients. This remedy worked. "I took it and Lay Still Near an hour after it: Being presently Eased and the Child Came from me in the after Birth all together and with verry Little pain." In Paschall's case, the intensive use of a variety of methods eventually succeeded. Abortion was not used for family planning but was necessary in order to cure "a violent Chollick Pain." She later used the same recipe to treat a "Could" and "Racking Torture" in "Every Single Joynt of my Back," also successfully. Her account, given as advice to her daughter, indicates the overlap between rheumatism, colds, and emmenagogues and also provides evidence of the interplay between professional and lay healers in the eighteenth century.[29]

Elizabeth Coates Paschall's intentions are fairly clear; Molly Drinker Rhoads's case is ambiguous. Drinker Rhoads was under investigation by her local Quaker meeting for her irregular marriage, was temporarily estranged from her father, and was without a home of her own. Only her mother's "*discourse* with the Doctor relative to Molly" revealed the pregnancy, and Elizabeth Drinker worried that her daughter was "very careless of herself which makes me much the more uneasy." Drinker Rhoads complained of colds in her third and fourth months of pregnancy. Her mother recorded that "she looked very pale and was in great pain in her bowels, she has been disorder'd and in pain for a long time past at times, oweing to taking colds—I gave her mint water etc." Peppermint and magnesia were the ingredients in mint water, given for intestinal complaints accompanied by "morbid depression." Mint water was also an emmenagogue. The hysteric symptoms reappeared two months later: "She then burst into tears and inform'd us how ill she had been most of the night—with pain, disorder'd bowels and a fluttering etc. and at times fainty—she took mint water and lavender compound, became rather easier towards morning—she was very much terrified." Lavender compound contained lavender and rosemary, both emmenagogues as well as cures for nervous complaints, plus alcohol and red dye (the red coloring might have been thought to encourage menstruation through sympa-

29. Paschall, Receipt Book, circa 1749–1766, College of Physicians of Philadelphia, 9. Contemporary medical texts defined clysters (glisters, enemas) as the anal insertion of liquids, but perhaps vaginal or uterine administration was practiced in this case and others. Coates Paschall was married for twenty-one years (1721–1742). She had nine children, only three of whom survived past infancy—the birthdates of these three are marked here with an asterisk (1723, 1726, 1727, 1728,* 1731, 1732,* 1735, 1738, 1740*); see "Extracted from the Paschall Family Bible by Isaac P. Morris, 11 month 9 [day] 1842," Paschall/Morris Bible Records, Genealogical Society of Pennsylvania.

thetic magic). At six months gestation, which should have been well past the point of quickening, a fluttering in the bowels was not identified with fetal movement by either mother or daughter. In the next month, however, preparations were under way for the expected delivery, which occurred two months later. The full-term fetus was stillborn. For the greatest part of this pregnancy, Molly Rhoads hesitantly treated her symptoms as an illness. Her condition was labeled a "cold" and medicated as if it were hysteria through the first six months. She did not, as she was expected to do, reduce her labor or watch her diet. She seems to have been as ambivalent about her pregnancy as she was tentative in coping with her physical and emotional symptoms.[30]

Enslaved women also sought to terminate pregnancies. We have no evidence directly from the women themselves, but slaveowners assumed their bondwomen's abortive intentions rather than casting these episodes in the more respectable and obscurantist category of health problems requiring emmenagogues. In September 1826, a New Jersey slaveowner recorded that during the previous night his slave, Peg, then three months pregnant, cried out that she "would die for ad[ministering a] dose of Copperine [perhaps either copperas, also called vitriol, ferri sulphas, or copper sulfate, an ancient abortifacient] etc. [which] Jo had Provided for her to Produce abortion. It Came near killing her." Some of the circumstances surrounding Peg's decision can be pieced together from her master's scattered, laconic comments. The previous April, Peg had borne a child, unnamed by the diarist. It had died in early July, when she must have been four to six weeks pregnant. It is possible that her second pregnancy had left her unable to nurse her firstborn, causing its death. Perhaps she resented the pregnancy; perhaps she was exhausted by two pregnancies within eleven months; perhaps she had been raped. Joe and Peg were described by their master as cooperatively "working Exsperiments to Produce abortion." Their master did not think that they were trying to preserve either her physical or emotional health, but Peg and Joe's own framing of the incident is unknown. Their experiments may also be an indication that they either did not know of traditional methods—I know of no other cases of the ingestion of vitriol, if that was in fact the substance used—or that Peg and Joe did not have access to more typical drugs. Their attempt to curtail the pregnancy failed, and Peg bore a son on April 11, 1827. The candor of this description and the absence of any comment other

30. Biddle, *Materia Medica*, 164, 180; Farnsworth et al., "Potential Value of Plants," *Journal of Pharmaceutical Sciences*, LXIV (1975), table 3, 550; Carson, *Synopsis of the Course of Lectures on Materia Medica* (1863), 180; Elaine Forman Crane et al., eds., *The Diary of Elizabeth Drinker*, 3 vols. (Boston, 1991), II, 873–874, 878, 897, 900, 904–932.

than the diarist's irritation at the disruptions to his family and the necessity of a doctor's visit confirm what we know about the slave system more generally: masters were concerned primarily about cost and convenience, not about morality.[31]

By the end of the eighteenth century, urban growth meant fewer Philadelphia women had access to kitchen gardens. The Philadelphia Dispensary, a charitable medical institution, provided outpatient services to the worthy poor who were either too sick to attend to themselves or too poor to afford private physicians. In the first six years of operation, from December 1786 to November 1792, the Dispensary treated eighty-two women for amenorrhea and cured 80 percent while relieving another 5 percent (Table 4). More patients were treated for four diseases in which amenorrhea was one of several symptoms: chlorosis (iron deficiency anemia associated with puberty); haematemesis (bloody vomiting associated with irregular menses—it was believed that the menstrual blood was diverted upward); hypochondria (a nervous disorder); and, overwhelmingly, hysteria (another nervous disorder, this one long associated with the uterus). In these four "diseases," 70 percent of cases were cured, but, of these patients with multiple physical and emotional symptoms, one in four was only relieved of her symptoms. These rates are substantially lower than those found in related disease categories as well as below the overall cure rates of 81 percent claimed at the Dispensary. Hysteria and hypochondria, the diseases associated with strong emotional symptoms as well as with amenorrhea, were particularly resistant to treatment and may indicate why some physicians were becoming critical of emmenagogues. The cure rate for amenorrhea alone, however, was much higher and virtually identical to the average cure rate for all diseases. The reason for these differences is unclear. It may indicate that emmenagogic drugs were specific to the condition of amenorrhea after all but unable to affect tangential or complex emotional complaints, or it may be that many of these patients' menses were only temporarily delayed and that they were "cured" by the passage of time and their underlying good health. The other patients might have had more serious conditions.[32]

31. Goodson, "Medical-Botanical Contributions of African Women to American Medicine," in Hine, ed., *Black Women*, 5; Stephen Vail, "Diaries," Sept. 9–10, 1826, Historic Speedwell, Morristown, N.J. Peg was manumitted in 1834. Copies of diary entries relating to "Peg" were provided by Dorothy Truman, research associate, Historic Speedwell. The diaries are the property of Historic Speedwell and are used by permission. My thanks to members of the staff in tracking down this information.

32. The records of the Philadelphia Dispensary allow a direct approach to the efficacy of contemporary medicine. From December 1786 through November 1792, a committee tabulated patient out-

TABLE 4.
Records of the Philadelphia Dispensary, 1786–1792

Disease	Cured	Dead	Relieved of Symptoms	Discharged, Disorderly	Remanded Elsewhere	Remaining under Care	Total
DISEASES ASSOCIATED WITH AMENORRHEA AND WITH WOMEN							
Amenorrhea	66	0	4	4	2	6	82
Chlorosis	1	0	0	0	0	0	1
Haematemesis	9	1	0	1	0	0	11
Hypochondria	14	0	10	2	0	0	26
Hysteria	174	0	59	1	0	12	246
Total (%)	72.2	0.3	19.9	2.2	0.5	4.9	100.0
DISEASES CONFUSED WITH AMENORRHEA APPEARING IN WOMEN AND MEN							
Dropsy	9	14	5	0	2	9	39
Rheumatism	428	2	107	6	7	35	585
Worms	219	3	1	1	0	7	231
Total (%)	76.7	2.2	13.2	0.8	1.1	6.0	100.0
OTHER DISEASES AND CONDITIONS OF WOMEN							
Abortion	8	0	0	0	0	1	9
Leucorrhea	27	0	5	1	1	4	38
Menorrhagia	43	0	1	0	0	0	44
Parturition	81	0	0	0	0	2	83
Prolapsed uterus	9	0	7	0	0	3	19
Puerperal fever	15	0	0	0	0	0	15
Swollen breasts	1	0	0	0	0	0	1
Total (%)	88.0	0.0	6.2	0.5	0.5	4.8	100.0
VENEREAL DISEASE							
Gonorrhea	145	0	1	3	0	5	154
Syphilis	499	6	25	32	13	82	657
Total (%)	79.4	0.8	3.2	4.3	1.6	10.7	100.0
ALL DISEASES TREATED AT THE DISPENSARY							
Total all diseases	7,915	439	614	151	77	521	9,719
Total (%)	81.4	4.5	6.3	1.6	0.8	5.4	100.0

Note: Patients were remanded either to Pennsylvania Hospital or to the House of Employment.

Source: Samuel P. Griffitts et al., "To the President and College of Physicians of Philadelphia [Tables of Diseases from December 1786 to December 1792]," College of Physicians of Philadelphia, Transactions, I, part 1 (Philadelphia, 1793).

Dropsy, rheumatism, and worms were all linked to amenorrhea by swollen abdomens and congested bodily fluids and so were treated with the same medications, but these diseases could appear among men as well as women. Of these cases, 76 percent were cured and 13 percent relieved. The figures give one indication why women avoided a diagnosis of dropsy in cases of amenorrhea—only 23 percent of those cases were recorded as cured, and 39 percent of patients died.

The venereal diseases, also affecting both men and women, had cure rates nearing the Dispensary's mean despite the difficulties of dealing with syphilis and the serious side effects of the mercuric substances most often prescribed for the disease. A portion of the clientele admitted for venereal disease proved unusually rambunctious, perhaps because officials discovered that these patients were prostitutes or otherwise ne'er-do-wells, rather than worthy, honest poor folk. More than one in twenty venereal cases were dismissed or transferred out by dispensary physicians, and about twice as many as the average for the institution were held for additional treatment.

The dispensary's record on other diseases and conditions of women—childbirth, uterine disease, and complaints involving the breasts—is particularly impressive, with reported cure rates approaching 90 percent and no deaths occurring even in the face of the contemporary dangers in childbirth, puerperal fever, menorrhagia, and uterine dysfunction. The gap between the experiences of women with these gynecological problems and those with amenorrhea alone is 8 percentage points. For those with hysteria, the gap is considerable—28 percentage points. Yet a reported success rate of even 80 percent in cases of amenorrhea and 60 percent in related diseases in the eighteenth century seems remarkable. How did doctors treat these diseases? Another source from the same city offers some clues.

The full billing records of partners Dr. Phineas Bond and Dr. Thomas Bond of Philadelphia give some indication of the course of treatment for women with amenorrhea. When called upon to treat Richard Edward's wife on October 17, 1753, the attending physician gave her pills for pain relief.

---

comes by disease. Annual totals were provided for the number who were cured, who died, who were relieved of their symptoms but not cured, who were held for additional treatment as well as those who were dismissed for disorderly behavior or were sent to Pennsylvania Hospital (a charity for the working poor) or the House of Employment (the local almshouse). These tabulations lack data on age, sex, and detailed diagnoses—categories that would now seem essential for analysis—and do not indicate the treatment supplied, but this record does permit a more direct measure of success and failure than other contemporary sources. See Samuel P. Griffitts et al., "To the President and College of Physicians of Philadelphia, a Return of the Diseases of the Patients of the Philadelphia Dispensary," College of Physicians of Philadelphia, *Transactions*, I, part 1 (Philadelphia, 1793).

The records show that he returned four days later to prescribe a liquid pain reliever, four emmenagogic pills, and then another pain reliever. Ludowic Cosser's wife had a similar course of treatment in 1755, although the doctor added a dose of four "Hyst[eric] Pills" of unknown composition. Thomas Bottom's wife appears to have had an adverse reaction to these emmenagogic treatments; she was subsequently treated with cordials for strength, styptics to stop bleeding, and Tincture Martis, a salt of iron used in cases of anemia. During the early fall of 1753, the doctor treated shopkeeper Robert Taigart's wife with Glauber's salts, which was a purgative and diuretic. Ten days later, she was given a drug to induce vomiting, the following day a refrigerant powder (which was an antipyretic used to reduce fevers), and five days later emmenagogic pills. In March and April 1754, she was treated with liniments, mercuric pills, and styptics, probably indicative of syphilis, but she also received two doses of emmenagogic pills during this latter period. In all these cases, treatment for hysteria or other illnesses preceded emmenagogic treatment. Amenorrhea was not treated as an isolated symptom. James White's wife was the only one given emmenagogues after her delivery, a difficult one. In this case, its likely use was to dislodge the placenta because emmenagogues were thought to remove various obstructions. Respectably married women with symptoms of emotional and physical distress account for the overwhelming majority of cases in the Bond casebooks—they were 67 percent of the twenty-four clients receiving emmenagogues, despite the claims by some historians that such activities were "the last resort of a particular segment of the unmarried: seduced, abandoned, and helpless women."[33]

But not all women treated by the doctors were married. The widow Robinson was given two rounds of emmenagogues in March and April 1752 as well as two mercuric pills. Because she traveled some twenty miles from her residence in the small town of Chester, Pennsylvania, to Philadelphia for treatment, there might have been some attempt at secrecy on her part, but no apparent reluctance on the part of the doctor. Another widow was from New Castle, Delaware. In all, three patients receiving emmenagogues were widows, another was an unmarried woman apparently living on her own (although a man paid her medical bill), and three were the daughters, nieces, or other relatives of a male head of household. Israel Pemberton's ward, Polly

33. Thomas and Phineas Bond Co-Partnership Ledgers, I–IV, College of Physicians of Philadelphia. These ledgers survive for 1751–1753, 1754–1755, 1756–1759, and 1764–1766. They are billing records, listing charges for attendance and medicines dispensed but not symptoms or disease categories. See also Marvin Olasky, *Abortion Rites: A Social History of Abortion in America* (Wheaton, Ill., 1992), 40.

Jordan, had a fever in October 1757 and was treated with emmenagogues as well as other medications. She was sick again the following July, when she was given two large doses of emmenagogues. An acquaintance described her "sickly mein" but erased some other comment about Jordan's health. Polly Jordan died late the following year of unknown causes. Just as puzzling is the case of an unnamed "N[egro] woman," undoubtedly a slave. During a doctor's visit to Mr. John Wallace in 1759, she received liniment, a bleeding, a cathartic, and then an emetic to induce vomiting. The following day, she was given a combination of emmenagogues and twenty pills for hysteria. Did she request this treatment, or was it was forced upon her? The records do not say. A servant's productivity would be reduced by pregnancy, and a pregnant slave could not be fired. The dosages this unnamed woman received for hysteria were unusually large, as was the final cost of £7 9s. 6d., nearly a third of the average price of an adult slave.[34]

Statistics indicate that eighteenth-century birthrates, particularly annual crude birthrates, were variable, not constant (see Appendix). If anxiety, grief, and distress were signs of pathology in married women, the birthrates should have been in decline during wars. J. P. Brissot de Warville thought that fewer births in wartime Philadelphia "was natural." But what is natural? Abigail Adams had politely shifted blame for infertility from women to the environment when she wrote about the city's "unfertile soil." Less circumspect was the Reverend Andreas Sandel, who, during a rumor of war that was designed to frighten Quakers in 1706, noted that "many women who were in delicate situations miscarried in consequence of their fright." The number of births recorded in the Friends meeting records dropped from twenty-six to four between 1705 and 1706. It is unlikely that simultaneous miscarriages could have accounted for the difference, since fear is not, in the twenty-first century, considered a cause of spontaneous miscarriage. Dr. Benjamin Rush found that "in 1783, the year of the peace, there were several children born of parents who had lived many years together without issue," even though he thought wartime rates were high "among the laboring part of the people." Emmenagogues should have been used more often in wartime if some women were deliberately curtailing fertility. There are no detailed medical records from the Revolutionary War. The Bond casebooks do give some indication of wartime practices during the Seven Years' War, although, because

34. Bond Ledgers, I, 210, III, 64, 94; Susan E. Klepp and Karin A. Wulf, eds., *The Diary of Hannah Callender: Sense and Sensibility in a Revolutionary Age, 1758–1788* (Ithaca, N.Y., 2009), July 1758, October 1759.

TABLE 5.

Drs. Thomas and Phineas Bond, Emmenagogic Prescriptions, 1751–1766

Years	No. of Active Clients	% Receiving Emmenagogues	Price per Dose	Price per Client
			Shillings/Pence	
1751–1753	149	4.0	5/10	7/10
1754–1755	173	2.3	6/0	7/6
1756–1759	198	7.0	6/1	8/3
1764–1766	190	1.0	4/9	4/9

Note: In 1756–1759, the emmenagogic dose was repeated for 35.7 percent of patients. In contrast, the total proportion of repeated doses in the pre- and postwar periods was 25 percent. The number of clients is the number of financially responsible individuals, not the number of patients. It is not always clear to whom these treatments were given: wives, daughters or other kin, or servants.

Source: Thomas and Phineas Bond Co-Partnership Ledgers, I–IV (1751–1753, 1754–1755, 1756–1759, 1764–1766), College of Physicians of Philadelphia. Records for 1760–1763 do not survive.

emmenagogues were also readily available from gardeners, pharmacists, and others, they cannot measure total demand for these items (Table 5).[35]

In peacetime, between 1 and 4 percent of the doctors' active clients were charged for emmenagogues. During the peak years of the Seven Years' War in North America, 1756–1759, this proportion jumped to 7 percent. Patients were also taking more medicine, with multiple doses rising from 25 percent of cases of emmenagogic use to 35 percent. Not surprisingly, the cost escalated as well. Before 1756 and after 1764, the average client cost for emmenagogues was 7s. 2d. Between 1756 and 1759, it was 8s. 3d. The immediate postwar period brought the lowest incidence of emmenagogic use perhaps because couples sought to compensate for the fewer births that occurred

35. J. P. Brissot de Warville, New Travels in the United States of America (1788), ed. Durand Echeverria, trans. Mara Soceanu Vamos and Durand Echeverria (Cambridge, Mass., 1964), 293; Charles Francis Adams, ed., Familiar Letters of John Adams and His Wife Abigail Adams, during the Revolution, with a Memoir of Mrs. Adams (New York, 1876), 129; Andreas Sandel, quoted in Andrew Rudman, "Transactions Relative to the Congregation at Wicacoa," 5, microfilm, Gloria Dei Lutheran Church Records, Genealogical Society of Pennsylvania; Benjamin Rush, "An Account of the Influence of the American Revolution on the Human Body" (1788), in Dagobert D. Runes, ed., The Selected Writings of Benjamin Rush (New York, 1947), 330–331; Sam Shapiro et al., Infant, Perinatal, Maternal, and Childhood Mortality in the United States (Cambridge, Mass., 1968), 47–77. Births are calculated from the records of the Philadelphia Monthly Meeting of Friends, Genealogical Society of Pennsylvania.

during the height of the war. These patients undoubtedly represent only a portion of the population — many Philadelphians could not afford doctors — and the changing demand for emmenagogues does not match changes in the crude birthrate for the city as a whole (see Appendix). For poorer Philadelphians, the war is credited with bringing full employment and opportunities to marry.

WOMEN'S CHILDBEARING EXPERIENCES reflected their circumstances. War, economic stress, or personal difficulties could produce anxiety. Anxiety was a sign of ill health that required medical treatment. When widespread, anxieties sometimes had dampening effects on the birthrate, even with medicinal failure rates in the range of 20 to 30 percent. Still, the reputation of these drugs as life threatening seems exaggerated, at least according to the records of the Philadelphia Dispensary. It would seem that eighteenth-century women were not entirely at the mercy of their biological nature, that they were not always beguiled by magical, dangerous, or ineffectual folk practice, but that they had some real influence over their fertility and could adjust childbearing in response to changes in their situations — reducing or attempting to reduce fertility during wars but less often turning to emmenagogues in peacetime.

The emmenagogic techniques in use in the eighteenth-century colonies allowed women to exercise some control over reproduction and also allowed both men and women to avoid, in reading, in writing, and in public and private conversations, any reference to indelicate topics. It should not, however, be seen as a golden age of women's power over reproduction. The failure rates were high, the methods painful, and the acceptable reasons for married women's employing emmenagogues were limited to conditions of emotional and physical ill health. These justifications for attempting to restore menstruation would need to be reexamined every month and weighed at the beginning of each pregnancy. Hysteria could be invoked by women in times of personal, political, or financial crisis in order to delay childbearing, but at a cost of succumbing to irrationality, overwhelming fear, and emotional excess — the very characteristics that were used to define women as inferior human beings, unfit for independence in marriage or in society. Other diseases like suppressed menses and the resulting colds, rheumatism, and pleurisy labeled women as physically weak and sickly by their very nature. In addition, notions of shame and propriety restricted access to such information as was available and could obscure appropriate procedures. Restriction of fertility as practiced in the eighteenth century allowed women limited control over their childbearing careers but, rather than liberating women, only helped confirm their separate and unequal status.[36]

The Emergence of Family Planning, Contraception, and Abortion

The emmenagogic techniques were most effective in lengthening the intervals between births; their primary use by married women during the eighteenth century was, insofar as can be determined, to allow health and well-being to return. Reducing family size was of little apparent interest to most women, since fertility rates tended to rebound once a crisis in health, security, or finances had passed. When, at the end of the eighteenth century, first women and then men began to express an interest in family planning, in limiting the number of children, or stopping childbearing after a predetermined number of children had been born, new techniques were tried.

Abstinence emerges for the first time as a part of marriage, although perhaps not as a common solution. In the 1790s, a Shaker accused Quakers of "gratify[ing] yourselves with your wives when they are not in a capacity of conception." This was, he argued, "fornication, as it is not for multiplying." The Quaker did not deny the practice, although he was troubled by the accusation. Elizabeth Willing Powel was exasperated with her pregnant sister. "What ails you all[?] why don't you exercise female Taste and love of veriety and fall on the Platonic system[?] you have really children enough in all reason." Although the recommendation of Platonic relations suggests celibacy, a "love of veriety" perhaps implies anal, oral, or other nonreproductive forms of sexuality. Powel might well have given detailed advice, but the next page of the letter is missing.[37]

Prolonged breast-feeding accompanied by abstinence seems to have proved a source of marital conflict. Alexander Hamilton was impatient with his wife's plan: "I shall be glad," he wrote to Eliza Hamilton on planning a

---

36. For a discussion of the character of women, see Vivian Jones, ed., *Women in the Eighteenth Century: Constructions of Femininity* (London, 1990). For a later period, see Carroll Smith-Rosenberg, "The Hysterical Woman: Sex Roles and Role Conflict in Nineteenth-Century America," in Smith-Rosenberg, *Disorderly Conduct: Visions of Gender in Victorian America* (New York, 1985), 197–216.

37. Joshua Evans Diary, 1794–1796, quoted in David Hackett Fischer, *Albion's Seed: Four British Folkways in America* (New York, 1989), 500; E. Willing to Mrs. Byrd, postscript, Aug. 15, 1768, Elizabeth Willing Powel Personal Papers, Outgoing Correspondence, 1763–1814, box 1, folder 1, Powel Family Papers #1582, HSP. My thanks to Niki Eustace for sending this addendum to the letter of Aug. 10, 1768.

trip home in 1802, "to find that my dear little Philip is weaned, if circumstances have rendered it prudent. It is of importance to me to rest quietly in your bosom." In the Hamilton household, sexual desire and prudence, a code word for family planning, were in conflict. Esther Bowes Sayre Atlee's husband had stayed away from home for months in 1788 but planned a short trip back to be with his wife. She promised to leave "our troublesome little folks" with friends but reminded her husband that "our little Het [aged eight months] must go where I go, as the leaving her behind might be a means of more trouble." Breast-feeding was unreliable, and separation was an awkward solution. Esther Atlee worried about local gossip concerning her husband's lengthy absence in 1778. Did neighbors think her an undutiful wife, failing to attend to her husband and driving him off? Had he unmanfully abandoned his family? She hoped his trip home would "show the world that I am not neglected by my husband." He, in turn, worried about his male acquaintances visiting her in his house in his absence, even though these colleagues were welcomed because they brought her news of him. He was firm: "I don't wish to see my home too much the resort of these gentlemen." His home and its occupants should remain under his control even in his absence. Esther Atlee and her husband were combining physical separation and prolonged breast-feeding in order to delay pregnancy. Still, she gave birth in 1780 to her ninth child, managing to achieve no more than a twenty-four-month interval between births. She wrote later, pregnant with her tenth child, "I cannot Account for a glooming which too frequently comes over me," but immediately added, "If I had some relief in my family affairs . . . I should be much easier." That relief proved elusive. For the Atlees, these stresses were a constant undercurrent of concern. In other marriages, there were more serious problems relating to sexuality, fertility, and contraception.[38]

Abstinence required a high degree of cooperation between wife and husband that could be difficult to maintain and that ran counter to the feme covert understandings of marriage. Mary Drinker Cope had her fourth baby in May 1798. Thirty months later her husband wrote in his diary:

38. Richard B. Morris, ed., *The Basic Ideas of Alexander Hamilton* (New York, 1957), 414; Esther Atlee to William Atlee, Oct. 7, 1778, and William Atlee to Hetty [Esther Atlee], Apr. 16, 1782, William Augustus Atlee Papers, 1759–1816, Library of Congress, Washington, D.C. My thanks to Frank Fox for sending a full set of photocopies of the Atlees' correspondence. See also Theodore Sedgwick to Pamela Sedgwick, June 24, 1786, Paul H. Smith et al., eds., *Letters of Delegates to Congress, 1774–1789* (Washington, D.C., 1976–2000), XXIII, http://memory.loc.gov/ammem/amlaw/lwdg.html (accessed September 2003); Norton, *Liberty's Daughters*, 232–234; Jan Lewis and Kenneth A. Lockridge, "'Sally Has Been Sick': Pregnancy and Family Limitation among Virginia Gentry Women, 1780–1830," *Journal of Social History*, XXII (1988–1989), 5–19.

A man of feeling has his wishes thwarted by childish opposition. His home is rendered uncomfortable by the peevishness and cold manners of his spouse. Indifference ensues. His spirits are broken and if he does not seek to forget his chagrin by dissipation and unworthy indulgences abroad, melancholy follows and some fit of maniacal desperation finishes the tragedy; and all perhaps for want of a little common prudence in his wife.

Marital rape was not a crime, and Mary Drinker Cope gave birth nine months later to a stillborn son. By 1805, Cope had borne six children, and the family was in severe financial straits. Her husband came home and found her nearly dead: "Her pains were excruciating, her pulse gone and a death-like cold, clammy sweat had seized her whole frame. Her physician gave no hopes of her recovery." Her husband diagnosed "rheumatism or gout in the stomach," but, as a contemporaneous visitor noticed, "American women divide their whole body in two parts; from the top to the waist is stomach; from there to the foot is ankles." Stomach complaints could stand for any internal disorder, and rheumatism could have amenorrhea as a prominent symptom. For days Mary Drinker Cope suffered with "paroxism," "spasm," and "nausea and vomiting," but she survived, contrary to the expectations of her doctor. Although Thomas Cope wrote in this same passage that "no two perhaps have in general harmonized more perfectly than we," he quickly proceeded on a long rant about a "'house divided against itself,'" about mothers indulging sons and even letting them choose their own careers, about women "greedily devouring the contents of novel after novel," and about mothers resenting their husbands' beatings of their wayward sons. It was not a happy marriage or even a cooperative one.[39]

Periodic abstinence does not work well even when the reproductive cycle is understood and basal temperatures can be measured; it could not work when a knowledge of basic physiology was lacking. At a somewhat later period, another doctor and his wife failed miserably in their attempts to limit births despite this rare record of their self-control, planning, and careful counting:

May 30th, 1848 — Daughter born . . .
Aug. 6th, Menstrua.

39. Eliza Cope Harrison, ed., *Philadelphia Merchant: The Diary of Thomas P. Cope, 1800-1851* (South Bend, Ind., 1978), 48, 172, 173, 174; Roberts and Roberts, eds. and trans., *American Journey of Moreau de St. Méry,* 287. See also Barbara Duden, *The Woman beneath the Skin: A Doctor's Patients in Eighteenth-Century Germany,* trans. Thomas Dunlap (Cambridge, Mass., 1991).

11th, " ceased.

29th, Coitus—first.

Sept. 6th, Menstrua.

12th, " ceased.

25th, First Coitus.

Feb. 14th, 1849—Quickening.

July 26th, Son born=282 days from September 12th to July 21st.

This anonymous couple waited three months after the birth of their second child in May 1848 to resume sexual relations, waited until late in the menstrual cycle to have intercourse (because the best medical authorities assured the public that menstruation would flush out any impregnated egg before it could attach to the uterine lining), and yet managed only a thirteen-month interval between births.[40]

Some men assumed (or tried to assume) control of fertility. Dr. Anthony Fothergill wrote a male friend in 1810, "5 Children already! after a 6th appears—Festina lente 'ne quid nimus.' Voluptatis commendat rarior usus." (Roughly: "Make haste slowly; nothing in excess; less frequent exercise of one's appetite will be rewarded.") Partial abstinence was the only technique that the doctor could or would promote even in the privacy of the Latin language, but he now assumed that men would make the decisions about childbearing.[41]

Two reports suggest that coitus interruptus was being practiced but with mixed results. Male withdrawal before ejaculation was an old but not very reliable practice. In the midst of war in 1779, Maria Muhlenberg Swaine gave birth to her firstborn son, George Washington Swaine, exactly nine months after an unexpected visit from her officer-politician husband. Her father noted with some surprise that this first child appeared after his daughter and her husband had "been married for almost five years." Spontaneity seems to have disrupted a previously successful strategy to delay starting a family. Other women faced similar problems. Isabella van Havre wrote to her sister

40. Charles D. Meigs, *Obstetrics: The Science and the Art* (Philadelphia, 1856), 183–184. Meigs, like many in the nineteenth century, believed that women were most fertile during or just after menstruation because even fertilized ova would "be lost by effluxion" late in the cycle. For another example of ineffective counting, see Janet Farrell Brodie, *Contraception and Abortion in Nineteenth-Century America* (Ithaca, N.Y., 1994), 9–37.

41. Anthony Fothergill, Letterbook, 241, APS. My thanks to Gil Kelly for the translation. See also G. J. Barker-Benfield, "The Spermatic Economy: A Nineteenth-Century View of Sexuality," in Michael Gordon, ed., *The American Family in Social-Historical Perspective*, 2d ed. (New York, 1978), 374–402.

in 1812: "You asked how we were managing not to have any more babies. Alas, that is one of those decisions that a moment of folly can do in. I've had experience and I am sorry to have to confide that I am five months pregnant. I am extremely downcast and rather ashamed. . . . I shall never again take a trip—each one unfailingly results in a baby." In this instance, two sisters, one in Europe and the other in America, hoped desperately to bring an end to continued childbearing. They had, it appears, no certain knowledge of how this might be accomplished, although a moment of spontaneity combined with the disruptions of routine while traveling played a part in bringing about this unwelcome pregnancy with its attendant depression and embarrassment. Male-controlled forms of birth control were problematic.[42]

Breast-feeding was under women's control. In the last quarter of the eighteenth century, advice on the contraceptive results of breast-feeding were spread from one woman to another along with new attitudes on family size. Margaret Izard Manigault told a married daughter in 1809, "I think it less fatiguing to the constitution to nurse this one, than to bring forth another." Another of her daughters had so imbibed the new ideas on family size that she criticized an aunt for becoming pregnant. Their "family is sufficiently large," she wrote in 1814. Other women, especially artisans' wives, took in strangers' babies to nurse just as their own child was ready to be weaned. The scanty evidence suggests that this age-old practice became more widespread in the early Republic. Elizabeth Owens's son was sixteen months old when she accepted a "foundling, found by the Watchman in a segar box and given to her for nursing." She could continue nursing for another year or more. Elizabeth Drinker had earlier advised her daughter that "she is now in her 39th. year, and that this might possible be the last trial of this sort, if she could suckle her baby for 2 years to come, as she had several times done heretofore etc." The "etc." may indicate that Drinker added other advice of a more private nature. And, although this passage indicates that health and welfare rather than family planning were the primary concerns, Elaine Forman Crane's reconstruction of the family history of Drinker and her daughters shows that "all three of Elizabeth Drinker's daughters appear to have nursed their children for longer periods than their mother did." "Even Nancy (who nursed her children for shorter periods than the others) breast-fed at least sixteen months." Elizabeth Drinker had 8 births between 1761 and 1781 (but only 1 after 1774) at an average interval of sixteen months and was forty-seven at

42. Henry Melchior Muhlenberg, *Notebook of a Colonial Clergyman*, ed. Theodore G. Tappert and John W. Doberstein (Philadelphia, 1959), 211; Callcott, ed., *Mistress of Riversdale*, 233 n. 2.

her last delivery, but her three daughters averaged 4.3 births at twenty-one-month intervals and bore their last child at age thirty-six—all between 1790 and 1807. Breast-feeding worked best in lengthening the intervals between births. The earlier cessation of childbearing probably resulted from the use of other techniques.[43]

Margaret Shippen Arnold wrote to her sister, Elizabeth Shippen Burd, near the close of the eighteenth century: "It gives me great pleasure to hear of your prudent resolution of not increasing your family; as I can never do better than to follow your example, I have determined upon the same plan; and when our Sisters have had five or six, we will likewise recommend it to them." The Shippen sisters made these decisions on their own, as women had throughout the century. Their husbands were not involved either in the decision or in the attempt to not increase the family. The Shippen sisters' "prudent resolution" to stop bearing children does not indicate what method they intended to follow. Sixty years later, the "delicately named, 'prudential considerations'" was a code phrase for abortion, linked primarily to "women distinguished for genius and intellectual attainments [who] have never as a class been prolific of offspring." That there could be an entire class of distinguished women in the nineteenth century was something new under the sun, not timeless. These and other womanly attainments owed much to the persistent drop in birthrates and family size that began in the previous century.[44]

Not all women were educated and knowledgeable. Some were isolated and ignorant of the available remedies. Joseph Leacock wrote to William Hall shortly after moving from Philadelphia to Barbadoes in 1796: "I must tell you a bit of news [my wife] begins to increase in sise [size] since my arrival,—I have got a fine Girl and two Boys, God knows how many more I am to have, I wish I had got a Receipt from Cousin Jinny to give to her that she might know when to stop." Here traditional emmenagogues were clearly being promoted as birth control—but the recipe never arrived, and Mrs. Lea-

43. Norton, *Liberty's Daughters*, 233; Virginia Armentrout and James S. Armentrout, Jr., eds., *The Diary of Harriet Manigault, 1813–1816* (Rockland, Maine, 1976), 51; Gloria Dei Lutheran Church, Baptismal Records, July 17, 1813, 1090, HSP; Elaine Forman Crane, "The World of Elizabeth Drinker," *Pennsylvania Magazine of History and Biography*, CVII (1983), 12. See also Stephanie Patterson Gilbert, "Pregnancy, Childbirth, and Family Limitation in an Eighteenth-Century Affluent Family: The Fertility Transition of Elizabeth Sandwith Drinker and Her Daughters" (paper presented at the Annual Meeting of the Pennsylvania Historical Association, Bethlehem, Pa., October 2004).

44. Randolph Shipley Klein, *Portrait of an Early American Family: The Shippens of Pennsylvania across Five Generations* (Philadelphia, 1975), 285 n. 105; Rev. I. W. Wiley, "Social Science," *The Ladies Repository: A Monthly Periodical, Devoted to Literature and Religion*, n.s. I (1868), 52.

cock bore twelve or more children, most of whom died young. Somehow the technology of family limitation was lost in migration, even if the desire to limit births persisted, suggesting again the importance of female networks in diffusing knowledge. For Julia Clark on the Missouri frontier, migration to "this wild Country" also left her without access to the usual medicines. She was about three months pregnant when she requested her sister-in-law back east to send "some Garden herbs dried, particularly time and Sage, as none is to be got in this place." These requests for medicinal herbs were repeated in several later letters and may indicate one reason why fertility was higher on the frontier.[45]

In 1794, Moreau de Saint-Méry began selling syringes in his bookstore in Philadelphia. "I wish to say that I carried a complete assortment of them for four years; and while they were primarily intended for the use of French colonials, they were in great demand among Americans, in spite of the false shame so prevalent among the latter. Thus the use of this medium on the vast American continent dates from this time." Despite these grandiose claims, retailing syringes was hardly new in the city. Nathaniel Tweedy, druggist, was advertising the availability of "small ivory syringes," along with Hooper's Female Pills and Fraunce's Female Elixir, at his store in 1760. It may be, however, that these devices were more acceptable and in greater demand by the end of the century. Moreau de Saint-Méry observed: "Syringes, when first imported by French colonists seemed a hideous object. Later they were put on sale by American apothecaries." It appears from his description of these syringes, "ingenious things said to have been suggested by the stork," that they were being used to dilate the cervix, not to douche, since the stork feeds its young by inserting its beak far down the throat of its fledglings. If so, this is the first evidence of uterine-intrusive abortion or contraception in Pennsylvania, although a case from Connecticut a half century earlier proves that surgical intervention was known and had been attempted earlier. Another hint that abortion technology was changing from botanicals to uterine intrusion comes from Dr. William Currie's listing of the distinctive diseases of particular occupational groups. The "ladies" of "the opulent and fashionable class" were especially subject to hysteria, according to Currie, but also suffered from menorrhagia, spontaneous abortion, and sterility. These latter conditions could have been the results of botched abortions: abortions that

45. Joseph Leacock to David Hall, Dec. 19, 1796, David Hall Papers, B H142.1, photocopy of original owned by Mrs. Simson, 1969, 1, APS; James J. Holmberg, ed., *Dear Brother: Letters of William Clark to Jonathan Clark* (New Haven, Conn., 2002), 143, 184, 197, 224, 225 n. 5. Julia Clark's health steadily deteriorated as the births mounted. She died in 1820 at age twenty-nine.

had perforated the uterus, had failed to expel the fetus immediately, or had produced infection. By the 1830s, the sale of syringes, rubber goods, pessaries, and other devices was brisk and began to arouse the opposition of the medical profession, certain religious leaders, and some politicians.[46]

Druggists at the turn of the nineteenth century continued to advertise drugs for women's "troubles." The Philadelphia Dispensary and other institutions offered emmenagogic treatments to the poor. Home health guides and herbals proliferated in the early nineteenth century, offering more detailed advice about familiar emmenagogic practices. Newer barrier techniques of fertility regulation might have been suspect because of their intrusive nature, because of their risk or discomfort levels, or because of their newness. In the meantime, older emmenagogic techniques were being redefined as contraceptives and abortifacients as women and men began to articulate a desire to reduce fertility permanently. A combination of an intensified use of older technologies with a gradual employment of douches, dilation, and barrier methods of birth control helped initiate a long-term decline in fertility levels.

WHEN COLONIAL-ERA WOMEN were motivated by ill health, the threat of war, or financial difficulties, they were largely successful in temporarily delaying childbearing, although failure rates were high. This control was achieved at a cost: the methods were painful and were limited to the treatment of severe physical and emotional weakness and distress. Only at the end of the eighteenth century and in the early decades of the nineteenth century is there evidence that family planning had become the primary goal of fertility regulation and only then is there a sustained decline in both family size and marital fertility rates. Prudent choice, not illness or anxiety, would henceforth justify fertility decisions made over the course of an entire lifetime. But whose choice was a question that would be debated by men, women, physicians, church, and state.

Control over fertility had been women's preserve in the eighteenth century, although the rationality of women's choices was hidden by reference to illness and hysterics. But as fertility goals shifted from a concern over

46. Roberts and Roberts, eds. and trans., *American Journey of Moreau de St. Méry*, 177–178, 314–315; advertisement in *Pa. Gaz.*, Sept. 25, 1760; William Currie, *An Historical Account of the Climates and Diseases of the United States of America* . . . (Philadelphia, 1792), 107; Mohr, *Abortion in America*, 3–45; Brodie, *Contraception and Abortion*, 233–237; Cornelia Hughes Dayton, "'Taking the Trade': Abortion and Gender Relations in an Eighteenth-Century New England Village," *William and Mary Quarterly*, 3d Ser., XLVIII (1991), 19–49.

immediate circumstances to long-range planning of an ideal family size, the separate spheres of women and men in fertility and gynecology collapsed. A new social norm of acceptable family size, pegged variously at two, four, or six children, replaced the less numeric, more lineage-oriented standards of earlier periods. Men were increasingly involved because they, too, had personal, social, and economic interests in reduced fertility and because male involvement made the new goals more attainable. Some women found the new technologies requiring male interference in gynecological matters to be offensive or oppressive. These women continued to stress the older, women-centered practices, or they denounced all contraceptive and abortive activities as shameful, preferring to advocate sexual abstinence. Some men, too, favored sexual restraint, either for all or for the lower sorts and outsiders. Other women turned to their husbands for help in achieving an end to lifelong childbearing through the employment of coitus interruptus or barrier methods of contraception. Some husbands followed their wives' wishes; other husbands asserted control over yet another aspect of their wives' lives. Some women turned to the medical profession for aid, but most obstetricians saw female-dominated medicine as an obstacle to professionalization, while pharmacists, druggists, and professors of material medica preserved traditional remedies and added some new plants to the lists of emmenagogues and abortifacients. There were other commercial and professional sources of aid, all requiring cash and most in the hands of men. The disappearance of the old rigid gender roles on gynecology produced a growing consensus on the desirability of substantial limitation of potential births, but there was no unanimity among men or among women on the appropriate technology. Still, where goals and methods were contested across a gendered divide, it was the men who had more power and authority. Women's direct control over reproduction eroded throughout the nineteenth century and much of the early twentieth century even as they were freed of the nearly continual childbearing of their grandmothers. By the middle of the nineteenth century, eighteenth-century gender roles had reversed, especially in middle class, urban America. Shame was attached to women's knowledge of reproduction, and professional men were supposed to be the experts who managed fertility decisions and births. Still, women's networks remained an important source of knowledge about gynecology, pharmacology, and the cooperativeness of particular medical doctors into the present.

6

Increase and Multiply

EMBARRASSED MEN

AND

PUBLIC ORDER

There was, once upon a time, a woman brought before the Connecticut court on bastardy charges—for the fifth time. She flummoxed the straight-laced judges in this most puritanical of colonies by insisting that she had done nothing wrong: "Can it be a Crime (in the Nature of Things I mean) to add to the Number of the King's Subjects, in a new Country that really wants People?" After all, she had expected that her first, faithless suitor would have married her. In giving birth then and later she was merely fulfilling "the Duty of the first and great Command of Nature, and of Nature's God, *Encrease and Multiply.*" She should not be punished, but, she insisted in an audacious finale, she should have a statue erected in her honor. The judges were dumb-founded. One, perhaps her original suitor, was so shamed by her speech that he soon married her, and she, according to some accounts, bore him an additional fifteen children. In retrospect, a future of yearly childbearing seems a high price to pay for the belated respectability of marriage. It was not the happily-ever-after ending expected in fairy tales, but then that was part of the joke. Not even the advocates of abundant childbearing promoted families of twenty children. The story appeared in print across the colonies and throughout Europe. Echoes of Polly Baker's speech even turned up later in tea-table chatter. Philadelphia wives, Eliza Stedman reported in a laughing mood in 1764, were about "to increase and Multiply in down right compasion as this is a young Country and wants peopling." It was a patriotic act to fill these underpopulated colonies with young colonials.[1]

The widely published and republished tale of Polly Baker and her many children was a fraud composed by Benjamin Franklin (himself the fifteenth child of his father) in 1747 just as he was beginning his investigations of the demographic relationship of family size, population growth, and the means of subsistence—work that would influence thinkers as diverse as Adam Smith, Robert Thomas Malthus, and Charles Darwin. This fake news item certainly played on the inherent tensions between, on the one hand, contemporary pronatalist state policies and biblical commandments to populate the earth and, on the other, the legal and religious insistence on institutionally sanctioned procreation. It mocked the double sexual standard that punished women for sexual failings and absolved men of responsibility. It played with both the older images of women as passionate and lusty creatures and the gradually emerging imaginings of female innocence or asexuality (so often portrayed as vulnerable to the melodramatic, vile seducer). And it broached in public gynecological issues that belonged properly and privately to women—hence the mute silence of the fictional judges, the naive willingness of newspaper and magazine editors to accept the story as fact, and the very few, flat-footed, real-life refutations of the tale's moral implications.

The British Empire and its constituent governments did have an interest in enhancing procreation, in enforcing the marriage bond, and in preventing fornication, sodomy, adultery, abortion, and infanticide. The growth and security of the Empire depended on having a large population. Social order depended on the family. It was primarily the family that provided policing, education, social welfare, and many other crucial social and economic functions. Most production was based in the family whether on farms or in artisanal households. The peaceable transfer of property from one generation to the next, the supervision and rearing of children, the obedience of servants— especially adolescent servants—and the disciplining of both wives and unmarried wenches all depended, it was thought, on the presence of a strong male householder who would enforce law and religious proscription while keeping dependents to their tasks.

1. Max Hall, *Benjamin Franklin and Polly Baker: The History of a Literary Deception,* rev. ed. (Pittsburgh, 1990), 157–167, esp. 161, 167; Eliza Stedman to Elizabeth Graeme, Dec. 16, 1764, in Simon Gratz, ed., "Some Material for a Biography of Mrs. Elizabeth Fergusson, née Graeme," *Pennsylvania Magazine of History and Biography,* XXXIX (1915), 277.

Most household activities were strictly gendered. There was a woman's world of sexuality and birth, rumor and reputation, nursing and burying, food and clothing production, potions and pills, legitimacy and bastardy. Men dominated households and fields, and elite men led in the professions, the church, the state, the militia, and much of the formal, monied economy. Although free, propertied men—voters, legislators, jurymen, prosecutors, and justices—negotiated and interpreted Anglo-American law codes on subjects that directly affected women's lives and shaped what few choices early American women had, their interference in women's realm was for the most part minimal and desultory, not interventionist and active. There was a window of opportunity for women in the late eighteenth century to experiment with new interpretations of marriage, sexuality, and childbearing. Judges showed considerable reluctance to punish women offenders, and physicians had not yet assumed preeminence in matters of gynecology and obstetrics.

Many English historians have used the anthropological term "taboo" to describe the traditional, strict division between English men's and women's roles in obstetrics and gynecology. Menstruation, childbearing, and fertility were under the control of women and appropriate only to women. Most men, with clergymen and physicians occasionally excepted, would not transgress these rigid boundaries of acceptable social roles. Barbara A. Hanawalt writes of the medieval period: "Folkloric sources are virtually the only ones with information on childbirth. They illustrate the taboo on having a man present and the anxiety of both sexes at breaking it." Patricia Crawford finds that "scriptural and medical taboo during the seventeenth century" warned against male contact with menstrual fluid. Angus McLaren labels the fertility-enhancing, abortive, and contraceptive activities of English women a "separate female sexual culture" in the sixteenth through eighteenth centuries. Even though these taboos lessened in the eighteenth century, considerable shame still attached to the transgressor of gender-appropriate spheres well into the nineteenth century.[2]

2. Barbara A. Hanawalt, *The Ties That Bound: Peasant Families in Medieval England* (New York, 1986), 216; Patricia Crawford, "Attitudes to Menstruation in Seventeenth-Century England," *Past and Present*, no. 91 (May 1981), 61–62; Angus McLaren, *Reproductive Rituals: The Perception of Fertility in England from the Sixteenth Century to the Nineteenth Century* (London, 1984), 111; William L. Langer, "The Origins of the Birth Control Movement in England in the Early Nineteenth Century," in Robert I. Rotberg and Theodore K. Rabb, *Marriage and Fertility: Studies in Interdisciplinary History* (Princeton, N.J., 1980), 271. Also pointing to male ignorance of contraception are the sources quoted in R. R. Kuczynski, "British Demographers' Opinions of Fertility, 1660 to 1760," in Lancelot Hogben, ed., *Political Arithmetic: A Symposium of Population Studies* (New York, 1938), 283–327;

These English ideas of proper male and female spheres were transported to the New World. Fertility and childbirth were women's concerns, and men stayed away whenever possible. A French visitor to Pennsylvania in the 1790s was surprised that, "when a Philadelphia woman bears a child, her husband is never present." Childbirth in Anglo-America was a female ritual from which husbands were normally excluded. Birthing women called together female friends and neighbors, as well as the local midwife, to assist at the birth. So customary was the exclusion of men that when watchmaker John Fitch assisted at a birth in 1789 because no one else was available, he fretted that he had been "obliged to degrade the man and become a nurse." Childbirth and other gynecological events, particularly menstruation, were shameful for men and were supposed to remain female secrets. Contact was emasculating. One consequence of this shame was that the available male techniques of contraception—condoms (used mostly to avoid venereal disease) and coitus interruptus—seem to have been little used or known by eighteenth-century colonists. Another consequence was a fitful attention by officials to bastardy, contraception, abortion, adultery, fornication, and other forms of sexuality customarily prohibited by legislatures and courts.[3]

Women's bodies might have been private and clothed in secrecy, at least ideally, but secrets are hard to keep. A German visitor to Philadelphia in 1765 was shocked—so shocked that he wrote in code—to hear "the young boys talk, all their talk is about nothing else but how they lost their virginity[?] and how girls and women are made." He continued, in plain German, "To sum it up, they are quite open about some things that cannot be told." There was certainly an underground male tradition of gossip about female anatomy and sexuality that was a sniggering bond of unity among adolescent males. Even older men joked. One example of colonial "wit" goes like this: a woman fell head over heels off her horse, and her upturned skirts revealed what "the whole Sex are very Solicitous about concealing." She exclaimed to a male bystander, "Did you ever see the like! [meaning the accident]—yes by God, said the fellow, a hundred and a hundred times over, my wife has got Just such another." These male gossipers and jokesters simply underscored men's nagging feeling that women knew much more than they, even as they

---

Marie Mulvey-Roberts, "Menstrual Misogyny and Taboo: The Medusa, Vampire, and the Female Stigmatic," in Andrew Shail and Gillian Howie, ed., *Menstruation: A Cultural History* (Basingstoke, Hampshire, 2005), 149–161.

3. Kenneth Roberts and Anna M. Roberts, eds. and trans., *Moreau de St. Méry's American Journey (1793–1798)* (Garden City, N.Y., 1947), 289; Frank D. Prager, ed., *The Autobiography of John Fitch,* American Philosophical Society, *Memoirs,* CXIII (Philadelphia, 1976), 126.

passed around ragged copies of the much republished seventeenth-century sex manual misleadingly entitled *Aristotle's Masterpiece*—a book with crude woodcuts of naked women, a gravid uterus, and monstrous births that promised to reveal the secrets of generation.[4]

When the unimaginative Samuel Keimer, printer of the *Universal Instructor in all Arts and Sciences: and Pennsylvania Gazette,* was desperate for news in 1729, he began printing an encyclopedia, article by article, starting from the beginning. He did not even get through the letter *A* when he thoughtlessly allowed the article on abortion to appear on the front page of his paper. The republished medical essay not only defined abortion, but it even included directions for inducing abortions ("immoderate Evacuations, violent Motions, sudden Passions, Frights, . . . violent Purgatives; and in the general, any thing that tends to promote the *Menses*"). This was shocking stuff that should have been available only to women and to a small, educated elite, not broadcast on the front page of the local paper to the general public. A young Ben Franklin immediately satirized these *"indecencies"* by crafting a feminine persona in the rival paper, the *American Weekly Mercury.* "Martha Careful" warned Keimer that, "if he proceed farther to Expose the Secrets of our Sex, in That audacious manner, . . . to be Read in all *Taverns* and *Coffee-Houses,* and by the Vulgar: . . . which ought only to be in the Repositary of the Learned," then he would be made a public example of "for his Immodesty." Men did have some knowledge of female anatomy and physiology, although not as much as women did, but to admit it so publicly was to invite ridicule, shame, and dishonor. Only men in the learned professions—clerics and physicians—were partially exempt from this taboo, and propriety dictated that even their knowledge of women's bodies be subsumed under the secrets of their professions, not publicly discussed.[5]

The aura of secrecy meant that men's knowledge of women's physiology,

---

4. Dieter Pesch, ed., *Brave New World: Rhinelanders Conquer America: The Journal of Johannes Herbergs,* trans. Angelika Orpin and David Orpin (Kommern, Germany, 2001), 129 (square brackets are published, indicating an obscure word in the manuscript); Alexander Hamilton, *The History of the Ancient and Honorable Tuesday Club,* ed. Robert Micklus, 3 vols. (Chapel Hill, N.C., 1990), I, 364. See the disconcerted reaction by Jonathan Edwards in 1744, in Ava Chamberlain, "Bad Books and Bad Boys: The Transformation of Gender in Eighteenth-Century Northampton, Massachusetts," *New England Quarterly,* LXXV (2002), 179–203; Mary E. Fissell, "Hairy Women and Naked Truths: Gender and the Politics of Knowledge in *Aristotle's Masterpiece,*" *William and Mary Quarterly,* 3d Ser., LX (2003), 43–74.

5. "Abortion . . . ," *Universal Instructor in All Arts and Sciences: and Pennsylvania Gazette* (Philadelphia), [Feb. 21, 1729], 1; Leonard W. Labaree and William B. Willcox, eds., *The Papers of Benjamin Franklin,* I (New Haven, Conn., 1959), 111–113.

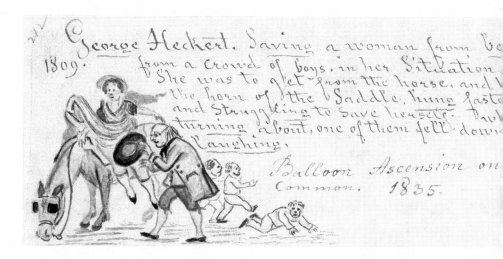

George Heckert. Saving a woman from be
1809. from a Crowd of boys, in her Situation.
She was to get from the horse, and
the horn of the Saddle, hung faste
and Struggling to save herself. Pul
turning about, one of them fell down
Laughing.

Balloon Ascension on
Common. 1835.

even after consulting medical texts or *Aristotle's Masterpiece,* was patchy and clothed in mystery. And the idea that, in this one area, at least, women might know more than men brought some married women enough respect that judges and juries would occasionally accept their opinions in cases involving pregnancy or accusations of rape, adultery, fornication, bastardy, infanticide, and other crimes needing judgments upon the physical state of an accused or violated woman. This experiential knowledge was so esoteric (from the viewpoint of officials), and yet so important, that women's testimony on female anatomy was considered authoritative, at least within the "conservative and supportive" role allotted to respectable women in maintaining the status quo. Still, it was men who made the final judgment about the value of women's testimony and the appropriateness of judicial access to their bodies.[6]

Not all women were considered to be respectable, of course. Unmarried camp followers, for example, received little or no consideration. In 1777, Captain Robert Kirkwood of the Continental army ordered that the "Weomen belonging to the Reg[imen]t be paraded tomorrow morning and to undergo an Examination from the Serjeon [surgeon] of the Reg[imen]t at his tent, except those that are married, and the husbands of those to undergo said examination in their Stead." In this instance, married women's coverture under male authority spared them from an invasive physical examination by a stranger. Their modesty was protected because their husbands served

6. Laurel Thatcher Ulrich, *Good Wives: Image and Reality in the Lives of Women in Northern New England, 1650–1750* (New York, 1982), 60.

PLATE 26.

George Heckert. 1809. Saving a Woman from Being Expose't. . . .
From the Sketchbook of Lewis Miller, I, 89. Permission,
Historical Society of York County.

The artist described the scene as follows: "George
Heckert. 1809. Saving a woman from being Expose't—from
a Crowd of boys. in her Situation, by his hat covering her She was
to get from the horse, and her close caught at the horn or the
Saddle. hung fastened against the horse And Struggling to
Save herself. while the boys were turning about, one of them
fell down. and all the rest began Laughing."

as medical proxies (although the wives were not spared the consequences
of their husbands' possible diseased states and their own presumed infections). Respectability here and elsewhere had less to do with women's behavior and more to do with their relationship to appropriate male authority.
Enslaved women could expect even less consideration. Phillis, the slave of an
Easton, Pennsylvania, shopkeeper, was ordered to go to the stable or to the
kitchen or upstairs with her master where he pulled up her clothes and "had
carnal knowledge of her," as she testified, "a great many times." Only when
his wife learned of Phillis's pregnancy did Phillis feel she could refuse these
commands. She had no authority over her body in her own right, and she
was assumed to have no reputation to protect. Married women similarly had
no control over their bodies—their bodies belonged to their husbands—but
there was some benefit in being considered respectable.[7]

Secret knowledge could also bring fear or contempt. One political allegory
from 1785 played on these fears of transposed power relations through an
elaborate, metaphorical depiction of a pregnant woman. The expectant wife
is imagined to claim, "I shall wax mighty, and become great." To be "great
with child" was a common enough description of late pregnancy, but here
it overlaps with a grandiose declaration of absolute female power. Probably
because feminine strength implied an overthrow of masculine control and
an unleashing of the animallike passions assumed to be innately feminine,

7. Joseph Brown Turner, ed., "The Journal and Order Book of Captain Robert Kirkwood of the
Delaware Regiment of the Continental Line," Historical Society of Delaware, *Papers*, LVI (1910), 94.
The deposition of Phillis is given in Francis S. Fox, *Sweet Land of Liberty: The Ordeal of the Ameri-
can Revolution in Northampton County, Pennsylvania* (University Park, Pa., 2000), 127–129.

the husband in this political piece suspects his wife of adultery and gives "her such a confounded thump, as immediately to bring on great distress, hard pain, and insupportable agonies." Miscarriage is threatened. The doctors had to be called. Medicines had to be paid for: "very long and learned recipes, which may be seen at large in the book, entitled, Diseases and Remedies." So during pregnancy husbands and physicians can be reduced to "Gentlemen in waiting," and, if the woman's condition is not appropriately handled, if her longings and demands are not fulfilled, "it will prove the destruction of the foetus." Pregnant women could become the centers of attention, reversing the orderly conduct of the household. Fecundity could become a source of malevolent female power.[8]

Men had more to worry about. The old belief that loss of sperm brought loss of strength still prevailed. As one almanac recounted in rough rhyme: "So Youth grown up to strength and Manly state, / His tender Beauty fades to procreate." Men could lose by gratifying both sexual desire and desire for an heir. Women might gain. Birthing metaphors in letters and essays occasionally bring male anxiety about women's procreative powers to the surface. Females were both creative and destructive. If men wanted male heirs, they might just have to truckle to feminine demands.[9]

Women's tongues could tell against male prerogative. John Fitch, nearly fifty years old in the early 1790s, was still worried about the jokes that gossips might have told at his birth, "I suppose the same cerimonies merryment and invidious talks were told as is common on such occasions but being then unacquainted with the world [I] did not notice them so as to recollect them at present." As a grown man he still resented the possibility that women might have taken advantage of his infancy to undermine his virility through, as often happened at birthing scenes, jokes about his penis. Fitch was perhaps unusually anxious, but it was common for men to demean wives and mewling, puking babies. Men rarely bothered to record their disdain, but again metaphorical flights of fancy do preserve a commonplace language of contempt. Congressman John Mathews wrote to Nathanael Greene in 1781: "Great events are in the womb of time. I hope Madam is so far gone, that she will produce soon, when we shall be able to judge what sort of brat it is." When a Mrs. F. was pregnant with her fourth child, after bearing three daughters, her husband "would walk up to her, seize her cranium with his

8. Tom Bumpkin [pseud.], "A Fable," New-York Journal, and State Gazette, Jan. 20, 1785.
9. Titan Leeds, The American Almanack for the Year of Christian Account 1714 . . . (New York, 1713), n.p.

fingers extended, and observe humorously, 'that if she presented him with another daughter instead of a son, thus he would pinch it in the head.'" Not surprisingly, she was horrified by this frequent "joke" about killing female infants. But the case of Mrs. F. was only one example of a society in which girls often counted for little. Even young boys, who were placed in a feminine sphere until they were five or six, were little noticed until they came under a father's care. This crucial shift was ritualized when their clothing switched from the skirts characteristic of infants and women to the pants, shirts, and jackets worn by men. Hannah Sansom noted her widowed friend's son's transition from the world of females to that of males: "Bill first clad in mans Attire. How pleasing to his father would this day have been." Females and their skirts, their leaky bodies, and their irrationality were to be avoided by men as were their skirted, crying, hungry, leaking infants. Most men kept their distance from such lesser, messier things — or tried to.[10]

It is not surprising, given this shame, resentment, and distancing, that eighteenth-century men seem to have been quite ignorant of gynecology, obstetrics, and contraceptive techniques, despite their surreptitious reading of midwifery manuals. Joseph Price, a farmer and carpenter, could have some "fat Jokes" with Granny Latch, the local midwife, but was earlier humiliated at being "44 years old and [with] a young Wife." He wrote in his diary that he was "almost ashamed to Show [his] face" by his wife's figure, "She is so very pregnant and only 6 or 7 weeks Married." His sexual transgressions, which consisted of bundling and "sparking" several women at once, were now exposed to public view, and he was deeply embarrassed. John Fitch abandoned his wife in 1769: "Fearing an increass of my familey urged my departure. And before I left that place my wife was with child with a daughter. Which had I known I should never have left her but worried thro' life as well as I could." Here, of course, Fitch's ignorance was self-interested and undoubtedly disingenuous. But other men seem to have been truly in the dark. Joseph Shippen wrote to his father in 1770, after the birth of a child, "If Events were always to correspond to our own particular Desires, I should have rather wished this to have been postponed a Year or two longer," a statement that assumes

---

10. Prager, ed., *Autobiography of John Fitch*, APS, *Memoirs*, CXIII (1976), 21; John Mathews to Nathanael Greene, Aug. 28, [1781], *Letters of Delegates to Congress, 1774–1789*, XVII, *March 1, 1781–August 31, 1781*, 567, Library of Congress, http://memory.loc.gov/ammem/amlaw (accessed May 2005); P. J. Stryker, "Case of Monstrous Birth," *Philadelphia Medical Museum, Conducted by John Redman Coxe, M.D.*, VI, no. 2 (Jan. 2, 1809), 145; Susan E. Klepp and Karin A. Wulf, eds., *The Diary of Hannah Callender: Sense and Sensibility in a Revolutionary Age, 1758–1788* (Ithaca, N.Y., 2009), Apr. 23, 1763.

that he did not know how the spacing of births might be accomplished. In 1781, Robert Barclay wrote to a friend that he "hope[d] his wife would wait for awhile before having any more children," as if he had nothing to do with the process. Because regulation of fertility focused on the regulation of the menstrual cycle, not on barrier methods of birth control, men were in a particularly helpless position. Even a compulsive libertine, like the anonymous Philadelphia sawyer who kept records of his liaisons in an accounting book, did not use prophylactics. Although he was certainly no naïf, he was surprised by his wife's pregnancy: "Molly informs me she is big again with child—oh my—how can I endure it." He did not use contraceptives in illicit encounters either. "She caused me much fright on asking me where I dwelleth and that in case increase from contact she would make known to me the fact—I said I live in the Carolinas—and fled." Nor did he use a condom to prevent the spread of venereal disease, although condoms were being used by London prostitutes and their customers to guard against infection. A belated six months after the first diagnosis, he resolved: "Clapp—Much itching in my flopper—must keep away from my Wife." Men could wish and hope, they could be frightened, but they had little direct, daily control over fertility except perhaps to escape the consequences by fleeing.[11]

In the colonies, month-to-month fertility decisions were left to women, although those decisions were made within a larger context in which high fertility and many sons were valued and promoted. Only late in the eighteenth century would the focus of fertility regulation shift away from a postcoital concern with menstruation. That shift would mitigate some male shame and allow men a more open role in fertility decisions (see Chapter 5).

Childbirth, menstruation, and fertility were rarely discussed by men in the eighteenth century. When gynecological problems occurred, it was the women who administered the treatment, provided medical advice, and attended the patient, sometimes in consultation with physicians. When some male physicians began to take a more active role in obstetrics at the end of the century, their role was initially confined to that of an assistant at the birth. Legislators and jurists tried to prevent illegitimate births by punishing

11. Joseph Price Diary, July 19, 1797, Sept. 4, 1804, Lower Merion Historical Society, http://www .lowermerionhistory.org/texts/price (accessed March 2003); Prager, ed., *Autobiography of John Fitch*, APS, *Memoirs*, CXIII (1976), 46; Randolph Shipley Klein, *Portrait of an Early American Family: The Shippens of Pennsylvania across Five Generations* (Philadelphia, 1975), 150; Judy Mann DiStefano, "A Concept of the Family in Colonial America: The Pembertons of Philadelphia" (Ph.D. diss., Ohio State University, 1970), 25; anonymous diary, June 3, Feb. 15, Dec. 22, James Wilson Papers, American Philosophical Society, Philadelphia. The author was probably a sawyer in Wilson's employ. Internal evidence places the yearlong record between 1792 and 1798.

some unmarried mothers after the fact but had little to say about married women's procreative lives. Nor did enslaved women's sexual lives concern authorities. The direct regulation of fertility was not usually a masculine prerogative through most of the eighteenth century.[12]

Gender and Gynecology in Political Life

In 1784, Elizabeth Wilson of Chester County, Pennsylvania, was convicted of the murder, by crushing, of her illegitimate twin children, some six to ten weeks old. To the end, she insisted upon her innocence and in her dying confession declared one Joseph Deshong, sheriff of Sussex County, New Jersey, as the father and killer. On the day of her scheduled hanging, her brother, William Wilson, having investigated Deshong's activities, was finally able to obtain a stay of execution from the state's Supreme Executive Council. He galloped from Philadelphia to Chester only to arrive twenty minutes after she had been hanged. She was immediately cut down, but all attempts to resuscitate her failed. Some accounts say her brother died soon after, others that he became a hermit, living for another nineteen years in a cave outside Harrisburg.[13]

The case became a cause célèbre, producing a flood of pamphlets, a versified broadside, a lightly fictionalized short story, and personal meditations. Charles Biddle, who signed the stay, later wrote an account of the case and concluded: "If death is the punishment of the mother, what punishment is too severe for the villain who seduces, and afterwards abandons the wretched mother?" Elizabeth Drinker called it a "sad tale" and stressed the truthfulness of Wilson's account of her innocence. The anonymous versifier, apparently a young woman, exclaimed, "Such cruelty [as Deshong's] sure

12. Judith Walzer Leavitt, *Brought to Bed: Childbearing in America, 1750 to 1950* (New York, 1986), esp. 58–60.

13. [Elizabeth Wilson], *A Faithful Narrative of Elizabeth Wilson . . .* (Philadelphia, 1786), reprinted in Daniel E. Williams, ed., *Pillars of Salt: An Anthology of Early American Criminal Narratives* (Madison, Wis., 1993), 271–281. Charles Biddle, who signed the stay of execution (called in other sources a pardon), recounts the event in *The Autobiography of Charles Biddle, Vice-President of the Supreme Executive Council of Pennsylvania, 1745–1821* (Philadelphia, 1883), 199–202. See also *The Pennsylvania Hermit; a Narrative of the Extraordinary Life of Amos* [sic.] *Wilson, Who Expired in a Cave in the Neighborhood of Harrisburgh (Penn.) after Having Therein Lived in Solitary Retirement for the Space of Nineteen Years, in Consequence of the Ignominious Death of His Sister* (New York, 1838); Daniel E. Williams, "Victims of Narrative Seduction: The Literary Translations of Elizabeth and 'Miss Harriot' Wilson," *Early American Literature*, XXVIII (1993), 148–170. The fullest and most recent exploration of the case finds Wilson guilty (Meredith Peterson Tufts, "A Matter of Context: Elizabeth Wilson Revisited," *PMHB*, CXXXI [2007], 149–176).

ne'er was known in our *America.*" The case was propelled into the spotlight not only because of its shocking violence, the dramatic race against time, and the tragic result but also because it touched on complex, and perhaps intractable, legal and ethical issues being debated in the new nation: republican virtue and sin, self-evident truths and seductive falsehoods, and individualized pursuits of happiness and self-control. And at base were questions about whether women were essentially irrational, turbulent beings in need of cool-headed masculine domination or whether they were innocent and passive, needing men's protection but, in turn, taming men's more impulsive, passionate natures.[14]

If colonial men were easily shamed when they were discovered trespassing onto women's procreative realms, they were similarly reluctant to interfere in childbirth and fertility in their roles as legislators and judges. Pennsylvania is the prime example here. The colony borrowed from the more thoroughly Protestant law codes of Scotland that other colonies similarly adapted to their situations and beliefs. The newly independent state of Pennsylvania, both because of Quaker influence and political radicalism, quickly reformed its laws to incorporate contemporary legal trends, particularly a less sanguinary criminal code and new gendered emphases in family law.[15]

Infanticide was an occasional transgression that colonial courts faced. Infanticide was prosecuted both directly as a felony and indirectly through the concealment statute. Infanticide was separate from murder because the usual perpetrator was female rather than male, the motivation was desperation rather than antagonism, and the victim was not clearly delineated as an independent, fully rational being. It was a capital offense to conceal the death of a bastard child in colonial Pennsylvania and elsewhere in the British Empire. Should an unmarried mother "endeavour privately" to conceal the death of a newborn by hiding the body, then she "shall suffer death, as in case of murder; except such mother can make proof . . . that the child . . . was born dead." An anomaly in English law, this enactment overrode the presumption of the accused's innocence by making the discovery of a dead bastard child presumptive evidence of murder by the mother. It was her responsibility to prove her innocence, not the government's duty to prove guilt. Only an unmarried woman was considered liable to commit infanticide and hide the fact, since the law assumed that respectably married women would not con-

14. *Elegy, etc., Fair Daughters of America . . .* (Boston, 1786?); Biddle, *Autobiography,* 202; Elaine Forman Crane, ed., *The Diary of Elizabeth Drinker,* 3 vols. (Boston, 1990), II, 918.

15. Compare colonial codes with John Erksine, *The Principles of the Law of Scotland* (Edinburgh, 1802) and with the writings of English jurists Edward Coke and William Blackstone.

ceal the death of a newborn because they need not fear prosecution for fornication, bastardy, or, presumably, for adultery. The legal concern was with the attempted cover-up of illegal sexual activity by unmarried women.[16]

There were just eight Pennsylvania women convicted under the concealment statute between 1718 and 1775. Only three of these women were hanged, however: an execution rate of 37 percent, compared to 74 percent for convictions of murder. Between 1779 and 1792, fifteen women were charged with the crime of concealment, but only three were convicted, two of whom were pardoned. As William Bradford, the attorney general of the United States, former attorney general of Pennsylvania, and judge of the state Supreme Court, commented after the Revolution, "Where a positive law is so feebly enforced, there is reason to suspect that it is fundamentally wrong." Given a choice between executing the mother and acquitting her, prosecutors failed to take suspects to court, juries overwhelmingly chose not to convict, and governors intervened to pardon.[17]

There was little support for the punishment of infanticide as murder and less for conviction of concealment. In Chester County in 1697, a woman accused of infanticide, together with her brothers and her sister, fought off warrant servers, apparently permanently. Prosecutorial standards became increasingly restrictive as standards of evidence changed to favor the accused. By the middle decades of the eighteenth century, the woman would not be convicted of concealment if she told anyone of her pregnancy, if she had assistance in childbirth, or if she had collected baby linen. These were taken to be proof that she had not intended concealment. In addition, it became accepted that the body of the infant had to show marks of violence sufficient to convict under the murder statute. Even with these qualifications,

16. *Laws of the Commonwealth of Pennsylvania, from the Fourteenth Day of October, One Thousand Seven Hundred, to the Twentieth Day of March, One Thousand Eight Hundred and Ten . . .* (Philadelphia, 1810), I, 113.

17. J. W. Ehrlich, *Ehrlich's Blackstone, Part Two: Private Wrongs, Public Wrongs* (New York, 1959), 397; Leon Radzinowicz, *A History of English Criminal Law and Its Administration from 1750* (New York, 1948), I, 430–436; William Bradford, *An Enquiry How Far the Punishment of Death Is Necessary in Pennsylvania; with Notes and Illustrations* (Philadelphia, 1793), 40; Lawrence H. Gipson, *Crime and Its Punishment in Provincial Pennsylvania: A Phase of the Social History of the Commonwealth* (Bethlehem, Pa., 1935), 14; G. S. Rowe, "Women's Crime and Criminal Administration in Pennsylvania, 1763–1790," *PMHB,* CIX (1985), 360, 365–366. Rowe, "Infanticide, Its Judicial Resolution, and Criminal Code Revision in Early Pennsylvania," APS, *Proceedings,* CXXXV (1991), 207–209, has uncovered cases unknown to Bradford for the period 1682–1800: of 73 women prosecuted for concealment and infanticide, 57 were tried, 24 convicted, and 8 executed. Although prosecutions remained stable after 1720 (1.2 per 10,000 population in 1700–1719, falling to 0.8 in 1720–1739, 0.7 in 1740–1759, 0.9 in 1760–1779, and 0.8 in 1780–1800), executions declined markedly over time.

the law remained unpopular. A case from western Pennsylvania in 1791 involved a widow who first "denied, but afterwards confessed having had a child.—She said she had buried her child, it having been dead born. Afterwards owned she had taken it up, and thrown it in the river." The jury found her not guilty in spite of her contradictory and self-serving explanations, her ultimate confession, the marks of violence on the corpse, and the evidence of concealment.[18]

Reforming the unpopular concealment law was a priority of the newly independent state of Pennsylvania. William Bradford's sentimental, breathless depiction of the pitiable, abandoned unwed mother made a strong, if emotional and sensational, plea not only for women's essential innocence but also for their appropriate passivity.

> May not the child perish from want of care, or of skill, in so critical a moment? A helpless woman, in a situation so novel and so alarming — alone, and, perhaps, exhausted by her sufferings. may she not be the involuntary cause of her infant's death? and, if she afterwards consults a natural impulse to conceal her shame, is not the penalty beyond the demerit of the offence?[19]

The law was revised in 1786 and 1790 to require proof that the child was born alive before the woman could be convicted. The burden of proof therefore shifted from the accused to the prosecution. In 1794, the legislature again revised the law to require proof that the mother "did wilfully and maliciously destroy and take away the life of such child," a belated legal recognition that newborn infants died of causes other than murder. The legislature, perhaps persuaded by Bradford, perhaps seeking more convictions in cases of suspected infanticide, also provided a legal category mediating between felony murder and acquittal by revising the concealment statute. The

18. Herbert William Keith Fitzroy, "The Punishment of Crime in Provincial Pennsylvania," *PMHB*, LX (1936), 268; Radzinowicz, *History of English Criminal Law,* 430–436; Bradford, *Enquiry,* 39–40; Alexander Addison, *Reports of Cases in the County Courts of the Fifth Circuit . . .* (Washington, Pa., 1800), 1–2. Joseph Price mentions a woman's attributing her bastard child's paternity to his brother and his brother's reluctance to marry her (Mar. 15–May 28, 1795), determining whether a bastard child's support would fall to her master or to the town (May 28, 1796), paying a grandmother to foster a presumably illegitimate child ("hope we Have go Read [rid] of it," Nov. 16, 1796), and threatening to arrest one man for begetting a bastard but letting him go "upon his Honour" when he promised to pay (Dec. 26, 1796). These four cases of bastardy were handled privately or civilly, without criminal prosecution. See Joseph Price Diary, Lower Merion Historical Society, http://www.lowermerionhistory.org/texts/price.

19. Bradford, *Enquiry,* 39.

1794 law fixed a maximum sentence of five years of imprisonment where the unwed mother concealed the death of her child. Thereafter, Pennsylvania women suspected of infanticide were usually tried for and convicted of concealment rather than being accused of infanticide or felony murder. In one indictment for murder, the district judge commented: "The circumstances were very strong, and might reasonably have been thought sufficient, to satisfy the mind of the jury. . . . However, the jury did not find the murder, but found the concealment." In general, Pennsylvania legislators, prosecutors, judges, and jurymen did not equate infanticide with murder, choosing to acquit the accused woman or, particularly after 1794, to convict her of the lesser charge of concealment rather than a felony.[20]

A few women were convicted of felonies nonetheless. Bradford had argued that pity was the appropriate and usual response of jurymen as long as the accused woman preserved her proper role by appealing to the court as a "helpless woman" or as one of those "unfortunate creatures." In those cases, the protective and compassionate male judiciary would view them "with compassionate eyes" and acquit. If the courts are a theater, then the woman who played the role of a weak, helpless supplicant allowed jurymen to enact a paternalistic, protectionist role and magnanimously pardon the poor female. The few convictions occurred when the woman showed no remorse. Women operating within the expected bounds of their gender were not to be punished, but brazen disregard or denial of their allotted roles brought conviction. Elizabeth Wilson, whose twins died violently and well after birth, who did not confess to infanticide nor plead humbly for mercy from male jurymen, and who instead insisted on her innocence, was convicted of the deaths of her infants and hanged. Circumstances and appropriate behavior were key factors.[21]

The reluctance on the part of jurymen to intervene in the private endeavors of women at childbirth, even when there was suspicion of crime, was part of a tendency to "view female sexual activity as a private matter." This tendency was also apparent in Pennsylvania's failure to adopt the British statute on abortion or to enforce its provisions. Pennsylvania legislators, as was true generally in the colonies, followed English precedent. The English anti-abortion law of 1623 had not been concerned with the fetus before quickening (the point at which the pregnant woman first felt fetal movement, usually in the third, fourth, or fifth month of gestation). Quickening

20. Ibid.; *Laws of the Commonwealth*, I, 113–114; Addison, *Reports*, 8.
21. Bradford, *Enquiry*, 39.

was believed to be the point at which a soul animated the fetus and was a crucial marker for women as well as jurists. A pregnant but unmarried servant was urged by her lover to take an abortifacient well after she would have quickened, but she was shocked and told him, "I might as well go in the bed and kill one of My Masters Childer." She threw the stuff away.[22]

There was a tripartite, schematic view of procreation. Conception, quickening, and birth corresponded to animal life, ensoulment, and reason. Interference in the first stage was outside the scope of the law, interference during the second stage was a misdemeanor, and felony murder charges could only be brought after the death of a live-born child. It was a neat, logical system combining gestational physiology, religious precept, and jurisprudence.

Although abortion itself was rarely prosecuted in the colonies, testimony on abortive practices surfaces incidentally in a small number of criminal cases, most from the seventeenth century. Five occurred in Maryland between 1652 and 1663. There was a case in Rhode Island (1683), two cases in Delaware (1679, 1688), and a few in Pennsylvania (1739, 1757, 1772). A handful of clear cases along with several suspicious cases occurred in Massachusetts. An especially well-documented case exists in Connecticut records (1745). A few have been recovered in Virginia (1635, 1714, 1792), and undoubtedly two or three or more times that number, if all surviving records in all colonies were searched. Yet, despite claims by some twentieth-century lawyers that the English statute on abortion was enforced in the colonies, most of the cases mentioning abortion came before the courts only incidentally during the prosecution of crimes such as infanticide, murder, rape, fornication, adultery, assault, perjury, and slander. Some women were battered in these attempts to end pregnancy. More often medications were employed. The Old World herb savin was most commonly named. The nine mentions of the drug occurred in illicit encounters. Most involved single women, but one married woman, accused of adultery, swore that she took savin as a vermifuge. The court was skeptical of her professed ignorance. Other medications included single mentions of steel powder, gum guaiacum, peppermint, pennyroyal, wormwood, and a combination of pennyroyal, horehound, nip, and marigolds. There was only one case of a surgical abortion that resulted in expulsion of the fetus, but that also, within a month, led to the woman's death, perhaps from septicemia or trauma. Virtually all these attempted abortions were

22. Rowe, "Women's Crime," *PMHB*, CIX (1985), 360, 367; Margaret Kain (1739), quoted in Jack D. Marietta and G. S. Rowe, *Troubled Experiment: Crime and Justice in Pennsylvania, 1682–1800* (Philadelphia, 2006), 86–87. Unmarried women had an interest in carrying the pregnancy to term, since the court might enjoin marriage or at least child support.

failures, although had they succeeded there might have been little public knowledge of the activities that brought those accused into court. It is clear from the surviving depositions at trial that knowledge of the abortive reputations of emmenagogic drugs was widespread among young and old, rich and poor, and, particularly by the eighteenth century, among married and unmarried. There was also a tendency in the very few eighteenth-century cases for women to proclaim that they were taking drugs that accidentally and unintentionally killed the fetus in utero.[23]

What brought these cases into court were not only the often gruesome details of the suspected or attempted abortions in the context of other, usually violent, criminal behavior (particularly rape, battery, and assault) but also the transgression of important social boundaries by the principals. These were not the usual fornicating teenagers. Cross-racial couplings appeared in two cases; another concerned the actions of a Jewish doctor in what was a predominantly Protestant settlement. In addition to racial and religious divides, the lines of social rank, authority, and deference were blurred in many of these cases. Servant women who acted out of their place were targets: some had previously come before the authorities as unruly, and some were involved with their masters. Anne Tayloe was a wealthy woman in a relationship with a substantially poorer man. Nancy Randolph was suspected of an incestuous relationship with her brother-in-law. It was gendered transgressions that particularly brought cases into court. The facts in at least seven cases found that men had forced abortifacients on unwilling women in order to hide evidence of sexual transgression. It was not so much that male sexual

23. Kathleen M. Brown, *Good Wives, Nasty Wenches, and Anxious Patriarchs: Gender, Race, and Power in Colonial Virginia* (Chapel Hill, N.C., 1996), 204, 306–313, 433 n. 38; Craig W. Horle, ed., *Records of the Courts of Sussex County, Delaware, 1677–1710*, 2 vols. (Philadelphia, 1991), I, 610–612, 879; Cornelia Hughes Dayton, "Taking the Trade: Abortion and Gender Relations in an Eighteenth-Century New England Village," *WMQ*, 3d Ser., XLVIII (1991), 19–49; Mary Beth Norton, *Founding Mothers and Fathers: Gendered Power and the Forming of American Society* (New York, 1996), 36–37, 265–268; Marvin N. Olasky, *Abortion Rites: A Social History of Abortion in America* (Washington, D.C., 1992), 20–25; Julia Cherry Spruill, *Women's Life and Work in the Southern Colonies* (1938; rpt. New York, 1972), 325–326; Roger Thompson, *Sex in Middlesex: Popular Mores in a Massachusetts County, 1649–1699* (Amhurst, Mass., 1986), 25–26, 58, 107–108, 182–183; Marietta and Rowe, *Troubled Experiment*, 86, 136; Cynthia A. Kierner, *Scandal at Bizarre: Rumor and Reputation in Jefferson's America* (New York, 2004), 56–57; Joseph W. Dellapenna, "The Historical Case Against Abortion," *Continuity*, X (1989), 73; Clare A. Lyons, *Sex among the Rabble: An Intimate History of Gender and Power in the Age of Revolution, Philadelphia, 1730–1830* (Chapel Hill, N.C., 2006), 97–99. As Lyons has discovered, the 1772 Pennsylvania case was a fraud. A woman and her brother thought that confessing to second trimester abortion would obscure evidence of infanticide. Useful is the full trial record at "The Grosvenor-Sessions Abortion Case, Pomfret, Connecticut, 1742," http://facultystaff.richmond.edu/~aholton/Dayton/index (accessed February 2007).

predation was of judicial concern; the double sexual standard meant that there were few prosecutions of male sexual offenses outside Puritan New England (and even there prosecutions had largely ceased by the early eighteenth century). The anxiety focused on the presumption that men were not normally supposed to meddle in gynecology or obstetrics — this was women's business. Shame, dishonor, and social transgressions offended community norms. Yet, despite the scandal, social anxiety, and revulsion in these cases, there were few convictions, particularly of men. Defendants were acquitted or they fled, sometimes with the connivance of prominent members of the community; they married the plaintiff; or they paid small fines.[24]

That abortion was connected to public discussions of women's menstrual cycles made state interference nearly as offensive to community norms as the presumed crime itself. Other than withdrawal before ejaculation (coitus interruptus), contraceptive techniques were little known in the colonies — probably why there were no laws against contraception. Most of the medicines that women and physicians resorted to in times of trouble were classed as emmenagogues — herbs and minerals that regulated a woman's health by restoring menstruation. These would now be classed as early term abortifacients (see Chapter 5). From the middle of the eighteenth century until the middle decades of the nineteenth, there would be little public interest in regulating the use of medicines, no matter what the circumstances. It was also in this period that birthrates began to decline.

Changing professional understandings of gestation and doctors' rejection of quickening might be a factor in the failure of Pennsylvania (or any other colony) to adopt or to enforce the English statute on abortion. Quickening was increasingly untenable as a distinct developmental stage by the late seventeenth century, at least for those who kept current with the latest developments in the medical literature. Popular belief, even among the well read, however, continued to cling to a staged view of fetal development, as did the contemporary legal and medical categories. Franklin has Polly Baker describe her contribution to the gestation of her children as passive: "the little done by me." Here she / Franklin reflects the ancient belief that a complete homunculus was contained in the sperm and only nurtured in utero. (Women could potentially harm the fetus through their irrational desires; a craving for strawberries, as just one example, was believed to be a possible cause of strawberry birthmarks.) The fictional Baker (whose last name undoubtedly hints at her bun in the oven) adds, "God has been pleased

24. Kierner, *Scandal at Bizarre.*

to add his Divine Skill and admirable Workmanship in the Formation of their Bodies, and crown'd it, by furnishing them with rational and immortal Souls." So women carry the fetus while God operates as an artisan—the Bible often likens God's role in gestation to that of a potter—working in stages from the most basic forming of the clay to the finishing touches: first the body, then the soul, animation, and reason. (The Bible also compares God's involvement to that of a cheese maker, "Hast thou not poured me out as milk, and curdled me like cheese?" [Job 10:10].) Frederick Whitehead referred in his 1795 autobiography to "my flesh and bones which nature collected and operated for my existence before I came forth from [the] womb." He omits God and, like Polly Baker, makes no reference to quickening, but Whitehead preserves the artisanal analogy of fetal development by likening gestation to the construction of a machine, first the assembly of the parts and then motion. Sally Hastings, in her early-nineteenth-century recasting of the creation story, contrasts the void of gestation to the life emerging postpartum:

> The new-made World, deep in its wat'ry bed,
> Formless and void, a dark embryo laid;
>
> . . . .
>
> The fields and meadows struggled into birth—
> God call'd the waters Sea—the dry-land Earth.

Just as Adam was first given a clay form by God, and only later had life breathed in, various popular, classical, and biblical models of gestational stages and birth prevailed in the eighteenth century.[25]

More detailed understandings of fetal development appeared by the nineteenth century. In 1832, Dr. William Dewees, the leading expert in the new field of obstetrics, rejected traditional understandings of gestation and insisted that "the latest information upon this subject [the development of the fetus] will almost necessarily be the best." He insisted that the stages of pregnancy can "only be elucidated by the experienced practitioner of midwifery," meaning medical doctors. Women, even midwives, were no longer to be consulted as the experts in gynecology, which is one reason that by this time juries of women were less and less likely to be impaneled. Man-

25. Hall, *Benjamin Franklin and Polly Baker*, 165; Susan E. Klepp, Farley Grubb, and Anne Pfaeltzer de Ortiz, eds., *Souls for Sale: Two German Redemptioners Come to Revolutionary America* (University Park, Pa., 2006), 115; Sally Hastings, "A Paraphrase of the First Chapter of the Book of Genesis," *Poems on Different Subjects to Which Is Added, a Descriptive Account of a Family Tour to the West* (Lancaster, Pa., 1808), 135–136.

midwives, who were presumed to be well-trained specialists, were the repositories of exact knowledge. Dewees discussed fetal development by quoting at length from his conversations with the unnamed author of a text on medical jurisprudence. According to the combined wisdom of these two experts, in the first two weeks the "produce of conception appears only as a gelatinous, semitransparent, flocculent mass, of a grayish colour, liquefying promptly, and presenting no distinct formation." At one month, the embryo is the size of "a large ant." At six or seven weeks, it is "equal in size to a small bee." Insect metaphors dominate the discussion of the first trimester. In the fourth month, the "external parts all develope themselves, with the exception of the hair and nails." The "brain is pulpy" in the fifth month, when the mother begins to feel movement. In the sixth month, the brain of the fetus "acquires more consistence, but is still easily dissolved." Sexual organs have developed. So in the second trimester the outward form takes shape, but the internal organs remain underdeveloped or nonexistent. Only in the seventh month does the brain begin to furrow and do the nails and eyes fully develop. It is finally in the ninth month that "the digestive apparatus, the heart, and the lungs, are in a state fit to commence extra-uterine life." Quickening no longer signaled a distinct stage in fetal development, but distinct stages persisted in popular and professional understandings of pregnancy. Full-term birth differentiated the incomplete fetus from completely developed humanity. This more complex understanding of gestation brought little or no change in the law. It would not be until the mid- to late nineteenth century that the legal status of abortion and contraception would change under a variety of social, professional, and religious pressures.[26]

Sex and Sexuality and the Law: Colonial and Metropolitan

William Penn and the early members of the Pennsylvania Assembly did their best to eliminate what they considered the worst features of a corrupt Old World. The "offenses against God" that promoted "wildness and looseness" were to be strictly prohibited. The foundational law code of 1682 forbade "swearing, cursing, lying, profane talking, drunkenness, drinking of healths, obscene words, incest, sodomy, rapes, whoredom, fornication, and other uncleanness (not to be repeated)" as well as "all prizes, stage plays, cards, dice, May games, gamesters, masques, revels, bull-baitings, cock-fightings, bear-

26. William P. Dewees, *A Compendious System of Midwifery, Chiefly Designed to Facilitate the Inquiries of Those Who May Be Pursuing This Branch of Study* (Philadelphia, 1832), 79, 81, 89.

baitings, and the like, which excite the people to rudeness, cruelty, looseness, and irreligion." Both the deviant act and the opportunity for sexual sin were forbidden. Yet just a generation later a popular almanac published this ribald ditty:

> The Weather's hot, days burning eye
> Doth make the earth in favour frye.
> *Dick* on the Hay doth tumble *Nell*,
> Whereby her Belly comes to swell.
> The Dog star now we hot do find,
> And some have Dog tricks in their mind.

Attitudes on sexuality were complex and contradictory but underlay contemporary views on marriage, childbearing, contraception, abortion, and family size.[27]

Popular and legal judgments of sexual activity were evolving over the course of the eighteenth century. Scholars currently offer widely differing assessments of sexual expression in the early Mid-Atlantic region. One view is that there was a Quaker-inspired pall of repressive asexuality; another view finds an expanding "pleasure culture," at least in Philadelphia. Since actual behavior, especially normative sexual expression, was little recorded, historians have looked at ideals, images, proscription, and prosecution for attitudes on sexuality. The colonial context of morals legislation throws some light on contemporary attitudes.[28]

Pennsylvania's Holy Experiment under Quaker rule was designed to eliminate the corruptions of the Old World. Certainly, colonial cities were not London. Sexuality saturates the visual images of Hogarth's London and reflects a general, if perhaps middling-sort, view of the dangers of urban life. Teeming London with some seven hundred thousand inhabitants in the early eighteenth century supported taverns, theaters, concert halls, molly houses, masquerades, places of assignation, and fashionable and popular resorts, especially Vauxhall Gardens. A multitude of meeting places provided

27. Jean R. Soderlund, ed., *William Penn and the Founding of Pennsylvania, 1680–1684: A Documentary History* (Philadelphia, 1983), 132 (see also 250–252); David H. Flahery, "Law and the Enforcement of Morals in Early America," in Donald Fleming and Bernard Bailyn, eds., *Law in American History* (Boston, 1971), 203–253; Leeds, *American Almanack*, n.p.

28. David Hackett Fischer, *Albion's Seed: Four British Folkways in America* (New York, 1989), 498–502, argues that the sexual asceticism of Quakers and German Pietists influenced "the official culture" of the Philadelphia region. Clare A. Lyons finds an urban pleasure culture emerging in the second half of the eighteenth century that freed sexual expression from traditional restraints (*Sex among the Rabble*).

anonymity and spaces where like-minded individuals might meet discreetly or openly depending on opportunity and inclination. Salacious prints, scatological cartoons, bawdy song sheets, and guides to local whorehouses graced the windows of print shops for all to observe. Prostitution was highly specialized as well as highly visible. Advertisements for condoms, for patent cures for venereal disease, and for discreet establishments for pregnant women appeared in newspapers. Sex was not only visible; it was commercialized.[29]

The supervision of morals was only beginning to be transferred from the church courts to the state in England, but neither church nor state could effectively police morality in a city the size of London, even if there had been a consensus on sexual propriety. Whether London was in fact more libertine or liberated than the rest of England is unknown. But the popular image was of urban decadence. This construction was in part predicated on pastoral fantasies of an innocent countryside peopled by ethereal shepherds and shepherdesses and in part on enlightened and early Romantic notions of noble primitives, those sturdy and hardy British yeomen living natural, healthy, productive lives in quaint rural villages. In contrast, the city's overcivilized fops, eviscerated clerks and writers, harried businessmen, and frivolous women of fashion and fortune assiduously and pointlessly cultivated artificial manners and absurd fads. They were the prime sources of decay and parasitism. Illicit and unnatural sexuality must, therefore, by these assumptions, be urban. Still, reputation need not be reality. John Gillis, looking at the large numbers of bound servants and apprentices living and working under a master's control and forbidden to marry, has called London the "celibate city" in the early part of the eighteenth century.[30]

By comparison to both the reality and the reputation of the English metropolis, Philadelphia through much of the eighteenth century was a very small town, provincial in its placement on the western edge of empire and rusticated in its lack of entertaining amenities. Pennsylvania's elite, such as it was, was far more concerned with upholding conventional Christian views of sexuality than England's far wealthier, more leisured, more pampered, and very powerful aristocracy. There would be no established church or officially sanctioned church courts in Pennsylvania to supervise morals, but there would be an expanded role for the state as moral watchdog.

Unlike secular courts, church courts could order neither corporal punish-

29. Sean Shesgreen, ed., *Engravings by Hogarth: 101 Prints* (New York, 1973), 18–24, 28–36; Roy Porter, *English Society in the Eighteenth Century* (London, 1982).

30. John R. Gillis, *For Better, for Worse: British Marriages, 1600 to the Present* (New York, 1985), 161–169.

ment nor confinement. Pennsylvania legislators, by placing morals offenses in the colonial courts, could, in theory, rely on both sectarian and secular supervision of sexual behavior. The history of the adultery law provides one example of Pennsylvania's attempt to legislate sexual morality. According to the 1682 law, a convicted adulterer was to be publicly whipped and imprisoned at hard labor for a year for a first offense: "to the behoof of the public." A second conviction brought life imprisonment—repetition indicated a corrupt individual best removed from society. The law was intended both to punish offenders and to educate the first-time perpetrator as well as the general public on the consequences of sexual immorality.[31]

In 1700, the Pennsylvania Assembly attempted to conflate fornication and adultery as equally heinous crimes, but this was overturned on review in England. After 1705/6, a first-time adulterer could be fined fifty pounds or whipped. A second offense could bring twenty-one lashes, seven years of hard labor, a fine of one hundred pounds, or branding on the forehead with the letter *A*. In addition, the aggrieved party could sue for divorce from bed and board, a stipulation indicating the legislature assumed most adulterers would be men and that their wives would want a legal separation and require financial support. After 1725/6, if the adultery involved interracial intercourse, a free person of African descent would be sold for seven years. The adultery law was harsh, even by eighteenth-century standards. The county courts of the seventeenth century document the prosecution of sex crimes, although it appears that wayward husbands and wives were more likely to be tried under the fornication laws than under the harsher adultery laws. Pennsylvania accused 188 people, mostly women, of adultery between the 1690s and 1790s and 664 of fornication, increasingly men. So, despite the assumption that most adulterers would be men, it was unfaithful women who were hauled into court. Men, married or not, were more likely to be charged with fornication. Conviction of fornication did not allow wives to sue for support through a divorce.[32]

31. Staughton George, Benjamin M. Nead, and Thomas McCamant, eds., *Charter to William Penn and Laws of the Province of Pennsylvania, Passed between 1682 and 1700, Preceded by the Duke of York's Laws in Force from the Year 1676 to the Year 1682 with an Appendix Containing Laws Relating to the Organization of the Provincial Courts and Historical Matter* (Harrisburg, Pa., 1879), 109.

32. Ibid.; James T. Mitchell and Henry Flanders, eds., *The Statutes at Large of Pennsylvania from 1700 to 1805*, II–XVII (Harrisburg, Pa., 1896–1915), II, 180, XIV, 133–134. On church courts, see Paul Hair, ed., *Before the Bawdy Court: Selections from Church Court and Other Records relating to the Correction of Moral Offences in England, Scotland, and New England, 1300–1800* (New York, 1972). Colonial Pennsylvania—predominantly Philadelphia—was much more likely to prosecute crimes against the person than were London and Middlesex County in England. In Pennsylvania before

Pennsylvania also punished other deviations from proper family order, even those not specifically named in the legal code. On the day after Christmas 1702, four cross-dressers—two men and two married women—went cavorting from door to door in Philadelphia and then danced and reveled at a tavern. They were presented by the grand jury and bound for trial. The foreman was appalled at the behavior of the men, "it being against the Law of God, the Law of this province and the Law of nature . . . and Incoridging of wickednes in this place," but excoriated one woman in particular for acting "contrary to the nature of her sects [sex], . . . to the grate disturbance of well minded persons, and in Coridging vice in this place . . . and other Like in ormities." Although few court records survive for early Philadelphia, it is certain that the local governments intended to eradicate sexual misconduct to defend the orderly patriarchal household. Men, and only men, should wear the pants.[33]

In addition to an expanded legal apparatus for the prosecution of morals offenses, Philadelphia offered few of the venues for assignation that London boasted. Taverns were unspecialized and served heterogeneous, although mostly male, populations. There were no public gardens, and even in the mid-eighteenth century there were few concerts, circuses, or theatrical performances. There was no demimonde in provincial Philadelphia. Elite women lived apparently virtuous lives around the tea table and, if Quaker, at the meetinghouse; or, if Anglican or Presbyterian, also at private dances and balls. But even the dances and balls were closely supervised, and admittance was by invitation only. Propriety seems to have reigned.[34]

---

the 1780s, between 20 and 30 percent of all convictions were for felonious crimes against the person (rather than against property); in London, it was less than 10 percent. The chances of proving one's innocence in accusations of rape, bestiality, sodomy, and other morals felonies were substantially lower in Pennsylvania. Of those charged with felonies, between 40 and 50 percent were convicted in Pennsylvania, compared to fewer than 15 percent in London. These imperfect statistics, which do not cover lesser charges or provide useful categories of accusations, do indicate the greater effort by the colony to prosecute and convict suspected criminals. Pennsylvania data for 1683–1775 is in Gipson, *Crime*, 10–12; for 1779–1792 and 1794–1815, see Philadelphia Society for Alleviating the Miseries of Public Prisons, *A Statistical View of the Operation of the Penal Code of Pennsylvania* . . . (Philadelphia, 1817), 8–9, 13. London and Middlesex data for 1689–1804 is in Great Britain, Parliament, House of Commons, *Report from the Select Committee on Criminal Laws* . . . (London, 1819), 146–163, 166. See also Horle, ed., *Records of the Courts of Sussex County, Delaware*, I, 17–19. Sussex County was under the control of Pennsylvania until 1704 and followed Pennsylvania law for several years thereafter (Marietta and Rowe, *Troubled Experiment*, table 2.4, 41, 87, 202–203).

33. Craig W. Horle, ed., "Ancient Records of Philadelphia," *Pennsylvania Genealogical Magazine*, XXXV (1987–1988), 220–222.

34. Peter Thompson, *Rum Punch and Revolution: Taverngoing and Public Life in Eighteenth-*

If illicit sexuality was to be regulated by state supervision, marital sexuality was unleashed from its Old World constraints. Marriage ages for both women and men were earlier in all the colonies than in the Old World. Birthrates soared. Celibacy was a rarity, and reproduction was celebrated. Eliza Stedman reported, "Mrs Smith taking under consideration that Mr. [John] Penn was a very good Freiend of her husband it was her duty as a return to add one more to his province." Smith was going to make sure she was impregnated as soon as possible—another young citizen would be a boon to the colony and to her husband's friend, the governor. Sexuality was visible everywhere and laughingly promoted, but it was not the extramarital, commercialized sex of London.[35]

But surface impressions of the triumph of married sex can be deceptive, and the efforts of early legislators to govern private morality often came to naught. Their attempts to constrain extramarital behaviors ran into the realities of early Philadelphia. The city might have been small and unsophisticated, but it was an important port in a wide Atlantic world. An anonymous flux of sailors, immigrants, and travelers passed in and out of the provinces and mingled with the resident population. These men and women helped create demands for illicit as well as licensed taverns and supported prostitution and other "riotous" behaviors. In 1685, Joseph Knight was among the first of many to be presented to the grand jury for allowing drunkenness and "evil orders" in his house. Philadelphians tried in vain to prevent the "riott and tumultuous manner" of the gatherings of the enslaved and worried about European "heathens" and ne'er-do-wells flooding the colonies.[36]

Little is known about the early history of prostitution in the city (too few of the early court records survive), but it undoubtedly flourished as Philadelphia expanded, even if theaters, pleasure gardens, and other public places of assignation did not yet exist. Benjamin Franklin certainly had no trouble finding "low Women that"—it just so happened—"fell in [his] Way." Philadelphia was also a frontier town that attracted the riffraff of the Empire,

---

Century Philadelphia (Philadelphia, 1999); Lynn Matluck Brooks, "Emblem of Gaiety, Love, and Legislation: Dance in Eighteenth-Century Philadelphia," *PMHB*, CXV (1991), 63–88; Karin Wulf, *Not All Wives: Women of Colonial Philadelphia* (Ithaca, N.Y., 2000), 53–84.

35. Stedman to Graeme, Dec. 16, 1764, in Gratz, ed., "Some Material for a Biography of Mrs. Elizabeth Fergusson," *PMHB*, XXXIX (1915), 277.

36. John F. Watson, *Annals of Philadelphia, and Pennsylvania, in the Olden Time* (Philadelphia, 1899), I, 171; Gary B. Nash, *Forging Freedom: The Formation of Philadelphia's Black Community, 1720–1840* (Cambridge, Mass., 1988), 14; Horle, "Ancient Records," *Pennsylvania Genealogical Magazine*, XXXV (1987–1988), 220–222.

or, as Gottlieb Mittelberger put it, a "gathering place for all runaway good-for-nothings"—some well-to-do individuals with shady pasts, some people temporarily down on their luck, some impoverished men and women—who were seeking to escape their reputations, their misdeeds, or their spouses. Deborah Read Franklin was only one of many bigamists in the city. Newspapers were filled with advertisements announcing runaway wives, and, to a lesser extent, absconding husbands. Marriage was not the permanent institution it would later become, especially for those below the level of the elite. Colonial Philadelphia was, in many respects, an ungovernable city.[37]

The decision of the founders to abolish church courts in the name of both religious liberty and a strengthened secular authority made the enforcement of morality doubly difficult. The state could impose harsher punishments on offenders than could church courts, it is true, but the secular courts did not have the latitude of the church courts in ferreting out criminal behavior. There was no police force to funnel cases into the secular courts in either the city or country. The Anglican Church courts in England could actively seek out offenders, and mere reputation might serve as proof of guilt in those religious hearings. The colony could only discover offenses when there was a complaint from a private citizen. Secular courts required witnesses, evidence. The accused could hire lawyers. Much of the legally and religiously unacceptable sexual behavior thus escaped prosecution.

Between 1682 and the 1720s, the colony of Pennsylvania wrote and rewrote its laws on sexual morality at least four times from a sense of failure, always moving in the direction of harsher and presumably more effective punishment. After the 1720s, Philadelphians largely abandoned the prosecution of morals offenses, although this was not the case in the outlying counties, particularly heavily Pietist, Quaker, and German areas. Mittelberger thought that "fornication as such . . . is not punished," and the court records bear out his observation. According to the work of Gail Rowe, there was only one fornication or bastardy charge brought against a Philadelphia woman between 1763 and 1775, and she was not convicted. In the rural portions of Philadelphia County, there were thirty-six accused women in the same time period, and in nearby Bucks County, ninety-eight. Yet between 2 and 3 percent of married couples in the city are known to have had their first child out of wedlock, and an unknown number of other bastards were never legitimated

37. Leo Lemay and P. M. Zall, eds., *Benjamin Franklin's Autobiography: An Authoritative Text* (New York, 1986), 56; Gottlieb Mittelberger, *Journey to Pennsylvania*, ed. Oscar Handlin and John Clive (Cambridge, Mass., 1960), 70.

by the marriage of their parents. The sexual sins of the city went unpunished while rural districts attempted to enforce the law, although the actual incidence of illegitimacy is unknown. The diary of Joseph Price in Montgomery County, a sometime overseer of the poor, suggests that criminal prosecution of bastard bearers was spotty in the late eighteenth century.[38]

For all the strangeness that the multiethnic, multiracial city presented, Philadelphia did not fall into the same category of sexual danger as London, in part because of the apparent moral probity of those in power. But it was also because the countryside was perceived to be more dangerous than the city. With fewer churches or schools and even less government, the hinterlands were as profane and lawless as any place in the Western world. Heterodox sects—the Woman in the Wilderness, the Moravians, the Ephrata Cloister with its charismatic leader, and many, many others—experimented with new forms of celibacy, marriage, and sexuality. A woman calling herself Mary the Abbess lived in Berks County as head of a household of three women. Maria DeTurk joined the New-Born sect, a group of German immigrants who rejected the church, the Bible, and the sacraments as earthly instruments of the devil. DeTurk claimed not only that she had been reborn free of sin but that, whatever she might do in the future, "I cannot sin any more." These and other unorthodox beliefs drew the curious and inspired wild rumors of debauchery and promiscuity from more mainstream critics of these radical religions.[39]

Rural areas were constantly in danger of drifting, not toward bucolic pastoralism, but toward uncivilized barbarism, in particular toward the "wild Indian." Said Mittelberger, "Young people especially grow up like Indians or savages." He saw unmarried men dressed in hides on May Day, calling themselves Indians while carousing with single women. A decade earlier, a British diplomat was horrified at the sight of rural Pennsylvania women who "danced wilder time than any Indians." A newly ordained minister thought

38. Mittelberger, *Journey*, ed. Handlin and Clive, 70; Rowe, "Women's Crime," *PMHB*, CIX (1985), 335–368; Marietta and Rowe, *Troubled Experiment*, 119; Susan E. Klepp, *Philadelphia in Transition: A Demographic History of the City and Its Occupational Groups, 1720–1830* (New York, 1989), 87; Joseph Price Diary, Lower Merion Historical Society, http://www.lowermerionhistory.org/texts/price (see Note 18 for examples).

39. United States, Bureau of the Census, *Heads of Families at the First Census of the United States Taken in the Year 1790: Pennsylvania* (Washington, D.C., 1908), 33; William T. Parsons, ed., *Mountain Mary Legends* (Collegeville, Pa., 1989). DeTurk's letter to family in Germany is translated in P. C. Croll, *Annals of the Oley Valley in Berks County, Pennsylvania: Over Two Hundred Years of Local History of an American Canaan* (Reading, Pa., 1926), 18.

western settlers as "barbarous, clownish, and ungospelized as the Indians." The colonial city was an outpost of civility, not a wen of sexual depravity.[40]

The Revolutionary War helped alter perceptions of sexuality. Many Philadelphians were shocked by the behavior of British officers during the 1777–1778 occupation of the city. The officers' encouragement of foreign, aristocratic liberties among local elite women called forth condemnation. A Quaker woman warned in meeting, "Women and girls are said to be exchanging visits with these warriors. . . . Some have made so light of their shame that they stroll about with these people in broad daylight. . . . These people have a wandering foot, . . . you cannot prosecute them under our laws when your daughters go too far." The unnamed preacher assumed that parents could exercise some control over young women, although this was doubtful in the face of the enticements offered. Becky Franks was one of several women who flaunted their independence. She urged a married friend to embrace the "gay life" and promised her "rakeing as much as you choose," while she bragged that she was "engaged [to dance that evening] to seven different gentlemen." These flirtatious women who passed from man to man at balls offended Philadelphians, particularly poorer Philadelphians and radicals.[41]

Both during and after the war, there were powerful reactions to wartime libertinism. Street theater by enlisted men attempted to humiliate the elite women who adopted British aristocratic manners by labeling them whores, bawds, and strumpets. There were raids on whorehouses in the city and countryside. Later, balls were strictly regulated, according to the marquis de Chastellux, so that at dances as in marriage "each lady [has] a partner, with whom she dances the whole evening without being allowed to take another." Monogamous behavior was promoted, at least for women.[42]

A new criminal code evolved in Pennsylvania after the Revolution that abandoned colonial efforts to protect the marriage bond. Instead, legislators tried to enforce female purity. In 1794, when all capital punishments were

40. Mittelberger, *Journey*. ed. Handlin and Clive, 80, 85; Brooks, "Dance in Eighteenth-Century Philadelphia," *PMHB*, CXV (1991), 69; F. Alan Palmer, ed., *The Beloved Cohansie of Philip Vickers Fithian* (Cumberland County, N.J., n.d.), 277.

41. Johann Ewald, *Diary of the American War*, trans. and ed. Joseph P. Tustin (New Haven, Conn., 1979), 118; Jacob R. Marcus, *The American Jewish Women: A Documentary History* (New York, 1981), 16.

42. Susan E. Klepp, "Rough Music on Independence Day: Philadelphia, 1778," in William Pencak, Matthew Dennis, and Simon P. Newman, eds., *Riot and Revelry in Early America* (University Park, Pa., 2002), 156–178; the marquis de Chastellux, quoted in Brooks, "Dance in Eighteenth-Century Philadelphia," *PMHB*, CXV (1991), 78.

abolished except in cases of treason and first-degree murder, conviction of rape brought the harshest penalty, ten to twenty-one years in the penitentiary, whereas the sentence for second-degree murder, next in severity, was five to eighteen years. The forcible loss of female sexual virtue was construed as intermediate between first- and second-degree murder, so the destruction of a woman's sexual respectability was the same as her death. Even married women had to meet an exceptionally rigid standard of sexual innocence. The divorce law of 1786 gave innocent wives protection from bigamists, adulterers, deserters, and wife beaters so long as they did not admit "the defendant into conjugal society or embraces" after learning of their husbands' transgressions. Sexual relations with impure husbands would have tarnished innocent wives. How these wives — still femes covert — might refuse their husbands was not considered. The divorce law also stipulated that any adulterous woman who moved in with her lover after a divorce would be declared legally dead. To partake of the benefits of the divorce law, women had to remain pure, with female purity defined entirely in sexual terms. The protection of female purity could even trump patriarchy and parental rights by the early nineteenth century: "In general a father is entitled to the custody of his children. But where both the father and mother are persons of immoral character, the court may order a *female child* to be delivered to a third person." By the 1850s, women would automatically gain custody of their children as the more moral caretakers. The morals laws in Pennsylvania had shifted from a defense of marriage and its channeling of sexuality to a defense of female sexual innocence. The shift is also apparent in the iconography of women's portraits. Philadelphia even began prosecuting women for fornication and bastardy in the 1780s. Fifteen women were hauled into court, more than in some of the older counties in the commonwealth.[43]

After the mid-eighteenth century, the spread of evangelical religions and republican ideals renewed attacks on debauchery and stressed self-control, marriage, and a certain degree of sentimentality — paralleling the redefinitions of fertility occurring at the same time. Respectability became a goal, particularly attracting large segments of the middling and working classes. One outward measure of respectability would be a small family — a visible sign of sexual restraint. The very chatty registers at Philadelphia's Gloria Dei

43. Mitchell and Flanders, eds., *Statutes at Large*, XIV, 175–176; Thomas I. Wharton, *A Digest of the Reported Cases Adjudged in the Several Courts Held in Pennsylvania . . .* , 4th ed., 2 vols. (Philadelphia, 1843), II, 3 (emphasis added). See Ruth H. Bloch, *Gender and Morality in Anglo-American Culture, 1650–1800* (Berkeley, Calif., 2003); Michael Grossberg, *Governing the Hearth: Law and the Family in Nineteenth-Century America* (Chapel Hill, N.C., 1985).

Lutheran Church between 1790 and 1830 are filled with supplicants looking for antedated marriage certificates to cover premarital intercourse, quick
marriages to save reputations, and false marriage certificates to gain entrance
into inns, suggesting both the force of new standards of decorum and the
difficulty many people had in complying with those more rigid standards.
The incidence of premarital pregnancy was half of what it was in the early
colonial period, and more bastards were apparently being legitimated by the
eventual marriage of their parents. The advertisements for runaway wives or
absent husbands that filled newspapers in the earlier period tapered off in
the nineteenth century, certainly because advertising noncompliance with
new standards was unacceptable, not respectable, and perhaps because marriages had become less flexible, trapping abused or just unhappy spouses
in miserable unions. The new romanticism, placing the emotional over the
physical, seems to have restrained manners. Bowdlerism began shaping both
the language and the publications of educated, respectable, and religious
readers, although salacious publications proliferated in cheap print forms.
Novels, in particular, warned against seduction and flirtation, albeit while
giving lessons in immodest deportment. Cheap religious tracts spread a doctrine of self-control. Sexuality was being constricted, especially before and
during marriage. Two men, a Quaker and a Shaker, agreed in the 1790s "to
marry but not to go into her but for propagation." But this was only one
view.[44]

If women were ideally sexually innocent after the Revolution, then some
interpreted men's sexuality as both naturalized and ungovernable. Judge
William Bradford thought that rape was "the sudden abuse of a natural
passion," caused by a "phrenzy of desire," but it did not indicate "any ir-
reclaimable corruption" in the rapist. Adultery, according to Judge Jacob
Rush, was the consequence of "the pleasure resulting from sensual indulgence, and the strength of temptation, arising, perhaps, from some constitutional bias." Male sexuality was reconfigured as both innate and essentially ungovernable. The adultery law, once so harsh, was reduced to a fine
not exceeding fifty pounds and the possibility of less than a year in prison.
There was no longer any attempt to educate either the perpetrator or the
public with harsher punishment for a second offense. The crime of sodomy,
too, was made noncapital, on the grounds that it was, in Bradford's words,

---

44. Susan E. Klepp and Billy G. Smith, "The Records of Gloria Dei Church: Marriages and 'Remarkable Occurrances,' 1794–1806," *Pennsylvania History*, LIII (1986), 125–151; Joshua Evans Journal, Sept. 28, 1795, quoted in Fischer, *Albion's Seed*, 500.

"dangerous" to "blindly" follow "Mosaical institutions." "Laws might have been proper for a tribe of ardent barbarians wandering through the lands of Arabia, which are wholly unfit for an enlightened people of civilized and gentle manners." Men's sexuality could be contained neither by law nor by religion but should be heterosexual or patriarchal: there was a feeble upsurge in sodomy prosecutions during and after the 1780s.[45]

The newly entrenched double standard was accompanied by a more public commercialization of sex in the city. By the 1790s, the growth of the city and the development of ideas of social exclusivity produced specialized taverns and brothels. By the 1830s and 1840s, there were published guides to local bawdy houses as well as slightly risqué publications like "Philadelphia by Slices," a series of cynical descriptions of the underside of the city. Crime stories and scandalous exposés countered the respectable and moralistic publications of literary and religious groups. Circuses, beer gardens, pleasure gardens, public dances, hotels, theaters, and other places of entertainment provided spaces to meet. There was an emergent demimonde as well, particularly during and after the 1790s, influenced both by British models and by ideological defenses of free love coming from France. Radical artisans like John Fitch set up irregular ménages à trois. Prominent merchant Stephen Girard openly lived with his mistress (after incarcerating his wife). Handsome daughters of downwardly mobile fathers held on to their former economic status by accepting valuable gifts from wealthy lovers.[46]

If married women were to be innocent, virtuous femes covert, and men were ungovernable but in control of the cash, then a separate world of commercial sexuality was, not too surprisingly, an adjunct to the new sexual system. "A woman in society must either be a mistress or a wife," wrote Thomas P. Cope in 1800 after forcing his wife to have sex. And a wife should take care to "anticipate [her husband's] wishes, administer to his best principles and even to his foibles." If she does not, Cope warned, he will surely seek "unworthy indulgences abroad." Not all men agreed with Cope's

45. Jacob Rush, *Charges, and Extracts of Charges, on Moral and Religious Subjects* . . . (Lenox, Mass., 1815), 98; Bradford, *Enquiry*, 21, 29.

46. George Rogers Taylor, ed., "'Philadelphia by Slices,' by George G. Foster," *PMHB*, XCIII (1969), 23–72; Susan Branson, *Dangerous to Know: Women, Crime, and Notoriety in the Early Republic* (Philadelphia, 2008); Prager, ed., *Autobiography of John Fitch*, APS, *Memoirs*, CXIII (1976), 124–129; Harry Emerson Wildes, *Lonely Midas: The Story of Stephen Girard* (New York, 1943), 85–89, 132–138. Public spaces were also political spaces, both open to all and selective: Thompson, *Rum Punch and Revolution*, esp. 182–185, 197–198; David Waldstreicher, *In the Midst of Perpetual Fetes: The Making of American Nationalism, 1776–1820* (Chapel Hill, N.C., 1997), esp. 78, 158.

purely sexualized vision of womanhood. The editor of the *Port-Folio* magazine argued that his wife should "not merely fill his bed" (although this was obviously a prime consideration), but, echoing earlier women's protests, she should be more than "a washing, baking, brewing, spinning, sewing, darning and child-producing *animal.*" Women could and should be entertaining, rational companions.[47]

Women were given contradictory messages. They were to be multifaceted, virtuous, pure, restrained, self-controlled, and asexual, but they were also to marry for love and stoke the fires of passion or lose their husbands to less reputable women. Contraception allowed both self-control and passion to coexist, and birthrates began to decline.

By the middle of the eighteenth century and into the nineteenth, evangelicalism and republicanism both stressed self-control in the service of the greater good. New ideas about freedom, masculine prerogatives, and sexual expressiveness further incorporated sexual preferences into personal identity. Loving, companionate marriages might unleash sexuality, but a desire for fewer children might favor sexual repression. In all these shifts, the clear trend seems to have been the further separation of sexuality from procreation, with a growing emphasis on comfort and pleasure, at least for men. Attempts to ensure the strength of the family unit in colonial Pennsylvania were replaced by laws designed to protect the imaginary sexual innocence of women. More than ever a double standard prevailed by the early national period. Obstetricians believed themselves more knowledgeable about female anatomy than midwives; men were casting off shame, and it was now women who were supposed to be ashamed of their bodily functions.

Legislators and jurists in the eighteenth century were little interested in regulating male sexuality or the childbearing patterns of married couples. Bastard bearers, adulterers, and fornicators only fitfully aroused the interest of the authorities. Most men were still embarrassed if required to pay public attention to gynecological matters—a state of affairs that was beginning to change at the end of the eighteenth century. Even physicians exhibited extreme discomfort well into the nineteenth century. The chair of midwifery at the University of Pennsylvania's medical school, Thomas Chalkley James, would blush and avoid looking at his students during obstetrical lectures so that it was "painful [for students] to witness his embarrassment." His suc-

47. Eliza Cope Harrison, *Philadelphia Merchant: The Diary of Thomas P. Cope, 1800–1851* (South Bend, Ind., 1978), 46–48; "Supplement to the Port Folio for July 1810, Female Education," *Port-Folio,* IV, no. 1 (July 1810), 85, 86.

cessor in 1834, William Potts Dewees, was far more self-confident and asserted his authority in matters of obstetrics: "No blush suffused his cheek in the lecture-room," recalled a student. Still, his patient's uterus remained "a forbidden territory." Taboos and embarrassment were deeply entrenched in the culture, continuing to limit legal and medical interference in the private actions of most individuals.[48]

State and federal governments were committed to population growth. They promoted policies that expanded the boundaries of the United States, encouraged access to the resources that promoted marriage among residents, and welcomed immigrants from Europe. But officials and physicians did not express any interest in promoting some vision of appropriate family size, even as preferences for "small" families began saturating common discourse. Doctors, by the early decades of the nineteenth century, were just beginning to expand their practices to include obstetrics and gynecology, but women usually decided if and when to employ a doctor. In the countryside, midwifery persisted. Family size, contraception, and abortion were of little interest to male government officials and of gradually developing interest to physicians in the colonial and early national periods. The state, the medical profession, and religious leaders largely left families—that is women in families—alone. It was a brief hiatus between the moral policing that had prevailed in the seventeenth century and the anxieties that would reemerge in the middle of the nineteenth—most spectacularly in the Comstock Law of 1873. There was a power vacuum accompanying the upheavals of the second half of the eighteenth century that allowed women, particularly when inspired by the rights talk of the Revolution, to translate political liberty into a revolutionary reimagining of the meanings attached to body, sex, gestation, birth, and birth control and then to put these new ideals into action.

48. Samuel Weissell Gross and Albert Haller Gross, eds., *The Autobiography of Samuel D. Gross*, 2 vols. (Philadelphia, 1887), II, 240, 247, 248.

7

Reluctant Revolutionaries

"I should be not a little surp⬚⬚⬚⬚⬚⬚⬚⬚⬚⬚⬚⬚⬚⬚⬚⬚iscussion of women's rights, "to hear of a ⬚⬚⬚⬚⬚⬚⬚⬚⬚⬚⬚⬚⬚⬚⬚president or senator. It would be hard to restrain a smile to ⬚⬚⬚⬚⬚⬚a popular assembly to discuss some mighty topic." This character, although imaginary, expressed a common belief, common even among radicals, that there were limits to human rights and individual freedoms. All men might have been *created* equal, but they assuredly did not remain equal. Women were almost certainly excluded. A politically active woman could only be ridiculous, laughable, and out of her proper sphere. Nothing she said on the issues of the day could be taken seriously. "I should gaze [at her] as [if] at a prodigy," the young man continued, "and listen with a doubting heart: yet I might not refuse devotion to the same woman in the character of household deity." The egalitarian impulses of the Revolution could be stretched only so far. Women's options should be severely restricted to a few strictly domestic roles. "As a mother, pressing a charming babe to her bosom; as my companion in the paths of love, or poetry, or science; as partaker with me in content[edness], and an elegant sufficiency, her dignity would shine forth in full splendour. Here all would be decency and grace." Women, at least decent women, stood by their men, bearing their babies and keeping their houses. "These emotions," concluded the man, "I should not pretend to justify; but such, and so difficult to vanquish, is prejudice." Not everyone could or would support the transformations involved when couples decided to restrict fertility. Prejudice had deep roots and not just in fiction.[1]

The events of the late eighteenth century were social as well as political upheavals and caused Americans to reassess old habits of mind and to consider new ideas. Independence and a rejection of "slavish" behaviors had challenged and begun to undermine inherited rigid social ranks and roles for women as well as for men. The revolutionary moment was not always supported, nor could enthusiasm for change always be sustained. New Jersey had been the only state to grant single or widowed propertyowning women the vote, an experiment that ended in 1807. In that year, the embarrassed legislature disenfranchised women of all races and African American men, claiming that "the safety, quiet, good order and dignity of the state" were threatened by the appearance of female and African American voters at the polls. Attitudes had hardened.[2]

The protests and warfare that produced thirteen independent republics neither solved the question of who would rule at home nor determined how far the guarantees of liberty should extend. Fractiousness, not unity, prevailed. Women did not differ from men in their conflicting allegiances. Not all women or men embraced new ideas about family size and women's options in marriage. Family limitation might have been difficult either practically or conceptually for some. Statistics show that in some places birthrates rebounded in the 1780s or 1790s even if the overall trajectory was downward. Some women or men rejected family limitation and its myriad unsettling meanings for marriage, parenthood, and self-definition. Still others sought to make the new standards of small family size less revolutionary, less egalitarian, less disruptive of contemporary assumptions.

Practically, given the limitations of available birth-control technology and the tug of tradition and duty, comparatively few women managed to achieve the family size they desired. Elizabeth Bayley Seton, who in the early years of her marriage "so dearly love[d] quiet and a small Family," subsequently had to "reconcile every decree of Fate" when she became the "Head of so large a Number" of both her own children and her deceased father-in-law's or-

1. Charles Brockden Brown, *Alcuin: A Dialogue*, ed. Lee R. Edwards (1798; rpt. New York, 1971), 39–40.

2. Preface to the 1807 Election Law, quoted in J. R. Pole, "The Suffrage in New Jersey, 1790–1807," New Jersey Historical Society, *Proceedings*, LXXI (1953), 57; Linda K. Kerber, *Women of the Republic: Intellect and Ideology in Revolutionary America* (Chapel Hill, N.C., 1980); Mary Beth Norton, *Liberty's Daughters: The Revolutionary Experience of American Women, 1750–1800* (Boston, 1980); Jay Fliegelman, *Prodigals and Pilgrims: The American Revolution against Patriarchal Authority, 1750–1800* (New York, 1982).

phaned children by his second marriage. She invoked a prison metaphor for her changed status: "Death or Bread and Water would be a happy prospect in comparison." For some women, the high hopes expressed as newlyweds might sooner or later give way to disappointment and failure. For others, the radicalism of the Revolution faded into a status-anxious conservatism. A young Elizabeth Willing Powel asked in 1786, was it not "wonderfull that Men, in all Ages, shou'd be so totally regardless of female Education?" But by 1819, having failed to produce a living male heir to perpetuate her husband's lineage, she wrote a complicated will that specifically excluded women from inheritance. Expectations of self-abnegation and marital duty—perhaps tinged with guilt over her failure to produce viable children—and pressure to maintain social status affected Powel.[3]

Old ideas lingered in often subtle ways. Anxieties about the consequences of smaller family size began to bubble up occasionally in the literature of the early nineteenth century. Popular novels and short stories presented readers with romantic, pathetic, and often tragic stories of families in which "one daughter was the only fruit of the marriage." There was the enormously popular "Charlotte Temple, who was the only pledge of [her parent's] love." Even Washington Irving created a rustic heroine, "an only child," who "appeared like some tender plant of the garden." These innocents are sometimes born to families in straightened circumstances. The birth of sons might have been productive of wealth. Nonetheless, these self-sacrificing fictional parents afford their sole offspring a fine education even if newfangled female academies further drain familial resources. Although extended female education imparted all the social graces to these innocent and unworldly young women, they were ill equipped to preserve the family's honor, and, of course, they could not preserve the family name. These conceits provide the basis for dramatic twists and turns as the guileless daughters fall in love, are seduced, and often die melodramatic, lingering deaths in their shame and disgrace. Occasionally, they marry in the knick of time. The popularity of these plot devices suggests widespread anxieties about family limitation, fears that it had proceeded too far, too fast. Patrilineality, even the simple reproduction

3. Elizabeth Bayley Seton to Julia Scott, July 5, 1798, in Regina Bechtle and Judith Metz, eds., *Elizabeth Bayley Seton: Collected Writings*, I, *Correspondence and Journals, 1793–1808* (Hyde Park, N.Y., 2000), 36. Seton acquired responsibility for the six youngest children of her father-in-law at his death in 1798. She and her husband already had two children, and she was about to give birth to a third. See also David W. Maxey, *A Portrait of Elizabeth Willing Powel, 1743–1830* (Philadelphia, 2006), 18, 57.

of the parental generation, was being threatened by low birthrates and an absence of sons. The transition to small families could be profoundly unsettling to traditional values, although organized opposition to family limitation among native-born, white, middling, and wealthy families would not appear until the middle of the nineteenth century. Female self-mastery, egalitarian marriages, and indulgent parenthood could be either unrealistic or unappealing to segments of the American population.[4]

Fiction was not the only source for expressing anxiety. Two prints by John Lewis Krimmel from 1820, in the moralistic style of William Hogarth, offer an explicit critique of the changes in gender relations (Plates 27 and 28). The first shows a modest young woman saying good-bye to her beau as she heads off to a fashionable boarding school. The young man is a central figure in this "before" image. An ominous foreshadowing of things to come, however, is that the beau shares center stage with the elegantly dressed schoolmistress, here to pick up her pupil in her coach. The new student's father counts the money for her tuition but has plenty more—not only is the first cash bag overflowing with coins, but his ironbound chest beneath his desk is full of additional bags. The farmhouse is simply furnished but tidy and neat. Pictures of cows and other farm animals adorn the wall, an indication of the source of this farmer's prosperity. But, oh, the difference when the daughter returns from school!

The "after" image shows the disasters caused by "the mistaken pride and fondness of her parents" in educating their daughter. The now imperious, elaborately dressed young woman has thrown over her hometown beau and carries the miniature of another man, no simple rustic but an officer in the army. A lapdog has even usurped the place of the faithful family pet. The new graduate sits in her father's stead—he has had to move to the table— and it is the daughter who holds a purse, an indication that she now controls the family fortunes. Feminine froufrou dominates the room. Over the fireplace there is a framed picture of a romantic pastoral scene, the kind of embroidery or watercolor picture favored in women's schools at the time, and sketches of fashionable women have been substituted for those placid cows. An obviously expensive piano has replaced the father's desk. There is a carpet on the floor (the old, handmade, braided rag rug is stored with other junk

---

4. Charles Miner, *Essays from the Desk of Poor Robert, the Scribe: Containing Lessons in Manners, Morals, and Domestic Economy* (1815; rpt. New York, 1930), 21; Susanna Rowson, *Charlotte Temple and Lucy Temple*, ed. Ann Douglas (New York, 1991), 22; Washington Irving, "The Pride of the Village," *The Sketch Book of Geoffrey Crayon, Gent.* (New York, 1961), 313.

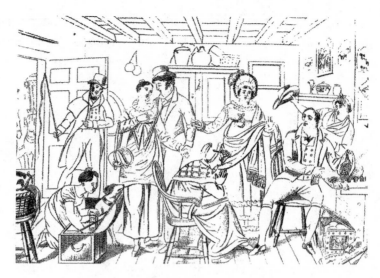

PLATE 27.

"Art. VIII—Going to Boarding School." By John Lewis Krimmel.
From the *Analectic Magazine*, II, no. 5 (November 1820), 421.

A modest young woman leaves her beau and departs for boarding school.

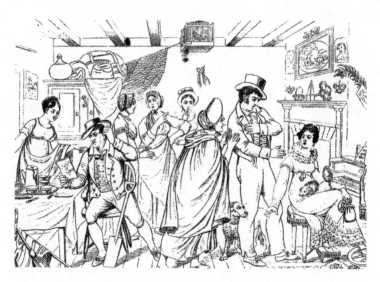

PLATE 28.

"Art. VI—Krimmel's Picture—'Return from Boarding School.'" By John Lewis
Krimmel. From the *Analectic Magazine*, II, no. 6 (December 1820), 507.

A haughty young lady returns from boarding school, rejects
her former beau, and bankrupts her father.

on top of the cupboard), and an elaborate tea service on a white tablecloth, a caged bird, a peacock feather, and more have altered the once plain and practical room. Meanwhile, a broom, scrub brush, and bucket of water have been carelessly left out, unused. The new graduate's foot treads on a spinning wheel. If women are educated, independent, who will carry on women's traditional tasks? Women now hold the center of the room and are inclined to imitate their genteel kinswomen. The contagion of female domination is about to spread. The displaced father worries that he will not be able to dig himself out of the financial hole all this useless extravagance has cost him. It is frightening stuff, this picture of a domestic world turned upside down.[5]

One way for men to avoid the changes occurring in eastern families was to move away from densely settled areas. Research on New England and New York State in the first half of the nineteenth century finds that western mountainous or isolated counties had the highest fertility. Moving west or into the mountains provided escapes from unwelcome changes. The poor ragman, George Erion, aspired to be a patriarch. When his first wife died in her fifth delivery, he noted, "she Diyd for me." His second wife, age sixteen at her marriage, bore him an additional eleven children. He began as a tenant farmer in Pennsylvania, then he moved south into the mountains of Virginia where he eventually acquired 180 acres of land purchased in installments for eighty pounds. He earned cash by collecting rags and selling them to paper mills and by sending his children into service. He expected his children to contribute to the family, and they, in turn, expected marriage settlements.[6]

George Erion had his hands full in the 1790s with his sixteen-year-old daughter, Babary, the eldest child. She was sent into service but was a "bade girl." He promised her twenty pounds as a dowry if she behaved. She did not. He therefore reduced this sum to eight dollars for a chest and a spinning wheel. Babary must have appreciated the penalty because she soon became more tractable. Her father was forced to renege on payment, however, so the following year he raised his future gift considerably: a cow, a bed and bedstead, a chest, a spinning wheel, and a good set of clothes, plus twenty pounds. But this promise seems to have been pie in the sky, and Babary was

5. "Art. VIII—Going to Boarding School," *Analectic Magazine*, II, no. 5 (November 1820), 421; "Art. VI—Krimmel's Picture—'Return from Boarding School,'" ibid., II, no. 6 (December 1820), 507.

6. Gloria L. Main, "Rocking the Cradle: Downsizing the New England Family," *Journal of Interdisciplinary History*, XXXVII (2006–2007), 35–58; Michael R. Haines and Avery M. Guest, "Fertility in New York State in the Pre–Civil War Era," *Demography*, XLV (2008), 358; "George Erion, the Ragman," *Der Raggeboge: The Rainbow*, XI, nos. 3–4 (1977), 3–17 (quotation on 15).

soon back to her disobedient ways. In retaliation, George Erion subtracted five pounds, the cow, and the bed and bedstead from her projected marriage portion, which brought her around again—so he added two sheep and a new hat and actually gave her a chest. A year passed, and he still could not provide the rest of his promised marriage portion; "I Will pay her as Soon as pasibel," he wrote on September 24, 1799. It was too late—by this time, Babary was pregnant with twins and unmarried. Did her partner balk at marriage when no dowry was forthcoming? Two years later, the still unmarried Babary finally received store goods worth three and a half dollars, but her father wrote angrily, "She tornd out to a Hor That is her name a Hor," circling the last word. There is no further mention of her in the diary.[7]

Meanwhile, George Erion was having similar trouble with failed promises to his occasionally rebellious eldest son, who would not be able to afford to marry until he was twenty-seven. As his other children reached late adolescence, they also raised his ire as he continually failed to provide them with a start in life. Erion had become a landowner when he moved into the mountains, but his attempts to control his children failed because his poverty continually undermined his control. Had he had fewer children, his authority and social status might have been more secure, but it seems not to have crossed his mind. Rebellious children who insisted on their rights provided an object lesson on the disadvantages of very large families in the wake of the American rebellion, even far from eastern cities.

Language and cultural barriers as well as isolation helped slow the diffusion of new ideas among Germans like Erion and particularly for his two wives. Unfortunately, no evidence from German-speaking women on their attitudes toward the pace and intensity of childbearing has been found, yet there are some hints from outside observers and in the press of the different circumstances of German women compared to British women. English-speaking women were beginning to laugh at the "Lords of Creation," yet German-language sources addressed women by repeatedly reminding them, "Your will shall be subdued by your husband's, he shall be your lord." This was a very different reading of Genesis than the one being developed by certain outspoken English-speaking women. Almanacs in German contained ditties like the following:

7. "George Erion," *Der Raggeboge*, XI, nos. 3–4 (1977), 6, 7, 9. Erion only once defined bad behavior. In 1805, sixteen-year-old daughter Christina was labeled a bad girl. "I am Not Willing to give her anny thing," he wrote; "she must arn me a Cow yet before She Comes homes." It seems she was not sending him her wages.

If only my house looks neat and clean
Then it equals palaces

. . . .

To be a Wife and a Mother
Is all that makes me happy.

These traditional attitudes were both patriarchal and pronatalist. What Benjamin Rush admired in rural Germans, and in himself as head of a large family, was "the ancient and patriarchal pleasure of raising up a numerous and healthy family of children, to labour for their parents, for themselves, and for their country." Rush's particular vision of Pennsylvania Germans remained, even in the 1780s, mired in male prerogative. "No dread of poverty, nor distrust of Providence from an encreasing family" hindered their procreative prowess, he thought, but he did not think to discover if the wives had different opinions about increasing their families.[8]

Benjamin Rush also stated, "The Germans are but little addicted to convivial pleasures." The snobbish Hessian doctor Johann David Schoepf concurred. Among the British colonists, tea parties and other social gatherings had been the source of a feminine civil society since at least the 1740s. Teatime gatherings provided frequent occasions for women and men to talk about the latest news, to gossip about friends and neighbors, and women could shape public opinion on subjects that included evolving ideals of femininity, individualism, liberty, marriage, and childrearing. Health, medicine,

8. "Form der Ehe-Einleitung [Forms for starting a marriage]" (1758), trans. and quoted in Christine Hucho, "Female Writers, Women's Networks, and the Preservation of Culture: The Schwenkfelder Women of Eighteenth-Century Pennsylvania," *Pennsylvania History*, LXVIII (2001), 122–123; *Spiegel der Eheleute* (1758), "Regeln and Grundlehren zur Beforderung derer ehelichen Guckseligkeiten," *Der Hock Deutsch Americanische Calendar* (1780), and "Hans liebt Grethe Hansen," ibid. (1793), trans. and quoted in Hucho, "Marriage, Migration, and the Enforcement of Gender Norms among German-Speaking Immigrants of Eighteenth-Century Pennsylvania," in Horst Pietschmann, ed., *Atlantic History: History of the Atlantic System, 1580–1830* (Gottingen, Ger., 2002), 469, 470; Benjamin Rush, "An Account of the Manners of the German Inhabitants of Pennsylvania," *Essays, Literary, Moral, and Philosophical* (Philadelphia, 1806), 233. Among Swedes, who had been in Pennsylvania for three or more generations at the time of a 1753 census, 90 percent of men could read English, whereas only 75 percent of women could. All the men spoke English as well as Swedish, but 10 percent of women could not speak English. Women were more isolated (Susan Klepp, "Five Early Pennsylvania Censuses," *Pennsylvania Magazine of History and Biography*, CVI [1982], 507). Gender relations in the German states were following a trajectory similar to that in other places. When there was no revolutionary movement rattling social hierarchies, enlightened ideals might offer men options while more firmly restricting women to domestic and reproductive roles; see Marion W. Gray, *Productive Men, Reproductive Women: The Agrarian Household and the Emergence of Separate Spheres during the German Enlightenment* (New York, 2000).

and the latest books were also topics for lively conversations. Although these gatherings are best known from elite sources, poorer women in the cities had their own, less elaborate tea ceremonies. Even in the almshouse, poor women could "sett by the fire and take their Tea and other refreshments in comfort." Urban women also had other social opportunities, including the practice of sitting before their front doors on summer evenings talking with their neighbors. It seems that German-speaking women or other rural women had less opportunity to participate in these conversational pastimes. In 1787, the elderly Reverend Henry Melchior Muhlenberg was sorely grieved that his daughter-in-law had "a first visit at her table from several neighboring women . . . [for] a glass of wine or a cup of tea and some cakes in the afternoon and evening and [to] entertain one another with vain conversations." But English-speaking women had been gathering together and conversing for decades by 1787. That "vain" talk included the issues that would revolutionize women's status and recast married life. Women without such a social network, women like George Erion's two wives, would have been cut off from the new ideas circulating elsewhere.[9]

German women's silence in the surviving record might have been due in part to limited education. According to Rush, "There is scarcely an instance of a German, of either sex, in Pennsylvania, that cannot *read;* but many of the wives and daughters of the German farmers cannot *write.*" Schoepf adds that German households had few books, most commonly just a Bible, a hymnal, and an almanac, less varied reading than English farmers who commonly owned some issues of the *Spectator* and other magazines, plus newspapers and dictionaries. This lack of formal education in writing and the absence of more varied texts for self-education meant that even in Philadelphia he met "only one or two agreeable and intelligent women of German origin, but they spoke German very little and did not owe their breeding to their own people." If these observations were approximately right, if many rural German women were unable to correspond with one another and if they did not gather sociably of an evening, then diffusion of new ideas would have been difficult. If there was also a stronger emphasis on patriarchy and

9. Rush, "An Account of the Manners of the German Inhabitants of Pennsylvania," *Essays,* 237; Johann David Schoepf, *Travels in the Confederation, 1783-1784,* 2 vols., ed. and trans. Alfred J. Morrison (New York, 1968), I, 103–104; David S. Shields, *Civil Tongues and Polite Letters in British America* (Chapel Hill, N.C., 1997), esp. chap. 4; Lillian B. Miller et al., eds., *The Selected Papers of Charles Willson Peale and His Family,* V, *The Autobiography of Charles Willson Peale* (New Haven, Conn., 2000), 242; Theodore G. Tappert and John W. Doberstein, eds. and trans., *The Journals of Henry Melchior Muhlenberg,* III (Philadelphia, 1958), 746.

propagation, then it is not too surprising that fertility rates remained high in Lancaster County and other predominately German communities. By 1818, however, a traveler reported that German women were "no longer willing to put up with the 'bossy tone' of German men." Changes might have come slowly, but they came nonetheless.[10]

Rural and German-speaking women's isolation could keep them uninformed of the emerging celebration of small family size. Other women were fully aware of these changing assessments of fertility but firmly rejected change. Martha Laurens Ramsay of South Carolina had waited out the Revolution in England and France and therefore missed the buzz of revolutionary conversation and contention. Her position as a mistress of slaves in a predominantly slave society might also have enforced a belief in the social necessity of cultivating unwavering deference and a fear of authority. In her world, underlings owed rigid subordination and unquestioning obedience to the head of the household. According to her husband, Laurens Ramsay had read Mary Wollstonecraft and "the plausible reasonings of modern theorists, who contend for the equality of the sexes." But, "in practice, as well as theory, she acknowledged the dependent, subordinate condition of her sex; and considered it as a part of the curse denounced on Eve . . . which led her to make all her conduct subservient to her husband's happiness." She accepted the patriarchal reading of the creation story. She bore eleven children, eight of whom survived childhood, perhaps because her conception of "conjugal duties" caused her to receive "the attentions of her husband as favours." She herself wrote, "Oh [Lord] let me be satisfied with whatever happens to the body." Laurens Ramsay struggled to achieve passivity and automatic obedience.[11]

If Laurens Ramsay rejected women's rights, she did not advocate sentimentalized childrearing either. Again, in her husband's words: "She was well acquainted with the plans of Rousseau, and other modern reformers, who are for discarding the rod . . . [but] believed that nothing injured the temper

10. Rush, "An Account of the Manners of the German Inhabitants of Pennsylvania," *Essays*, 233, 244; Schoepf, *Travels in the Confederation*, ed. and trans. Morrison, I, 104, 105; Hucho, "Marriage, Migration, and the Enforcement of Gender Norms," in Pietschmann, ed., *Atlantic History*, 465. Against this idea of limited communication among German women is the widespread knowledge of medicinal herbs and their uses, even if the surviving record was almost entirely authored by males.

11. David Ramsay, *Memoirs of Martha Laurens Ramsay* . . . (Philadelphia, 1845), 156, 249–251. The slave system was "patriarchy writ large" and "represented hierarchy, discipline, and corporate control" (Ira Berlin, *Many Thousands Gone: The First Two Centuries of Slavery in North America* [Cambridge, Mass., 1998], 3–4).

less, or more effectually promoted the proper end of punishment in young subjects, than corporal pain." Her own writings consistently confused punishment and suffering with loving attention. Hierarchical marriages, bodily subservience, high birthrates, and authoritarian childrearing were linked in Ramsay's life, just as they were linked—but rejected—in the thinking of many of her revolutionary-era contemporaries, especially those from areas where slavery was gradually being abolished and birthrates were falling. A potentially transformative mix of egalitarian, sympathetic—even sentimental—family relationships, mental and corporeal independence, self-restraint, and family limitation had emerged and was embraced by many American women after the 1760s. But revolutionary ideals were not universal, and many, for one reason or another, were unconvinced. Another southerner did adopt the language of limited childbearing and tokens of affection as something quite original. Ella Gertrude Clanton Thomas of Georgia declared, "I do not wish [to have] an only child, yet I should not object to long intervals," adding that her husband agreed with her new determination. Like other rural women, she chose a spacing strategy. This was a radical move, however, and she "mentioned this to no one but himself [her husband]." She felt that "rational, calm trusting happiness" could occur in a marriage of near equals. "[W]hat a strong cord of love to bind two hearts together is the birth of a child." But these plans for the future and sentiments of the binding power of birth, so similar to the languages of pledges and tokens of love invoked farther to the North, were made in 1854, eighty years and more after northerners made similar declarations. The diffusion of ideas, symbolic language, and fertility goals was uneven and often painfully slow.[12]

Other women did not themselves alter traditional childbearing patterns. They continued to bear children every two years or so as had their mothers and grandmothers, but they assisted in creating a new climate of opinion by expressing sympathy and sorrow for the similar childbearing experiences of their peers, as Elizabeth Drinker's diary indicates. Still other women likewise accepted their traditional lot in life but worked to assure a different fate for their younger sisters and daughters by giving them explicit birth-control information, as did, for example, some of the Shippen women.

The fertility transition was a radical break from tradition and produced many different reactions. Many eighteenth-century women and many more nineteenth-century women were moved to restrict their own family size

12. Ramsay, *Memoirs of Martha Laurens Ramsay,* 89; Virginia Ingraham Burr, ed., *The Secret Eye: The Journal of Ella Gertrude Clanton Thomas, 1848–1889* (Chapel Hill, N.C., 1990), 148, 154.

despite the pull of tradition and anxiety about self-interested, self-assertive womanhood. Women's letters, diaries, commonplace books, favorite novels, poems, and gossip diffused new ideas, sometimes openly, more often subtly. Margaret Van Horne arrived in the barely settled territory of Ohio and wrote to her best friend back east about meeting her cousin and his wife, "They have 3 children, and appear to be very well off, (you understand me) and happy." Here was the key: a small family, prosperity, felicity, and a hint to the wise. Dwight's later life did not follow this pattern, another instance of the often painful gap between early hopes and lived realities. She would later die a month after her thirteenth delivery.[13]

The radicalism of family limitation could be mitigated, not by rejecting the new goals, but by infusing these new standards of marital relations with old elitist, hierarchical notions. The coterie of ideas expressive of restraint and self-control were coming to be opposed by terms suggestive of a wild, brutish, and threatening nature. By the turn of the nineteenth century, large numbers of children were simultaneously represented by many Americans as a sign of and a cause of the backwardness and poverty of outsiders. It is hardly surprising that racialized assumptions, so prevalent in the dominant culture, were also attached to fecundity. Back in the 1730s, a bound woman's fertility had been a selling point, as in the advertisement offering "a Likely young breeding Negro Woman fit for Town or Country Business." It was thought to be "practically advantageous to have negro women," because "the children are all your slaves." Or, depending on the whim of the master, the resulting "blackamoors" could be "sold in their turn." Slave women's fecundity produced a cash crop of vendible babies and made them especially valuable.[14]

13. Max Farrand, ed., *A Journey to Ohio in 1810: As Recorded in the Journal of Margaret Van Horn Dwight* (Lincoln, Nebr., 1991), 63.

14. *Pennsylvania Gazette* (Philadelphia), July 25, 1734; A. B. Benson, ed., *The America of 1750: Peter Kalm's Travels in North America*, 2 vols. (New York, 1964), I, 206; Gottlieb Mittelberger, *Journey to Pennsylvania*, ed. and trans. Oscar Handlin and John Clive (Cambridge, Mass., 1960), 81. Did masters encourage or force enslaved women to bear children against their will? The evidence is mixed. Some slaveowners, particularly in areas like the late-eighteenth-century Chesapeake with its exhausted soils and a reduced market for plantation crops, recognized the profit to be made by wholesaling human beings. Other masters resented the loss of labor caused by pregnancy and so attempted to prevent frequent births. See Marie Jenkins Schwartz, *Birthing a Slave: Motherhood and Medicine in the Antebellum South* (Cambridge, Mass., 2006), chap. 1; Jennifer L. Morgan, *Laboring Women: Reproduction and Gender in New World Slavery* (Philadelphia, 2004); Philip D. Morgan, *Slave Counterpoint: Black Culture in the Eighteenth-Century Chesapeake and Lowcountry* (Chapel Hill, N.C., 1998), 87–92; Sharla M. Fett, *Working Cures: Healing, Health, and Power on Southern Slave Plantations* (Chapel Hill, N.C., 2002), 185.

This positive valuation of childbearing by slaveowners faded from Mid-Atlantic slave advertisements by the 1760s, well before any significant anti-slavery movement appeared. An enslaved woman's "breeding fast" commonly became "the only Reason of her being sold." Almost no one stipulated that the mother and child be sold together or that the fathers be considered. One woman was sold simply because "she is likely to have a Child." Success in "breeding" was no longer commended in slave sales. In fact, masters or mistresses advertising their human property sometimes emphasized the contrast between the enslaved woman's behavior and their own supposedly more restrained family size: variations on some bound woman's "too frequent bearing Children being inconvenient and disagreeable to her present Owner" appeared after the middle of the century. "Too frequent" in this case referred to just two children. Another master or mistress wrote, "She breeds fast, [two children again] which is disagreeable to the small family with which she lives." Ironically, these enslaved women's bearing of two children was far less than the average free woman's childbearing experiences, still hovering between an average of five to seven children. Facts did not get in the way of prejudice, however. Enos Ewing wrote his fiancée that his four slaves "work so well . . . that [he] may allmost turn Gentleman farmer" but criticized the enslaved woman for being "not yet Eighteen tho she is the mother of the [year old] child." Others chimed in on this theme. Pennsylvania African Americans with their "swarms of helpless children, and big-bellied women" were said to threaten their masters' livelihoods. The "uncommon fruitfulness" of slaves became a sign of an innate pathology to physicians. But enslaved women and men might see the importance of extended family ties as buffers against the dehumanization of the slave system—grandparents, sisters, brothers, aunts, uncles, cousins, and more could provide a support system for children, even if parents died or were sold away. The instability of families under slavery might be partially countered by creating an extensive network of kin. Force might also have been a factor. There is no hint of desires and goals of the enslaved people themselves regarding their family size in the writings of slaveowners or in the observations of travelers.[15]

15. Charles Varley (Varlo), *The Unfortunate Husbandman: An Account of the Life and Travels of a Real Farmer in Ireland, Scotland, England, and America*, ed. Desmond Clarke (London, 1964), 111; Benjamin Rush, quoted in Winthrop D. Jordan, *White over Black: American Attitudes toward the Negro, 1550–1812* (Baltimore, 1968), 519; *Pa. Gaz.*, Apr. 23, 1761, Mar. 3, 17, 1763, June 28, 1786. Some of these advertisements bemoaning the fruitfulness of female slaves might have been a backhanded advertising ploy to shift attention from want of skill or an unyielding demeanor or to highlight the future profit in offspring while seemingly deploring it—yet at least one master offered to exchange a "breeding woman" with a young child for another woman "of equal value" (*Pennsylvania*

If white children were no longer perceived as a source of wealth and profit, then black children were resented as costly, valueless, and excessively troublesome by owners and employers, especially after gradual abolition laws were passed in the North. Whites were imagined to be restrained and prudent and white women to be no longer engaged in breeding. African American women were presented as the embodiment of rejected values and their offspring as a social burden. These accusations say more about the accusers than the accused.

Maternity among African American women was valued only in the service of employers. Advertisements calling for "Negroe Wench[es]" who were "fond of children" or who might be a "good nurse among children" began appearing by the end of the century. White children were to be coddled by paid employees; the servant's children were to be invisible—neither seen nor heard, and preferably nonexistent. As one commentator put it, "Negroes just born, are considered as an incumbrance only," and even antislavery advocates chimed in. An investigator for a New Jersey group was relieved when "Grace's child died young," because she then had "no incumbrance." The sentimentalized language of birth and infancy did not apply to African Americans. Elizabeth Drinker groused: "Black Mary is gone home again sick, she is breeding I believe. a world of trouble." She also "dismist" one of her servants only because she "could not be here but when it suited herself, being a married woman," rather than putting her employer's family first. Drinker concluded, "So much for Negros, who are usefull to us, when they behave well." New attitudes on fertility absorbed and were shaped by older attitudes on race and became even more entrenched in the following century.[16]

Class provided another source of prejudice by the late eighteenth and early nineteenth centuries. Middling and elite commentators began asserting that the poor, "like vegetables ... shoot up wherever nourishment is the

---

Packet [Philadelphia], Jan. 29, 1784). Southern slaveowners did not mask their keen interest in the profitability of their enslaved women's childbearing; see Schwartz, Birthing a Slave; Enos Ewing to Susan F. Beatty, Apr. 31, 1799, Document E14, 1748–1830 Collection, Cumberland County [New Jersey] Historical Society, http://digilib.clueslibs.org/virt_lib/documents/index1748-1830.html, 3 (accessed January 2007); John W. Blassingame, The Slave Community: Plantation Life in the Antebellum South (New York, 1979); Herbert G. Gutman, The Black Family in Slavery and Freedom, 1750–1925 (New York, 1976).

16. Pa. Gaz., Sept. 22, 1778, Aug. 16, 1780; "Another Letter to a Clergyman in the Country, on the Question, Whether the Children of Slaves Ought to Be Held in Bondage," Pa. Packet, Jan. 1, 1780; William Poole to Robert Smith, Jr., Jan. 15, 1798, in Clement Alexander Price and M. M. Perot, eds., After Freedom (Burlington, N.J., 1987), 2; Elaine Forman Crane et al. eds., The Diary of Elizabeth Drinker, 3 vols. (Boston, 1991), II, 1239, 1313.

most copious" and that they "swarm like locusts in the land." In 1804, one farmer feared that millworkers were becoming a majority: "So many Imployed at the paper mills their is 7 of them in Less than 3 miles, Give bread to a number, and Great Many of they Journeymen have wifees and the hills Swarm with Children." Poverty, a loss of control, and large numbers of children were linked. And, even though more conservative Pennsylvanians seem to have been most vocal in asserting these essentially Malthusian assumptions, by the 1820s labor radicals also talked in terms of "the fruitful parent of misery and want." Within a generation, the new antagonism toward high fertility had become widespread. The multiplication of pests—swarms, locusts, weeds—and a lack of prudence or self-restraint were associated with high fertility after about 1780, not the comfortable, domesticated, agricultural images of previous years. Nature was not benevolent; it needed to be conquered. Respectable folk were disciplined, sacrificing, and, yes, better than the careless, thoughtless ones with their large families and lazy ways.[17]

The shift initiated by women during the Revolution to produce possible self-images beyond that of childbearer and to achieve certain equitable relationships within marriage proved equally useful after the Revolution in elaborating a new race consciousness and in defining the parameters of new class relations that might be crudely sketched as upper-class refinement, middle-class rectitude, and working-class respectability. These new class identities involved varying definitions of self-control and of superiority to mere nature and the profligacy of others: elite decadence, worker's thoughtlessness, and the presumptuousness of the middle classes. It was an invention of the late eighteenth century to assume that high fertility was uncontrolled fertility and to link uncontrolled fertility with a lower stage of social or economic development—something only irresponsible, thoughtless sensualists engaged in. Many children now meant poverty and moral laxity or indulgence and immorality, not wealth and divine blessing. Restricted fertility became one measure of group identity and personal virtue. Whatever the social definition, the insiders were civilized, virtuous, rational, prudent, restrained, and foresighted, in contrast to their inferiors, who were brutish, thoughtless, improvident, wasteful, and extravagant—even if these assessments could not be supported by actual numbers.

17. Eliza Cope Harrison, ed., *Philadelphia Merchant: The Diary of Thomas P. Cope, 1800–1851* (South Bend, Ind., 1978), 176, 311; Joseph Price Diary, Sept. 9, 1804, Historical Society of Pennsylvania, Philadelphia; The Philadelphia *Mechanic's Free Press*, Sept. 25, 1830, quoted in Edward Pessen, "The Working Men's Parties Revisited," in Pessen, ed., *New Perspectives on Jacksonian Parties and Politics* (Boston, 1969), 203.

In the middle of the nineteenth century, a majority of the voting population came to believe that abortion and contraception might be approved for people like themselves but must be generally condemned, since neither abortion nor contraception would give other people — usually seen as poorer, less educated, foreign, or female — the necessary restraint; it would only further sap the weak sense of morality in those less worthy sorts of people. So it was that the birthrate fell at the same time that large segments of the population embraced the goal of sharply restricted fertility, and yet voters, clergymen, doctors, judges, and legislators demanded more and more restrictions on contraception and abortion.[18]

Most of these examples of the fear of large numbers of children of the wrong sort were from men, but women, too, learned the lessons of the new virtues of refinement, rectitude, or respectability, albeit with less contempt for the "swarms" of poor children. In 1817, a guide to the new science of political economy, written by a woman for a female audience, linked the concerns over affectionate families, reproductive choice, and health with national economic and social goals.

CAROLINE. I declare I always thought that it was very desirable to have a great population. . . .

MRS. B. The birth of helpless infants . . . born merely to languish a few years in poverty, and to fall early victims to disease . . . can neither increase the strength, the wealth, nor the happiness of the country. . . . Yet such is the fate of thousands of children wherever population exceeds the means of subsistence.

CAROLINE. What a dreadful reflection this is! . . .

MRS. B. A large family of young children would require the whole of a mother's care and attention. . . . A delicate or an infirm woman requires repose and indulgence which she cannot command. . . . Those who have not reflected on the subject, have . . . with you, considered a great population under all circumstances as the cause of prosperity. Hence the most strenuous efforts have been made, not only by individuals, but even by the legislature, to encourage early marriages and large families. . . .

CAROLINE. This is a most unfortunate error.

18. There is a large literature on social-cultural change in the early nineteenth century, including analyses of working-class respectability, middle-class sincerity, the spread of genteel refinement, nationalism, racism as ideology and identity, and American variations on imperialism.

Caroline learned her lessons quickly. The Malthusian anxiety about the re-productive capacities of the poor was combined with the fictional women's concern over the proper care of children who required a mother's full atten-tion, a sympathetic interest in the welfare of others, and an assertion of the special needs of delicate (that is, pregnant) womanhood.[19]

Women had learned these attitudes without the book. Sally Hastings sar-castically described a rustic Pennsylvania farmer who in 1800 "has blessed the Community with fifteen hopeful Sons, and one Daughter." "I presume it is uncertain how many more such Tokens of Regard he may bestow on his Country." Harriet Manigault wrote in 1814: "Our poor Aunt Claudia intends to present her beloved with a tender pledge in four or five months. I should not suppose that the prospect would delight him much, for his family is sufficiently large." Excessive fertility was deplorable. The backwoods farmer burdened the state with his progeny, just as "poor" Claudia Smith Izard ac-quired a reputation that her financial situation did not merit. Conformity to new cultural norms was expected. Women's reproductive capacities were to be curtailed just as they were to have been enhanced several decades earlier. Competing interests sought control over women's pregnant bodies in the name of religion, family status, and the prosperity of the state. Women stressed voluntary motherhood, shared decision making, and a degree of liberty but were hardly immune to the demands of their racial, religious, ethnic, social, or political identities.[20]

Family planning emerged from the social, economic, religious, and politi-cal upheavals of the late eighteenth century. It was bound up in new ideas of womanhood that did not so much attempt to reduce the many attributes of masculine virtue (disinterestedness, honor, autonomy, authenticity, sincerity of expression and action, generosity, wisdom, courage) to virginal asexu-ality, as has sometimes been asserted by historians, but to extend the bodily integrity of virtuous free men to self-possessed, self-controlled, consenting

19. [Jane Haldimand Marcet], *Conversations on Political Economy; in Which the Elements of That Science Are Familiarly Explained* (Philadelphia, 1817), 118–120, 123. My thanks to Scott Stephen for finding this attribution in *History of Women*, microfilm, 995 reels (Woodbridge, Conn., 1975–1979), reel 116, no. 772.

20. Sally Hastings, *Poems on Different Subjects; to Which Is Added, a Descriptive Account of a Family Tour to the West; in the Year, 1800; in a Letter to a Lady* (Lancaster, Pa., 1808), 194. Hastings's confidence in 1800 would soon be replaced by a melancholy religiosity caused, at least in part, by her inability to sue for divorce. Traditional outlooks could have remarkable pulling power. See Mary E. Karnes, "Sally Anderson Hastings: A Poetic Diary," *Journal of the Lancaster County Historical Society*, XCIX (Spring 1997), 30–44; Virginia and James S. Armentrout, Jr., eds., *The Diary of Harriet Manigault, 1813–1816* (Rockland, Maine, [1976]), 51.

females. Without first acquiring self-possession, none of the other attributes of the virtuous individual could be achieved. A critical part of that achievement of bodily control would be the rational planning of childbearing within egalitarian, loving marriages. Both sisters and brothers would have more equal and enhanced claims to whatever resources their family could command. Wives might cultivate interests outside the domestic realm. Women were struggling to escape feme covert status by ceasing to be "the Sex" and becoming responsible, fully human adults. Control over fertility helped accomplish that revolutionary goal. A small family became an outward and visible sign of an inward and otherwise invisible virtue.

So, despite regional and social group variations in adopting new standards of appropriate family size and despite the occasional triumph of snobby or conformist impulses over the liberating intent of these original decisions, the commitment to limited fertility was well established by the first decades of American independence. Birthrates and family size might have fallen more rapidly in the East than in the West, in the North than in the South, among city folk before country folk, and among English speakers rather than German speakers. There might have been temporary and mild reversals in a few places after the Revolution; there are some suggestions, based on imperfect numbers, that this was true of some Presbyterians in York County, Pennsylvania, among Schwenkfelders, and among the Welsh in Radnor, Pennsylvania. The very rich were apparently slower than the middling sorts to adapt to changing expectations, as were the enslaved. The free poor generally had small families with or without the deliberate restriction of fertility. But rejection of or hesitation about limited childbearing was less common than an enthusiastic embrace of new possibilities. Ideas spread, behaviors changed, and a domestic revolution was under way.

Into the Nineteenth Century

The religious revivalism of the early nineteenth century returned Americans to the emotional, anti-authoritarian, and reformative strains of the first Great Awakening but offered women more institutionalized roles for expressing their faith than had been considered acceptable in the 1740s. Women now had time for extrafamilial activities. They were marrying later, concentrating births into the first years of marriage, and stopping childbearing sooner. Women's church-based activities expanded and included writing and distributing religious tracts, leading Bible study groups, forming missionary aid societies, and founding Sunday schools. Women took to the streets, seeking to redeem the fallen. In 1800, the Reverend Henry Boehm, a self-proclaimed patriarch, did not consider the childless state of Harry Ennalls's unnamed wife the misfortune it would have been seen a century earlier but rather an opportunity to advance Methodism. In fact, it was her "wise counsel" that "shaped [Boehm's] destiny for life." Boehm rationalized her religious influence as comfortably maternal; she, however, cast him in a fraternal and slightly inferior role, addressing him as "my young brother."[21]

Women had become the majority of congregants in many denominations by this period, although they were still denied access to the ministry and governing boards. No one yet advocated full rights for women—propriety, not equality, was promoted. Nonetheless, women had expanded opportunities and newly institutionalized roles by the early nineteenth century.[22]

It was not long before women's groups looked beyond their congregation or parish and undertook larger social and political reforms. Women turned their attention to missionary outreach for backsliders and non-Christian groups. They organized against the immorality of prostitution, illiteracy, Indian removal, alcohol abuse, poverty, maltreatment of the insane, illiteracy, war and violence, and slavery. One of the most active, Isabella Graham, warned of the dire consequences of the uncontrolled appetites of uninstructed American men, living as if in a state of nature. There are, she wrote, "in this new world, thickly settled in many places with natural men *eating and drinking, marrying and giving in marriage,* while the flood of wrath is hastening to overwhelm them." Marriage needed to be regulated and undertaken only by self-controlled, god-fearing individuals. If men would not act, then women needed to spread the word of God in a civilizing campaign.[23]

Some women were developing career options that provided alternatives to marriage. Carolyn Hyde, impoverished and a servant from the age of nine, found the care of infants to be "exceedingly trying" and "little adapted to expand the mind or cultivate the heart." So, despite her poverty, she left a paid

21. Henry Boehm, *The Patriarch of One Hundred Years; Being Reminiscences, Historical and Biographical, of Rev. Henry Boehm,* ed. J. B. Wakeley (1875; rpt. Lancaster, Pa., 1982), 60–61; Paul E. Johnson, *A Shopkeeper's Millennium: Society and Revivals in Rochester, New York, 1815–1837* (New York, 1978); Mary P. Ryan, *Cradle of the Middle Class: The Family in Oneida County, New York, 1790–1865* (New York, 1981).

22. But some of these women did come to advocate women's rights; see Lori D. Ginzberg, *Untidy Origins: A Story of Woman's Rights in Antebellum New York* (Chapel Hill, N.C., 2005).

23. Devotional Exercise, Sept. 10, 1811, in *The Power of Faith: Exemplified in the Life and Writings of the Late Mrs. Isabella Graham of New York* (New York, 1816), 163. There is a huge literature on these topics; for one example, see Jean Fagan Yellin and John C. Van Horne, eds., *The Abolitionist Sisterhood: Women's Political Culture in Antebellum America* (Ithaca, N.Y., 1994).

position and found more congenial work distributing tracts and working with older students, the sick, and prisoners. Her monetary loss contributed to her regimen of prayer and bodily control through fasting. Jarena Lee never remarried after the death of her husband. She found caretakers for her one surviving son and followed her calling to preach the gospel. Religious belief was not the only possible career. Lucretia Maria Davidson's "whole soul was absorbed in literary pursuits," so she decided never to marry because she "could not do justice to husband or children." Her mother actively supported her career.[24]

The choices available to women in the nineteenth century are often portrayed as limited to permanent spinsterhood or traditional marriage. There were intermediate positions: raising children could be combined with membership in church societies and reform organizations or with various self-improvement activities, especially if women spaced births widely or ended childbearing earlier. This juggling of social and familial duties became more feasible if childbearing was confined to a stage in life. Most women did not want to forgo parenthood but did want to limit childbearing and do a better job of providing for daughters and sons while developing interests outside the family. The expansion of women's activities and the restriction of childbearing worked in tandem.

The marital fertility rates of native-born northern women continued to decline. Native-born women in rural upstate New York who married in the 1810s and 1820s, for example, had an average of five to five and a half children, two fewer than the national average. Those native-born New York women who married in the 1830s and 1840s had just three and a half offspring, a figure not reached by the average American woman until 1900.

Large-scale analysis is only possible on the national level after 1830 when the U.S. census first offers sufficient detail on age and sex to calculate child-woman ratios. These figures, 1830 (the first U.S. census with adequate details on age and sex) to 1860, show that the fertility transition was well under way by the second quarter of the nineteenth century. The trends that had first emerged in the 1760s persisted and intensified into the antebellum period.

A comparison of child-woman ratios for the oldest and more recently

24. Charles Hyde, *Memoir of Caroline Hyde, Who Died in Philadelphia, March 7, 1832* (New York, [1836]), 20 (the author was not related to the subject of the tract); Jarena Lee, "The Life and Religious Experience of Jarena Lee . . ." (1836), in William L. Andrews, ed., *Sisters of the Spirit: Three Black Women's Autobiographies of the Nineteenth Century* (Bloomington, Ind., 1986), 45–46; [Margaret Miller Davidson], ed., *Poetical Remains of the Late Lucretia Maria Davidson . . .* (Philadelphia, 1843), 48.

FIGURE 10.

Regional Child-Woman Ratios, 1830–1860

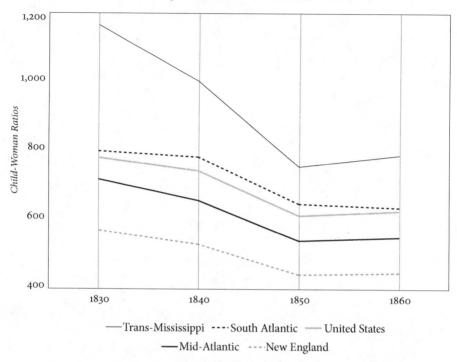

—Trans-Mississippi ----South Atlantic ~~~~ United States
—Mid-Atlantic ---New England

Drawn by Kimberly Foley. Figure shows the number of children from birth to age four per
one thousand women ages fifteen to fifty by selected regions. U.S. censuses as analyzed in J. Potter,
"The Growth of Population in America, 1700–1860," in D. V. Glass and D. E. C. Eversley, eds.,
Population in History: Essays in Historical Demography (Chicago, 1965), table 10, 674–676.

settled regions shows fertility decline well established in the East by 1830, followed by the Mid-Atlantic region, the south Atlantic seaboard, and the trans-Mississippi River western edge of American expansionism (Figure 10). In general, the higher the fertility levels in 1830, the more rapid the decline over the following forty-year period. The slight uptick in child-woman ratios between 1850 and 1860 reflects the impact of massive immigration after 1848 as Irish, Germans, and others escaping famine and political repression in Europe entered the United States (Figure 11). The fertility transition was already under way when the federal census began collecting relevant data.[25]

The censuses from 1830 to 1860 also reveal major differences between

25. Herbert S. Klein, *A Population History of the United States* (Cambridge, 2004), chap. 3, 69–106.

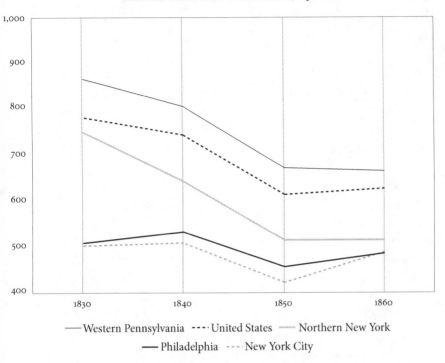

FIGURE 11.

Rural and Urban Child-Woman Ratios, 1830–1860

——Western Pennsylvania ----·United States ——— Northern New York
—— Philadelphia ---- New York City

Drawn by Kimberly Foley. Figure shows the number of children from birth to age four per
one thousand women ages fifteen to fifty by selected regions. U.S. censuses as analyzed in J. Potter,
"The Growth of Population in America, 1700–1860," in D. V. Glass and D. E. C. Eversley, eds.,
Population in History: Essays in Historical Demography (Chicago, 1965), table 10, 674–676.

large cities and distant rural places. The impact of immigration was felt most
strongly in the cities after 1848. Meanwhile, northern New York was swept by
a democratic, reformist religious fervor that involved women to an unprece-
dented degree and by 1848 saw the world's first women's rights convention at
Seneca Falls. That region shows a particularly steep decline in fertility levels
between 1830 and 1850—another indication of the dethroning of patriarchal
"lords of creation" by self-assured wives who wanted to place reasonable limits on their marital commitments. Women's rights, women's opportunities,
and fertility decline were linked.

The Mid-Atlantic states were particularly attractive to immigrant families
who either sought to preserve the traditional large family as a positive good
or who were forced by economic necessity to expand the number of potential
wage earners by bearing more children. Sarah Hoding, an Englishwoman

who lived for many years in Philadelphia, advised her countrymen "who have large families, and who do not know what to do with them" to immigrate to the United States. Rebecca Burlend did migrate from England to a farm in Illinois with her husband and some of her fourteen children. She attributed their ultimate success—twenty head of cattle, seven horses, a well-furnished house, and ownership in fee simple of 360 acres—to "having a family," since the children "greatly assisted in the culture of our land, without having so much [labor] to hire as we should otherwise have been obligated." This was the same unsentimental calculation of children's labor value that colonial Americans had once held dear but that had since been discarded in many places on this side of the Atlantic.[26]

In the city, mill owners gave hiring preference to "parents who could supply the greatest number of laborers." Prolific fathers would be paid a single "family wage" for their own labor and that of their children; wives usually stayed home, taking in boarders and presumably producing more factory hands. Few native-born parents were willing to take positions with such draconian requirements. Instead, Irish and English immigrants dominated in the factories that gave preference to fecund parents and their offspring. John West, an immigrant shoemaker, wrote back to Corsley, England: A "man can do better here with a family than with none. For children at 6 years old can work and get some money. A man nor woman need not stay out of employment one hour here." This was a different communication network than the one espousing an overthrow of the "lords of creation." This one spread information on the value of large families in the labor markets of the industrializing United States and might have brought a self-selecting immigration flow as a consequence. But within a generation or two, the children of immigrants came to adopt the ideal of small families too.[27]

The intentions, conditions, and compromises of immigrants and the persistence of a frontier are among the factors that kept national rates from falling even faster than they did. By the middle of the nineteenth century, there were worries that foreigners would out-reproduce Americans; the 1873

26. Sarah Hoding, *The Land Log-Book; a Compilation of Anecdotes and Occurrences Extracted from the Journal Kept by the Author, during a Residence of Several Years in the United States of America; Containing Useful Hints to Those Who Intend to Emigrate to That Country* (London, 1836), 212; Rebecca and Edward Burlend, *A True Picture of Emigration,* ed. Milo Milton Quaife (1845; Secaucus, N.J., 1974), 152.

27. Cynthia J. Shelton, *The Mills of Manayunk: Industrialization and Social Conflict in the Philadelphia Region, 1787–1837* (Baltimore, 1986), 61–63, esp. 61; G. Poulett Scrope, ed., *Extracts of Letters from Poor Persons Who Emigrated Last Year to Canada and the United States* (London, 1831), 32–33.

Comstock Law, which equated contraceptive information with pornography, was one attempt to roll back the clock by enforcing maternity. It did not work. The ideal of small families and greater choices for women had become entwined in the cultural values of the United States. Women's demand for lower fertility prevailed.[28]

28. Main, "Rocking the Cradle," *JIH*, XXXVII (2006–2007), 35–58; Ryan, *Cradle of the Middle Class*, 155; Johnson, *A Shopkeeper's Millennium*; Bruce Dorsey, *Reforming Men and Women: Gender in the Antebellum City* (Ithaca, N.Y., 2002).

CONCLUSION

Fertility and the Feminine in Early America

The adoption of family limitation was revolutionary: a sudden, sharp break with a long tradition of promoting high fertility within marriage. There could be no halfway measures. Starting in the swirl of revolutionary assertions of inalienable rights, individualism, foresight, and independence, wives or couples either quantified their ideal family size, or they did not. They favored restraint, or they continued to celebrate abundance and redundancy. Couples anticipated the future and carefully invested to secure the best possible outcome for each child, or they accepted the decrees of fate, whatever those might be. Couples or wives either employed delayed marriage, sexual restraint, prolonged breast-feeding, herbal remedies, and other methods to achieve their goals, or they let nature take its course. Women eagerly spread the word, or they were out of the loop, rejecting or never hearing what friends and neighbors were advocating.

There were radical changes in family relationships, too. Parents might insist that children owed labor and services to their superiors, or they might regard childbearing as a heavy fiscal responsibility that nonetheless provided emotional satisfaction and a shared domestic tranquillity. Parents either favored their eldest sons, or they treated all their children nearly equally. Americans could believe that the Bible commanded that all women suffer for Eve's sins, or they could insist that the faithful practice selfless compassion for the weak and a mitigation of human suffering. Women were either "the

Sex," those childish, passionate creatures tied inexorably to their biology, or they were adults capable of virtue, reason, and responsibility—at least in a domesticated sphere. Feminine beauty could be found either in women's fruitful bellies or in their heads, minds, and virtues. Women were loving companions to their husbands, or they were the vessels necessary for the breeding of male heirs.

There was no middle ground: high or low fertility, passivity or planning, patriarchy or companionship, lineage or individuality, innovation or more of the same. The women and men who began to break with the past during the last decades of the eighteenth century were as radical as any in this age of revolutions. There were no bold public declarations, no torch-lit marches through the streets, but there was plenty of excited conversation as women encouraged and admonished their friends and kin, often with bouts of nervous laughter at the audacity of the enterprise. Most men were slower to see the economic and personal benefits of reduced family size, but they, too, eventually promoted the new values entailed in family limitation.

Or, maybe that's wrong.

The fertility transition was a slow, gradual process that began in the late eighteenth century; its assumptions about family, women, and children are still being contested and the consequences are still unfolding nearly 250 years later. The shift to smaller families required a coalescing of many long-term changes in the economy, politics, gender relations, and religion in order for family limitation to succeed. Deeply entrenched ideas about masculinity, femininity, sexuality, the family, duty, and individualism could only be changed gradually. One generation's small family was another generation's excessive number of children.

The diffusion of new ideas was slow and uneven. Linguistic and cultural barriers in particular slowed the acceptance or even the knowledge of innovative beliefs and behaviors. Couples or just husbands or just wives might begin a marriage with high hopes for family planning only to find their hopes dashed by limitations in technology, by finances, or by opposition from spouses, relatives, friends, clergymen, or doctors. Other wives or husbands came to favor family planning late in their marriages and only after a train of sicknesses and female debility or heart-wrenching infant deaths made the rounds of births, ill health, and deaths unbearable. Some women might imbibe various potions if they were considered emmenagogues but perhaps not if they were reclassified as abortifacients or contraceptives. At the same time, others eagerly sought new methods of preventing births. Experimentation with various pills and potions sometimes succeeded but as often offered only elusive hopes of finding reliable methods of fertility control in the eighteenth and early nineteenth centuries.

Fertility could have very different meanings for enslaved women and men than for free couples. High birthrates might strengthen the community of enslaved people while providing personal satisfactions and a sense of belonging not otherwise available to bound individuals. But producing children also benefited the master's pocketbook. Masters could manipulate parents by threatening to separate, beat, or sell their children. Pregnancies could be forced on unwilling women. For the enslaved, childbearing might be both a blessing and a curse.

Even among the nominally free, there might be quite varied reactions to pregnancy and birth. Ethnic or religious minorities might be torn between communal survival and individual choice. The economic circumstances of the poorest free Americans, both black and white, seem to have suppressed childbearing to levels well below contemporary ideals.

Innovative attitudes on childbearing that made sense in the oldest settlements of the Northeast during and after the Revolution were initially of less interest or abhorrent elsewhere in early America: among free and bound in the slaveholding states, on the frontier, in isolated rural areas, and among the very wealthy. These were all populations where growth might counter the presence of upstart commoners, labor shortages, the perceived threat of neighboring enslaved or uprooted populations. In particular, the fringes of settlement where labor was scarce and land available, where profit could continue to come from an increase in human resources, where alien cultures threatened either the survival of tradition or outright war: these were also places where family limitation made less sense than in more sheltered and densely populated regions. There is some evidence that women in underpopulated regions embraced the image of the patriotic, heroic mother who sacrificed herself for the good of the whole through her abundant childbearing.

It was also the case that women's support networks often failed to survive the move west and were difficult to reconstitute in newly acquired territories. Communication with neighbors and kin back east was difficult. Favored herbs might not grow in new environments. Midwives might not live nearby. Pharmacists, druggists, and cooperative physicians might be scarce in newly settled, rural areas. Only slowly could those sources of women's knowledge be reconstructed in new settlements.

Revolution or evolution, which is it?

The fertility transition was a sudden and radical change for those first generations of individual women and men who made a conscious decision to disavow past practices and switch to various family-planning strategies. It was also, for American society as a whole, a drawn-out, contested, checkered, hesitant social and political process that gradually changed gender and family ideals. In its earliest stages, coequal with the disavowal of the monarch, the promotion of political independence, and the creation of a Republic, these very private individual decisions seem to have provoked relatively little public response or anxiety. The private nature of these family-planning efforts and the gradual spread of innovation meant that the earliest stages of the fertility transition have been overlooked or consigned to forces beyond individual control — an aging population, rising land prices, or urbanization, as examples — not to women's efforts to gain some control over their bodies, to limit matrimonial obligation, and to institute more equitable treatment for their daughters.

The transition drew on themes, ideals, and language circulating around the Atlantic world in novels, plays, travel accounts, news items, philosophical treatises, advertisements, prints, and sermons. The economic, material, religious, literary, and social currents of the eighteenth century were necessary, although not sufficient, causes for the shift to family planning, fewer children, birth control, and the increased options and respect for many women. The reluctance and embarrassment of men regarding gynecology provided an opportunity for a woman-centered reformation that did not yet exist in other areas of women's lives: in education, politics, the economy, the law, or the professions.[1] This female-centered gynecological sphere allowed women to seize the opportunity to devise and put into practice new goals, often to the belated surprise of husbands. The disruptions of the Revolution allowed

1. Indeed, in all these areas, women experienced setbacks in the early Republic. See Elaine Forman Crane, *Ebb Tide in New England: Women, Seaports, and Social Change, 1630–1800* (Boston, 1998), for the declining economic status of urban women. Carole Shammas, *A History of Household Government in America* (Charlottesville, Va., 2002), 53–82, stresses the persistence of patriarchy among the founders. Rosemarie Zagarri, *Revolutionary Backlash: Women and Politics in the Early American Republic* (Philadelphia, 2007), finds women increasingly isolated from political decision making. Nancy Folbre makes a cogent point, however. She finds that women's "struggle for individual rights took a different shape than men's, with more emphasis on sexual liberation and more immediate implications for demographic change." She discusses the early twentieth century, but American women first began to apply individual rights to bodily integrity and control over childbearing — although they would, no doubt, have been shocked by twentieth-century ideas of liberation — in the late eighteenth century ("Sleeping Beauty Awakes: Self-Interest, Feminism, and Fertility in the Early Twentieth Century," *Social Research*, LXXI [2004], 344).

the coalescence of preconditions, tied together formerly disparate ideas and experiences, stimulated conversations that survive only in manuscript, print, and visual remnants of a richer, if ephemeral, discussion among women and sympathetic men. These radical decisions stirred little reaction at first. There was, after all, nothing particularly original in the component elements of the arguments in favor of family limitation. Sensibility, enlightened thought, a religion of the heart, humanitarianism, numeracy, comfort, status considerations, fear of foreign and domestic enemies, a rejection of slavery for oneself, and a desire to assert order on an unstable economy through careful planning were not unique to America or to families planning their childbearing careers. What was exceptional was that these various threads became intertwined during an American Revolution that, at least in part, overthrew the inherited prerogatives of lords and masters, that promoted the bodily integrity of the free individual as the basis for white, male, taxpayer citizenship, and that spoke in universal, self-evident terms about both inalienable human and civil rights. If political leaders had blinkered visions of citizenship, women were also beginning the long labor of working out what an inclusive vision of natural rights and civic responsibilities might look like.

It was, as far as can now be recovered, the women of the middling and moderately wealthy ranks of society—women reared and married to artisans, shopkeepers, farmers, professionals, and some merchants—who led in the movement to restrict births within marriage during and after the Revolution. These women were literate, even if their spelling was often atrocious. They could afford books and magazines, could pay the postage that kept friends informed of new developments, and had sufficient leisure time (perhaps because of the labor of a household slave or servant) to become engaged in church, politics, and reform activities, among other outlets for their energy and intellect. Their descendents also preserved at least some of their papers. Urban women, eastern women, and women in long-settled areas tended to support family limitation by the last third of the eighteenth century. So did women from mainstream religions: Anglicans, Methodists, Quakers, Unitarians, urban Lutherans, Reformed, and Presbyterians. In the regions where slavery was being gradually abolished, free women were more inclined to assert control over their bodies.

Others resisted. Husbands were more reluctant than wives. Minority groups—the very wealthy, Pietists and Dissenters, slaveowners, the enslaved, and some immigrants were more hesitant or adamantly opposed to family limitation. The Quakers, with their long tradition of educational and reli-

gious opportunity for women were an exception among minority groups—
they were among the most successful in reducing family size. Language barriers were especially important in blocking, or at least delaying, the diffusion
of new ideas. German women in the countryside seem to have been especially isolated from the developments embraced by their English-speaking
neighbors. On the other hand, women of Swedish and Dutch descent, most
of whom were bilingual or English-speaking by the early national period,
appear to have behaved like their British neighbors. Community survival
might also have been a strong disincentive to restricted population growth
among minority groups, especially when perceived enemies were near. Many
men and some women placed a high value on the perpetuation of patriarchy,
lineage, and male preference in children.[2]

All groups deserve more study, since the most detailed statistics are based
on very small numbers. There is also much that is unknown. It looks as if the
urban poor and free people of African descent had the smallest families. Low
birthrates, low life expectancy, and hindrances to marriage all seem to have
played a part. Were these couples also exceptionally successful at contraception, or were family sizes depressed below the ideal level by poverty and ill
health? Little is known, either quantitatively or qualitatively, about laborers,
about the struggling—but not destitute—artisans in the cities, about Catholics, Baptists, and some other religious groups, about rural cottagers and the
landless in the countryside, or about possible ethnic differences. What international comparisons can be developed?

When this study ends, in the 1820s, abortion services had become commercialized, openly advertised in newspapers, and apparently profitable. Explicit contraceptive advice appeared in print and was sometimes followed by
the arrest of the authors, shocking not only for the open discussion of nonreproductive sex and the publicity of the trials but also because these were
men—Robert Dale Owen, John Humphrey Noyes, and Charles Knowlton,
among others—advocating birth control; they were unashamed trespassers
on still taboo spheres of knowledge. Surreptitious methods of family limi-

---

2. The rural Quakers were also deliberately becoming ever more of a minority in other areas,
withdrawing from government after 1756 and disowning slackers in large numbers from the middle
decades of the eighteenth century (Jack D. Marietta, *The Reformation of American Quakerism, 1748-
1783* [Philadelphia, 2007]). Quakers were moving from what biologists call an r-strategy, high fertility coupled with high infant mortality owing in part to inattentive childrearing, to a K-strategy,
low fertility with heavy parental investment in each offspring. Human strategies were, of course,
culturally determined and reversible.

tation and encoded language spread knowledge of birth-control techniques in spite of the well-publicized arrests. Women continued to write and advise their friends, and men increasingly did so as well.[3]

It would not be until the middle decades of the nineteenth century that any serious public debate on reproductive policy emerged, and this is where most research on fertility change has begun. It was particularly in the wake of the Civil War, when so many young men of marriageable age had been killed, that public anxieties about the separation of sexuality and reproduction emerged to a hailstorm of condemnation. The result was an attempt to ban contraceptives, to reassert the primacy of marriage, to promote the "right" kind of babies by redomesticating educated, Anglo-Saxon, Protestant women. The Comstock Law of 1873 equated contraception with obscenity. The result was not a suppression of contraception and abortion but a further multiplying of the euphemisms for family limitation goals and techniques. Despite the best efforts of segments of the medical profession, the police, the judiciary, the clergy, and eugenicists to reverse the trend toward small families by reconnecting sex and reproduction and by reasserting male control over lineage, American birthrates continued to decline. Pharmaceutical companies' catalogs contained all sorts of equipment under the rubric of providing for women's health. If women knew the code words and had access to pharmacies, often big "ifs," then resources were available for those wishing to limit fertility. Many women, particularly the poor and immigrants, were unaware of the code words and commercial outlets that gave access to the most effective and least harmful means of contraception. Class and ethnic disparities in family size, child survival, maternal mortality, and educational attainment became apparent to the general public by the nineteenth century. Sex education and contraceptive access became major issues for radical reformers around the turn of the twentieth century. For the first time, a very few women — Victoria Woodhull, Emma Goldman, and Margaret Sanger — spoke publicly on reproductive physiology and women's sexual and reproductive rights. Suffrage activists spoke more circumspectly of voluntary motherhood. Between the 1930s and the 1970s, the Comstock Laws were gradually dismantled through the development of a constitutionally protected right to privacy. New technologies made birth control more accessible, safer, and more certain than it had ever been while economic changes, an expanding consumer culture, and rising educational expecta-

3. James. C. Mohr, *Abortion in America: The Origins and Evolution of National Policy, 1800–1900* (New York, 1978).

tions made childbearing ever more expensive. Families became even more child-centered and sentimentalized. Suburban developments helped foster those ideals. The baby boom of the post–World War II period was an anomaly caused in large measure by the severely suppressed birthrates between 1930 and 1945 that had resulted from the Depression and large-scale military conscription.[4]

By the end of the 1960s, the long decline in births resumed. This time decline was aided by major advances in contraceptive technology. Substantial segments of the American population were still uncomfortable with the implications of seemingly unregulated sexuality, of the authority women gained over their bodies, or of the apparent undermining of the authority of the family, husbands, and parents that emerged in the 1960s. A smaller number were adamantly, occasionally violently, opposed to these changes. The heated politics over abortion, federally funded birth-control clinics, childcare centers, sex education in schools, no-fault divorce, births outside wedlock, and the rights of lesbian and gay couples embroiled elections in the second half of the twentieth century and into the next century. Once again, fertility goals became entangled with racial stereotyping. Birthrates continued to decline, despite the political prominence of "family values" platforms. These political successes in keeping certain values in the national spotlight had virtually no effect on personal behavior. Family limitation had emerged from the ideals of the nation's founding—from ideals of life, liberty, equality, virtue, individualism, and the pursuits of happiness; the attempts to revert to an imagined past of close-knit families, commanding men, domestic wives, and grateful, obedient children sometimes slowed, but did not stop, women's expanding control over reproduction.

Minor variations in births and fertility levels still occur. In 2007, a booming economy led to a record number of births. This was accompanied by an aesthetics of pregnant female beauty that had, for some years, touted tight-fitting maternity clothes and naked, late-term pregnant bellies on magazine covers. Celebrity magazines and their electronic ilk blared "news" of the pregnancies and adoptions of movie stars and popular entertainers. There

---

4. Among the many fine discussions of this later history are Andrea Tone, *Devices and Desires: A History of Contraceptives in America* (New York, 2002); Rickie Solinger, *Pregnancy and Power: A Short History of Reproductive Politics in America* (New York, 2005); Leslie J. Reagan, *When Abortion Was a Crime: Women, Medicine, and Law in the United States, 1867–1973* (Berkeley, Calif., 1997); Linda Gordon, *Woman's Body, Woman's Right: A Social History of Birth Control in America* (New York, 1976); Janet Farrell Brodie, *Contraception and Abortion in Nineteenth-Century America* (Ithaca, N.Y., 1994).

was a new language of "the bump" and "baby moma" that supported this very minor boomlet. The average American woman, however, still had 2.1 children over the course of her life, despite the temporary increase in births. By the end of 2007, the economic recession brought an end to the enthusiasm for births. The bizarre instance of "Octomom," an unmarried woman who gave birth to octuplets through fertility treatments, became the new symbolic representation of changed attitudes and filled old and new media with messages urging restraint and small families. Still, the United States no longer leads the world in limiting fertility. Japan, Italy, Germany, France, and former Soviet bloc countries are among the nations currently experiencing below replacement total fertility levels. As a result, their populations are aging, and labor forces and consumer markets are shrinking.[5]

Although the adaptation of family limitation was on the whole a positive achievement for women and children, there were costs. Men might assume control over reproductive goals even if, in most cases, women and children were the beneficiaries of smaller families and limited childbearing. The spontaneous, celebratory, and exuberant physicality of colonial wives was for many Victorian-era women and their daughters replaced by a repressive and anxious fear of the body. These anxieties, disappointments, and frustrations were one consequence of personal goals that outpaced the technological means for implementing those goals. Although it appears that traditional emmenagogues and contraceptives did work about 70 to 85 percent of the time, the failure rate was high by modern standards. Douches, suppositories, and other technologies associated with sexual intercourse trespassed on traditional gender boundaries. Abortion provided an alternative, at least for women in the largest cities, but even where available raised safety, moral, and financial issues. In theory and often in practice, family limitation helped promote companionate, loving marriages. But frustration and failure could also produce new sources of marital stress. Pride in parenthood remained an important social and personal value, but the ticking of "biological clocks" and the constraints of educational and career paths modeled on male experience were other sources of anxiety—there remains to this day precious little integration of family obligation and economic obligation. The twentieth- and early-twenty-first-century refusal of the United States to support child-

5. Mike Stobbe (Associated Press), "Boom! 2007 Record Year for Births," Mar. 26, 2009, http://www.nbcwashington.com/health/women/Boom-2007-Record-Year-for-Birth.html (accessed May 2009); Erik Eckholm, "'07 U.S. Births Break Baby Book Record," *New York Times*, Mar. 18, 2009; Raina Kelley, "Octomom Hypocrisy: Four Reasons Nadya Suleman Drives Us Crazy, and Why We're Wrong," *Newsweek*, Mar. 3, 2009, http://www.newsweek.com/id/187344.

care centers, after school programs, universal health insurance, and parental leave policies, among other forms of familial support common in industrialized nations, was an indication of an underlying callousness toward children that was coupled with a misguided and oversimplified sentimentality about stay-at-home (white, middle-class) motherhood. These fantasies could be a product of making childrearing so central a feature of family life and maternal obligation. Poorer mothers, even more illogically, should not stay at home, but should go to work or lose benefits, a legacy of late-eighteenth-century suppositions about the unthinking physicality of servile people.

Although labor and childbirth had long been equated with sickness in Western culture, the medicalization of childbearing was furthered by making childbearing exceptional. Increasing reliance on male doctors gradually diminished the roles of women — midwives, gossips, and parturient hosts — in the birthing process. Physicians' array of instruments and medications seemed to offer more aid in a time of denaturalized crisis, and late-eighteenth- and early-nineteenth-century women often chose male midwives, even if in reality these men were less experienced. Birthing moved from the home to the hospital by the twentieth century. Insurance policies often affected hospital stays and treatment. Fee structures and hospital regulations often favored cesarean births, producing another area where the U.S. experience differs from those of women in other nations. Yet midwifery has made a comeback, and birthing centers offer a less clinical setting for births. Reproduction may be power, but who will exercise control is still not settled.

Finally, the new doctrine of family limitation, which made small families respectable and a badge of moderation and rationality, eventually played into the existing racist, anti-immigrant, or elitist beliefs of significant numbers of white Americans. Limited childbearing was used by the upper and middling sorts to denigrate outsiders for their backwardness and thoughtless physicality. Most recently, it has been Roman Catholics, southern African Americans, rural whites, "welfare queens," Hispanics, Mormons, and Muslims, among others, who have been targets of fear-mongering. That these oft-repeated charges of irresponsible childbearing were typically not supported by any reputable evidence did not prohibit their widespread circulation or their practical effect on citizenship, the administration of social services, or other rights and benefits.

AT THE BEGINNING of this book, a number of current explanatory models were briefly described; many are not supported by the evidence compiled here — indeed, one conclusion must be that any monocausal explanation is inadequate. There is no direct support for the contention that diminishing land availability or rising land prices in agricultural regions made the cost of establishing many sons in farms of their own prohibitive, forcing a presumably unwelcome restraint on family size. Certainly, it is a plausible explanation, and the increasing cost of land through generations of settlement might have had some effect. Still, falling fertility was enthusiastically welcomed, not—for the most part—forced by financial pressures and regretted. And, as Gloria Main has suggested, family size might have fallen in long-settled regions because couples preferring large families for their labor value selectively moved westward where the unpaid labor of adolescents might bring the greatest rewards and where extensive schooling and its costs might be less necessary than in more commercial, bureaucratized settings. Embedded in the usual argument for the effect of the price of land is an assumption that parents wanted their married sons to settle nearby the paternal estate, that they valued rootedness. There is no evidence that this assumption is true for most Americans. Men, and to a lesser extent women, showed little disposition to stay put—U.S. censuses consistently show that Americans were and are highly mobile. We need more detailed studies of migrants and nonmigrants and their motives, and we must rethink the linkages, if any, between land and large families.

Another common explanation for the introduction of family limitation relates to industrialization, the market revolution or modernization and its many effects, including the possibility of decreasing productive contributions by children in the shift from agriculture to manufacturing or increasing participation by women in the labor force. The fertility transition in the United States began well before industrialization, just as industrialization in Britain occurred well before the fertility transition is considered to have begun. There is no sign that more women were working for wages in the early Republic than in the colonial era. Between 1820 and 1870, when a few newly created occupations were gendered female—shirtmakers in sweatshops, box makers in factory settings, teachers in elementary schools, retail clerks in shops, and clerical workers in offices, among others—these positions were filled almost entirely by young, unmarried white women who left the labor market as soon as they married. Economic explanations are not useless, however. The market revolution, consumerism, and new expectations of comfort and fashion played a role in family limitation by diverting funds from childrearing to more comfortable housing, genteel furnishings, and certain indulgences, like magazines and books. But the reverse was true as well. Childrearing was becoming more expensive. Greater concern for each individual child required more extensive outlays for toys, books, clothes, bedrooms, education, and more, especially if daughters were to get equal treatment. The consumer revolution and an increasing distaste for exploiting the labor of children seem to be among the key elements of innovations in marital fertility.

Other explanations for the fertility transition fail to find support in the experiences and writings of women and men in the Mid-Atlantic colonies. Limitation of births did not follow rising life expectancy and falling infant mortality levels. If anything, infant mortality rates were rising for the majority of Americans living in rural areas, and life expectancy in cities and on farms might have been falling. There was no expansion of social services or other governmental policies that would have replaced kin-based care. There were no technological breakthroughs providing reliable birth control devices. At the end of the period under consideration, in the 1820s and 1830s, there was greater access to abortion providers for urban women, but these commercialized services cannot be seen as a cause of family limitation but as a response to growing demand.

Urbanization is frequently given as a factor in the move to limit births. Before 1930, most Americans lived in rural areas, but those living in large cities, even in the eighteenth century, led the way in promoting small families—perhaps by as little as ten years, perhaps by nearly a generation. What is it about early cities that promoted family limitation strategies? Was it the cost of housing, the greater weight of middling-sort attitudes in the formation of public opinion, the greater literacy and skill sets needed for employment? Or was it the density of women's social networks that allowed conversation, debate, and novel linkages that drew on enlightened, revivalist, and sensible discourses during a series of political, economic, and military crises? The surviving documentation points to the latter. It was women in a revolutionary age who transformed their own and their daughters' lives.

Domestic feminism, as Daniel Scott Smith has characterized the goals of nineteenth-century wives, was not new in the antebellum period. The assertions of female inviolability and maturity and the adoption of numeracy and planning for the future first appear in the middle of the eighteenth century, not the middle of the nineteenth. These new values show up in some surprisingly public as well as domestic settings. Certainly, newspaper advertisements for employment, real estate, and slave sales were touting preferences for small families and low reproduction rates occasionally from the 1760s and commonly by the 1790s. Novels, satires, and portraits carried the new messages to audiences large and small. And there had to be a new masculinity as well, one measured by citizenship rather than lineage.

Reproduction marks the point of the greatest biological difference between women and men. Birth control makes childbearing a rational decision, not a punishment for Eve's sin, and erases some of that physiological difference. Family limitation and feminism are intertwined. As women gained greater control of their bodies, they gradually gained more authority in the family. Such advances were, of course, more easily acquired if they were lucky enough to have cooperative husbands and harder to obtain if they did not. The ending of childbearing at ever earlier ages bought women some release from familial responsibilities and more freedom to engage in church, social clubs, reform groups, and self-improvement activities.

Secularism is often given as a force behind the fertility transition, but women in the Mid-Atlantic states drew on theology as well as or perhaps even more than on secular sources. Their reading materials and writings were most often grounded in the Bible. Yet women began to read the Bible in ways that stressed the worth of each individual and that elided hierarchical messages. A few women read more deeply into history, science, ethics, and politics, but most seem to have found inspiration in the exhortations about love and companionship, sociability and sensibility, empathy and sympathy, and friendship and forbearance in the sermons of George Whitefield, in Hogarth's visual satires, or in the novels and poems that women wrote into their commonplace books. Almanacs and comic sayings also carried new messages that drew on religious as well as secular assumptions. Patriarchy and hierarchy were undermined by heartfelt religious beliefs that cannot be separated from declarations of universal civil rights and political independence.

The American revolutionaries and republican and emergent democratic ideologies have sometimes been criticized for failing to extend full civil and political rights to women, for failing to make the economic changes that could have led to women's control over wages and property, and for further restricting women to limited domestic roles. During the Revolution, some women began to assert control over their bodies, to determine when and how often they would bear children, to rationally and responsibly plan, like reasoning adults, the best possible futures for those children. Once they could hope to determine their futures, they might turn to the determination of career, of political candidates, or of public presence.

One of the discoveries of this research has been the full weight of the physical and cultural constraints on early American women as "the Sex." It was no surprise that women faced considerable hostility when they aspired to be educated, to take public roles, or to assert opinions. They were demeaned when they were outspoken or when they turned down men's offers of marriage. But the depth of the negativity women faced, even in their nominally celebrated roles as childbearers and mothers, was surprising. Before they could dream of the vote, women had to prove that they were rational, that they were, not childish, but grown-up, that they could be responsible and virtuous. They even had to prove that they were fully human beings and not animals controlled by their appetites and valued solely for breeding purposes. Women could instead be characterized as carriers of a progressively expanding, enlightened civilization. Family limitation opened opportunities for women by improving their and their children's health through later starts, longer intervals, and earlier ends to childbearing. To help promote the benefits of new family relationships, women emphasized the helplessness of infants and the intensive parenting that such unformed creatures needed through the long stage of childhood. Childrearing, rather than childbearing, became the core role in women's lives. It brought greater respect for motherhood and childrearing and promised their daughters a better future. That women also had more free time for self-education, church, and reform was yet another indication of women's essential humanity. It is an unfortunate, but telling, aspect of the transition to planned childbearing that many women and men did not entirely reject negative female attributes but shifted irrationality, sexual excess, and unrestrained appetites from white women to women of color. There is little evidence that this movement engaged large numbers of either the poorest women or the wealthiest women, although there is precious little record of poorer women's voices on any subject. By the nineteenth century, some textile mills and mines hired only men with large families, mostly immigrants. At the other end of a superimposed sociological hierarchy, property considerations, lineage, and family connections limited the assertiveness and independence of wealthy women. Middling women in the cities and then in the country led the way.

Fertility is power. It affects all aspects of human life. States seek military prowess, the market economy demands growing numbers of consumers, employers want workers, workers want jobs, and religious, political, and ethnic groups often seek more adherents. Women and some men in revolutionary America began a transformation whose origins are still obscure in many important details but whose outline is now clearer. Understanding the effects of the revolutionary decisions to limit family size is crucial for understanding the origins of the American Republic. Nor did the influence end there. Our lives continue to be shaped by both realistic and mythic under-standings of women's roles, parental responsibilities, economic possibilities, and political policies that emerged from those early personal decisions of women and men on the nature of the family, gendered equity, and the future of children.

This appendix contains more detailed statistics than could be included in Chapter 1.

Philadelphia's Annual Birthrates

Only the city of Philadelphia has a long-time series of annual baptismal and birth records that allow the calculation of birthrates over the course of the eighteenth and nineteenth centuries for the free white population. The calculations of crude birthrates for other populations are based on sampling techniques, life tables, or back projection rather than on direct observation (see Figures 2 and 10).

Figure 12 shows Philadelphia's annual crude birthrates, smoothed by calculating five-year running averages, for 1740–1850. Philadelphia's birthrates were generally high in the 1750s but dipped on the eve of the French and Indian War (1754–1763, in its European and naval phases called the Seven Years' War, 1756–1763). Philadelphia was fortunately spared direct engagement in warfare. Instead of suffering the damages of battle, the city's inhabitants profited from military spending. It is probably no accident that birthrates surged during the war, since the combination of prosperity and security could create a positive environment for marrying and having children. Anxiety about underpopulation in a global conflict could be another factor. Birthrates peaked in 1762 as the war wound down. But the formal peace did not bring either security or prosperity. Perhaps it was the brief threat of the armed and angry Paxton Boys' abortive march on the city in 1763 that triggered a downward trend, but there were more long-lasting changes that undoubtedly furthered this particular decline in births. A postwar economic downturn helped to fuel increasingly divisive protests against British taxation and parliamentary interference in local affairs. Birthrates tumbled from 1763 into the 1770s. Violence and inflammatory speech were accompanied by a particularly sharp drop in births in 1775, the year the Revolutionary

FIGURE 12.
Crude Birthrates in Philadelphia, 1740–1850

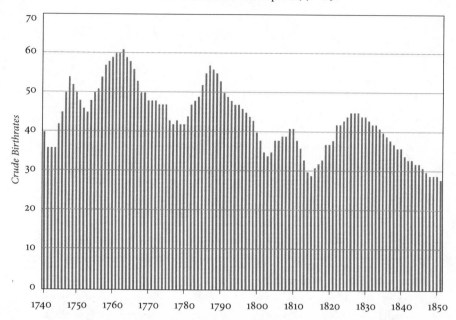

Drawn by Kimberly Foley. Susan E. Klepp, "Demography in Early Philadelphia, 1690–1860," in Klepp, ed.,
The Demographic History of the Philadelphia Region, 1600–1860, American Philosophical Society,
Proceedings, CXXXIII (Philadelphia, 1989), table 2, 104–107.

War commenced. The nadir in this fertility cycle was reached between 1776 and 1779. As the capital of the rebellious nation, Philadelphia was an obvious military target. Control over the city passed from the Americans to the British in 1777 and back again to the Americans the following year. Inflation was rampant. The total population fell from some thirty-two thousand in 1775 to about twenty-seven thousand in 1778 as men left for military service or from fear of the enemy. Women and children also abandoned the city. Some families became refugees, continually on the move as the fortunes of war threatened their security.[1]

It looks as if J. P. Brissot de Warville was right about the effect of war

1. Susan E. Klepp, "Demography in Early Philadelphia, 1690–1860," in Klepp, ed., *The Demographic History of the Philadelphia Region, 1600–1860,* American Philosophical Society, *Proceedings,* CXXXIII (Philadelphia, 1989), table 2, 104–107, as revised by the author; John J. McCusker and Russell R. Menard, *The Economy of British America, 1607–1789* (Chapel Hill, N.C., 1985), table 3.4, 62–63; Marc Egnal, "The Economic Development of the Thirteen Continental Colonies, 1720 to 1775," *William and Mary Quarterly,* 3d Ser., XXXII (1975), 193.

on urban birthrates, although perhaps for the wrong reason. If he assumed separation of husband and wife owing to military service was the cause, it is unlikely that the short tours of duty that were common for married men in the local militias and the proximity of these militiamen to their homes would have produced any significant impact on birthrates. Charles Willson Peale was as warm a patriot as any. Deeply involved in the Philadelphia militia and local radical politics from the start of the war in 1775 until 1779, he nonetheless was able to go to the assistance of his wife and children whenever they needed to move from the enemy's path. He and Rachel Brewer Peale had five children before the start of the war (in 1763, 1765, 1770, 1772, and 1774) and then, even though he was attached to the militia, a daughter in December 1775 and sons in 1778 and 1780. His military service does not seem to have inhibited the growth of this family (Peale was no advocate of family limitation, having seventeen children by his first two wives). In the revolutionary era, armies were small, soldiers had some discretion concerning their service, and the longest-serving men in the rank and file were commonly single. Other men and many officers brought their wives with them or, like Peale, left frequently to see them. These factors suggest that military service in the eighteenth century had little impact on birthrates. Factors other than separation must have been involved in the falling birthrates.[2]

As the combatant armies moved to distant battlefields after 1778, Philadelphia's residents slowly returned. Birthrates rose, jumping higher particularly in 1781, the year the British army surrendered at Yorktown, and in 1784, the year after the signing of the treaty of peace. Significantly, this postwar peak in births did not reach prewar levels of sixty-one births per thousand population. The postwar high point of fifty-seven births per thousand was reached in 1786, three years after the peace. Immigration from abroad and in-migration from the countryside also affected birthrates.

Crude birthrates began a sharp decline in 1787, the year of the Constitutional Convention, a decline that was similar in pace to the wartime decreases that had occurred two decades earlier. This time there was no war. The economy was generally strong, and the city was growing despite yellow fever epidemics between 1793 and 1805. It seems that, for once, birthrates were not responding to immediate political crises or economic cycles. New fertility goals based on long-range planning might be behind this decrease, and increasing numbers of American women and some American men

2. Lillian B. Miller et al., eds., *The Selected Papers of Charles Willson Peale*, V, *The Autobiography of Charles Willson Peale* (New Haven, Conn., 2000), xxxix–xl, 40–85.

were promoting family planning in their correspondence. This decline looks as if it stopped in 1802 but probably only because that year record keeping was transferred from Christ Church to the newly constituted Philadelphia Board of Health. The Board of Health provided far more complete coverage of the contiguous suburbs in its annual reports than had earlier records, and women in those suburbs, still rural in many areas, had higher birth-rates than those in the city proper. For several years, the Board experimented with various formats, which undoubtedly accounts for much of the apparent volatility in birthrates. Although changes in birth registration were the main factors in this bump, a net gain of thirty-four thousand in-migrants from the countryside and immigrants from abroad occurred between 1790 and 1809 (compared to a net gain of twenty-nine thousand immigrants during all of the ten previous decades stretching from 1690 to 1789). This massive influx of young adults probably encouraged marriages and childbearing, but, even with the influence of these factors, birthrates once again failed to reach the heights previously achieved.[3]

Another war in 1812 halted any upward tendency. Birthrates plummeted, particularly in 1814, and remained relatively low through the war and the Panic of 1819, a severe postwar depression. A brief but partial recovery of birthrates reached its peak in the mid-1820s as the last effects of the Panic faded. Net immigration kept the urban population young during these decades: 25,000 migrants were added to the city's residents in the 1820s, 33,000 in the 1830s, and 119,000 in the 1840s, but births per thousand residents continued their downward movement.

Despite the striking wartime and postwar swings in birthrates between 1750 and 1825, the overall trend was for urban birthrates to fall after 1762. Between the 1780s and the 1820s, these urban birthrates began the continuous, steady decline that would not be interrupted until the baby bust of the 1930s and the early 1940s, a sharp drop in births owing to depression and war, and the baby boom of the more prosperous, although not war-free, post–World War II period. With those much later exceptions, birthrates had stopped responding to current conditions in the early Republic. Family planning and

3. Susan E. Klepp, *"The Swift Progress of Population": A Documentary and Bibliographic Study of Philadelphia's Growth, 1642–1859* (Philadelphia, 1991), 13–14; Klepp, "Demography in Early Philadelphia," in Klepp, ed., *The Demographic History of the Philadelphia Region*, APS, *Procs.*, table 4, 111. Net gain is the difference between the births minus the deaths and the decadal increase in population. It differs from the number of arrivals at the port—these people might seek residence anywhere. Net gain also includes internal migrants.

family limitation were coming to dominate reproduction as married couples focused on future goals rather than immediate circumstances.

International Comparisons

The higher fertility of the British American colonies was not just an artifact of a younger population and earlier marriages. Age-specific marital fertility rates show that couples in both the city of Philadelphia and its hinterland produced more children than the couples in the small towns and parishes of England or in the rural districts of northwestern France. The prolific birth-rates of the Mid-Atlantic colonies, although famous at the time and exaggerated by later Victorians worried about the fertility of immigrants, did not reach the maximum registered by the Hutterites even during their height in the 1750s and 1760s.

During and after the American Revolution and the French Revolution, birthrates began to decline, but even in the city of Philadelphia overall rates did not fall quite as far as those in northwestern France. The urban Americans and these Frenchwomen were alike in concentrating childbearing into the earliest years of the marriage and limiting births after age thirty-five even if American women had more children over their life course. Rural Mid-Atlantic fertility fell at a slower pace and with less change in the proportion of births before age thirty-five than either Philadelphia or French rates, at least according to existing studies. Two of these studies of rural populations, it should be remembered, employ methodologies that raise the number of births, particularly at older ages. Still, the revolutionary Americans and the revolutionary French were beginning to achieve the family patterns that other nations would only adopt in the second half of the nineteenth century.

England had a different experience. English rates reveal increased childbearing especially among teenagers and to a lesser extent among young adults and some older women. Although Englishwomen had fewer children between ages twenty and forty-nine than did women in the early United States, both urban and rural American women were better able to concentrate their childbearing into the first years of marriage. English increases in fertility correspond to easier access to marriage brought about by the spread of wage employment and a subsequent decline in servitude and apprenticeships. The economic change sometimes called the Industrial Revolution produced consequences that differed from the effects of the political revolutions of the French and Americans (at least those Americans in the urban North).

At a minimum, city folk and Quakers in the countryside were in step with, although lagging somewhat behind, the French in reducing the size of families through delayed starts, prolonged spacing, concentration of births before age thirty-five, and early stopping.[4]

Montesquieu had written in his very influential *The Spirit of the Laws* (1748): "The females of brutes have an almost constant fecundity. But in the human species, the manner of thinking, the character, the passions, the humor, the caprice, the idea of preserving beauty, the pain of child-bearing, and the fatigue of a too numerous family, obstruct propagation in a thousand different ways." American women did revolt against being equated with breeding stock. And readers and writers reimagined the cultural, personal, and economic meanings of fertility as well as the aesthetics of the female body in the Revolutionary last third of the eighteenth century. Revolutionary republican thought in the late eighteenth century provoked a reevaluation of attitudes toward fertility, and the behaviors of married women and men were changing.[5]

Infant Mortality

Before leaving statistics behind, the question of infant mortality rates should be discussed, if only briefly. One explanation for the fertility transition posits that lower fertility was a consequence of falling rates of infant mortality. As life expectancy for the young increased, the argument goes, it was no longer necessary to have many children in the hope that at least a few would survive to carry on the family name and to care for the parents in old age or infirmity. In the mid-Atlantic region, the evidence is mixed. In Philadelphia, births began to outnumber deaths in the 1760s. In addition, infant mortality rates fell by 8 percent between the colonial and early national periods for the upper sorts. For the middling sorts, infant deaths fell slightly (2 percent), and for the lower sorts infant death rates rose—again slightly (2 percent) and probably imperceptibly. There were, however, substantial differences by occupational ranking. In the early Republic, the upper sorts could expect 85 percent of newborns to survive until their first birthday. For the middling

4. Rudolph Binion, "Marianne au foyer: Révolution politique et transition démographique en France et aux États-Unis," *Population* (French ed.), LV (2000), 81–104.

5. [Charles-Louis de Secondat], baron de Montesquieu, *The Spirit of the Laws*, trans. Thomas Nugent, 2 vols. (New York, 1949), II, 1.

sorts, it was 80 percent, and for the poor 75 percent. Still, despite higher infant mortality, the urban poor had lower fertility than other groups, according to the available studies. In rural areas, it appears that a surplus of births over deaths existed from at least the early decades of the eighteenth century, if not earlier. In Lancaster County, infant death rates were rising more substantially than in the city—up 13 percent for boys and 25 percent for girls between the early eighteenth century and the early nineteenth century, which might be one reason why the countryside lagged in the limitation of births. Overall, the number of infant deaths were (from a twenty-first-century vantage point) almost unimaginable—between 15 and 25 percent of all live-born infants failed to see their first birthdays. There is, however, no indication that people at the time perceived any changes in infant longevity. Crowded conditions and international shipping brought epidemics of childhood diseases to the city in unpredictable waves. Meanwhile, improvements in transportation, increasing population density, and the development of schools and other institutions that brought rural people into contact led to frequent but equally unpredictable bouts of deadly diseases in the countryside. Everywhere, some years were healthy, some were deadly. Some families were spared, some were not, and no one clearly understood why. Parents were simply not in a position to predict whether their children would live through childhood or die young in the eighteenth and early nineteenth centuries.[6]

Certainly, the loss of children could cause couples to reevaluate their fertility goals. Sarah Sansom Perot and Elliston Perot had five children in the 1780s and early 1790s—the same number that her mother had borne. Only one of Sarah's siblings had died in infancy, but four of her own babies died at young ages. Two sons succumbed to putrid sore throat (diphtheria), a daughter was accidentally suffocated by her wet nurse, and another son died during the yellow fever epidemic of 1793. Their surviving child, Hannah, was joined in rapid succession by brothers in 1794, 1796, 1799, and 1800. Sarah Perot did have a family of five children, but only after giving birth to nine.[7]

6. Susan E. Klepp, "Malthusian Miseries and the Working Poor in Philadelphia, 1780–1830: Gender and Infant Mortality," in Billy G. Smith, ed., *Down and Out in Early America* (University Park, Pa., 2004), table 1, 68, table 4, 77. The Lancaster County rates are based on the work of Rodger Craige Henderson; see his "Comparative Mortality Rates and Trends: Eighteenth-Century Lancaster County, Pennsylvania, British North America, and the Caribbean" (paper presented to the Philadelphia Center for Early American Studies [currently the McNeil Center for Early American Studies], Apr. 15, 1983).

7. Elaine Forman Crane et al., eds., *The Diary of Elizabeth Drinker*, 3 vols. (Boston, 1991), I, 511; Susan E. Klepp and Karin A. Wulf, eds., *The Diary of Hannah Callender: Sense and Sensibility in a Revolutionary Age, 1758–1788* (Ithaca, N.Y., 2009).

The declining fertility revealed by birthrates, censuses, and family re-constitutions cannot be linked to better survivorship among newborns. If anything, causation ran in the opposite direction as shrinking family size produced better and more intensive care of each child. These fewer children were now especially precious. Mothers-to-be switched from midwives to doctors because they felt they offered better obstetrical practices. Swaddling disappeared, bathing was promoted, and the use of wet nurses was discouraged. Guidebooks on rearing children proliferated. Not all of these changes were in fact beneficial—the childcare books, in particular, spread all sorts of dubious advice—but they indicate a new investment of familial resources in each child.[8]

Age-Specific Marital Fertility: Sources and Limitations

Reconstituted families are more likely to have been urban and relatively wealthy or belong to those religious denominations that kept careful records. Quaker and Jewish families, for example, have been thoroughly investigated by genealogists, but these relatively small minorities might not reflect the experiences of the general population. An interest in genealogy has tended to be confined to wealthier or politically prominent families. Church records provide another source for reconstituting families. Denominations that had been state-sponsored back in Europe—the Anglican, Lutheran, Reformed, and Presbyterian faiths—tended to keep good records of vital events. Their ministers were accustomed to bureaucracy. These groups dominate histori-cal studies of early American populations because of their fuller, more com-plete registers of births, marriages, and burials. These denominations are also representative of at least the majority of the free, white, churchgoing population. Baptists, Brethren, Methodists, Mennonites, Roman Catholics, and members of other faiths have been more difficult to trace and still await study. The nonchurched population has also not been investigated because of the limitations of the surviving records.

8. Sylvia D. Hoffert, *Private Matters: American Attitudes toward Childbearing and Infant Nurture in the Urban North, 1800–1860* (Urbana, Ill., 1989).

TABLE 6.

Colonial Urban Age-Specific Marital Fertility Rates, circa 1680–1780

| | BIRTHS PER 1,000 WOMAN YEARS | | | | | |
AGE	Upper (N=10)	Middling (N=26)	Poor (N=12)	Jewish (N=140)	Gentry (N=42)	Average (N=230)
15–19	411	556	457	400	—	456
20–24	459	355	270	637	546	453
25–29	447	429	333	443	480	426
30–34	514	326	319	431	418	402
35–39	431	308	267	400	336	348
40–44	204	197	133	128	198	172
45–49	0	18	67	40	38	33

SUMMARY AND SUPPLEMENTAL DATA

Total fertility, ages 15–49	12.3	10.9	9.2	12.4	—	11.4
Total fertility, ages 20–49	10.3	8.2	6.9	10.4	10.1	9.2
% total fertility (ages 20–49) by age 35	69.1	68.0	70.4	72.7	62.3	69.8
Actual no. of children	7.7	5.4	4.2	6.4	7.5	6.2
Mean age at marriage	18.6	23.3	24.1	20.6	20.8	21.5
Mean age at last birth	39.7	39.3	41.4	39.4	40.3	40.0
Childbearing years	21.1	16.0	17.3	18.8	20.8	18.5

TABLE 7.

Age-Specific Marital Fertility Rates of the Eighteenth-Century Poor

	BIRTHS PER 1,000 WOMAN YEARS			
AGE	African-Dutch, New York & New Jersey (N=25)	Colonial Poor (N=12)	Revolutionary Poor (N=53)	Total Poor (N=90)
15–19	400	457	419	425
20–24	391	270	511	391
25–29	312	333	400	348
30–34	236	319	332	296
35–39	212	267	200	226
40–44	169	133	186	163
45–49	49	67	44	53

SUMMARY AND SUPPLEMENTAL DATA

Total fertility, ages 15–49	8.8	9.2	10.5	9.5
Total fertility, ages 20–49	6.8	6.9	8.4	7.4
% total fertility (ages 20–49) by age 35	68.6	70.4	74.3	71.7
Actual no. of children	4.8	4.2	4.4	4.5
Mean age at marriage	23.6	24.1	21.8	23.2
Mean age at last birth	38.5	41.4	37.9	39.3
Childbearing years	14.9	17.3	16.1	16.1

TABLE 8.
Colonial Rural Age-Specific Marital Fertility Rates, circa 1680–1780

| | BIRTHS PER 1,000 WOMAN YEARS | | |
| | Quaker | Lancaster | Average |
AGE	(N=86)	(N=260)	(N=346)
15–19	443	524	484
20–24	466	535	500
25–29	419	506	462
30–34	400	470	435
35–39	309	380	344
40–44	145	204	174
45–49	[28]	27	28

SUMMARY AND SUPPLEMENTAL DATA

Total fertility, ages 15–49	11.0	13.2	12.1
Total fertility, ages 20–49	8.8	10.6	9.7
% total fertility (ages 20–49) by age 35	72.7	71.2	71.9
Actual no. of children	6.7	7.2	7.0
Mean age at marriage	22.0	21.3	21.6
Mean age at last birth	38.9	—	38.9
Childbearing years	16.9	—	17.3

TABLE 9.

Revolutionary Urban Age-Specific Marital Fertility Rates, circa 1760–1820

AGE	BIRTHS PER 1,000 WOMAN YEARS					
	Upper (N=67)	Middling (N=135)	Poor (N=53)	Jewish (N=110)	Gentry (N=46)	Average (N=572)
15–19	476	415	419	425	—	434
20–24	484	420	511	516	483	463
25–29	470	410	400	412	478	434
30–34	382	354	332	346	404	364
35–39	258	226	200	294	335	263
40–44	159	148	186	151	160	161
45–49	14	35	44	17	22	26

SUMMARY AND SUPPLEMENTAL DATA

Total fertility, ages 15–49	11.2	10.0	10.5	10.8	—	10.7
Total fertility, ages 20–49	8.8	8.0	8.4	8.7	9.4	8.6
% total fertility (ages 20–49) by age 35	75.6	74.3	74.3	73.4	72.5	73.7
Actual no. of children	6.4	5.6	4.4	5.1	7.9	5.9
Mean age at marriage	22.7	22.4	21.8	23.8	21.2	22.4
Mean age at last birth	38.1	37.9	37.9	39.5	39.1	38.5
Childbearing years	15.4	15.5	16.1	15.7	17.9	16.1

TABLE 10.

Revolutionary Rural Age-Specific Marital Fertility Rates, circa 1760–1820

AGE	BIRTHS PER 1,000 WOMAN YEARS		
	Quaker (N=65)	Lancaster (N=363)	Average (N=428)
15–19	446	546	496
20–24	408	508	458
25–29	410	486	448
30–34	322	454	388
35–39	182	385	284
40–44	159	233	196
45–49	[11]	30	20
SUMMARY AND SUPPLEMENTAL DATA			
Total fertility, ages 15–49	9.7	13.2	11.4
Total fertility, ages 20–49	7.5	10.5	9.0
% total fertility (ages 20–49) by age 35	76.4	69.1	72.1
Actual no. of children	5.7	7.3	6.5
Mean age at marriage	22.8	21.3	22.4
Mean age at last birth	37.3	—	37.3
Childbearing years	14.5	—	14.9

TABLE 11.

Nineteenth-Century Urban Age-Specific Marital Fertility Rates,
circa 1800–1870

AGE	BIRTHS PER 1,000 WOMAN YEARS		
	Jewish (*N*=140)	Gentry (*N*=61)	Urban (*N*=201)
15–19	369	—	369
20–24	470	454	462
25–29	411	377	394
30–34	421	303	362
35–39	297	211	254
40–44	194	70	132
45–49	19	12	16
SUMMARY AND SUPPLEMENTAL DATA			
Total fertility, ages 15–49	10.9	—	9.9
Total fertility, ages 20–49	9.1	7.1	8.1
% total fertility (ages 20–49) by age 35	71.8	89.7	75.2
Actual no. of children	6.4	5.3	5.8
Mean age at marriage	20.6	23.2	21.9
Mean age at last birth	39.4	35.8	37.6
Childbearing years	18.8	12.6	15.7

TABLE 12.

Nineteenth-Century Rural Age-Specific Marital Fertility Rates, 1800–1870

	BIRTHS PER 1,000 WOMAN YEARS				
AGE	Cumberland, 1800–1829 (*N*=93)	Cumberland, 1830–1859 (*N*=89)	Quaker (*N*=125)	Lancaster (*N*=507)	Rural (*N*=963)
15–19	340	220	347	562	367
20–24	384	354	351	545	408
25–29	397	394	340	492	406
30–34	367	347	265	456	359
35–39	365	330	180	375	312
40–44	233	229	86	210	189
45–49	[6]	[6]	[6]	32	12

SUMMARY AND SUPPLEMENTAL DATA

Total fertility, ages 15–49	10.5	9.4	7.9	13.4	10.3
Total fertility, ages 20–49	8.8	8.3	6.1	10.6	8.4
% total fertility (ages 20–49) by age 35	65.5	66.0	77.8	70.8	69.6
Actual no. of children	6.8	6.2	5.0	7.1	6.3
Mean age at marriage	22.3	22.4	23.4	22.6	22.7
Mean age at last birth	—	—	37.6	—	37.6
Childbearing years	—	—	14.2	—	14.9

TABLE 13.

Comparative Age-Specific Marital Fertility Rates

AGE	Hutterite	France, 1680– 1769	Eng., 1700– 1774	France, 1770– 1819	Eng., 1775– 1824	U.S., 1900	U.S., 2004
			BIRTHS PER 1,000 WOMAN YEARS				
15–19	623	306	406	322	526	502	39
20–24	549	448	417	454	424	368	88
25–29	502	423	371	386	376	273	99
30–34	447	378	318	312	306	201	94
35–39	406	262	248	214	246	153	42
40–44	236	139	128	90	145	49	13
45–49	63	16	22	10	20	12	1

SUMMARY DATA

Total fertility, ages 20–49	11.0	8.3	7.5	7.3	7.6	5.3	1.7
% total fertility (ages 20–49) by age 35	67.6	75.0	73.5	78.6	72.9	79.7	85.8

Note (Tables 6–13): A woman year is the amount of time married women spent in each age category. If a woman was married throughout her thirties, she spent five woman years in categories 30–34 and 35–39. If she died at age 36.5, she spent 2.5 years in category 35–39. The number of births per 1,000 woman years provides the basis for both age-specific and total fertility rates.

Total fertility is the number of births married women might have had if they all married on their twentieth birthdays and remained married until the eve of their fiftieth birthdays, giving birth at observed rates. It allows fertility to be studied independently of differences in nuptiality and mortality. The actual number of births does not attempt to compensate for earlier or later marriages or for the early deaths of wives or husbands.

Childbearing years indicates the number of years from marriage to last birth.

Sources (Tables 6-13): Philadelphia, urban: Louise Kantrow, "Philadelphia Gentry: Fertility and Family Limitation among an American Aristocracy," *Population Studies,* XXXIV (1980), 21–30; Robert Cohen, "Jewish Demography in the Eighteenth Century: A Study of London, the West Indies, and Early America" (Ph.D. diss., Brandeis University, 1976). African-Dutch: Rates are calculated by the author from Henry B. Hoff, "A Colonial Black Family in New York and New Jersey: Pieter Santomee and His Descendants," *Journal of the Afro-American Historical and Genealogical Society,* IX, no. 3 (Fall 1988), 101–134; and Hoff, "Additions and Corrections to 'A Colonial Black Family in New York and New Jersey: Pieter Santomee and His Descendants,'" ibid., X, no. 4 (Winter 1989), 158–160; Susan E. Klepp, *Philadelphia in Transition: A Demographic History of the City and Its Occupational Groups, 1720–1830* (New York, 1989), table 3.18, 217–220. Rural: Robert V. Wells, "Family Size and Fertility Control in Eighteenth-Century America: A Study of Quaker Families," *Population Studies,* XXV (1971), 73–82; Rodger C. Henderson, *Community Development and the Revolutionary Transition in Eighteenth-Century Lancaster County, Pennsylvania* (New York, 1989), table 32, 85, table 72, 157, table 104, 221; Kristin Senecal, "Marriage and Fertility Patterns in Cumberland County, 1800–1859," *Pennsylvania History,* LXXI (2004), 191–211. France: Louis Henry and Jacques Houdaille, "Fécondité des mariages dans le quart nord-ouest de la France de 1670 a 1829," *Population* (French ed.), XXVIII (1973), table IX, 889. England: E. A. Wrigley et al., *English Population History from Family Reconstitution, 1580–1837* (Cambridge, 1997), table 7.1, 355. United States: Michael R. Haines, "American Fertility in Transition: New Estimates of Birth Rates in the United States, 1900–1910," *Demography,* XXVI (1989), 140; Jane Lawler Dye, "Fertility of American Women: June 2004: Population Characteristics" (December 2005), table 1, http://www.census.gov/prod/2005pubs/p20-555.pdf; Robert Vale Wells, "A Demographic Analysis of Some Middle Colony Quaker Families of the Eighteenth Century" (Ph.D. diss., Princeton University, 1969). Hutterites: Charles Wetherell, "Another Look at Coale's Indices of Fertility, I_f and I_g," *Social Science History,* XXV (2001), 589–608; Barbara A. Anderson and Brian D. Silver, "A Simple Measure of Fertility Control," *Demography,* XXIX (1992), 343–356.

INDEX

Page numbers in italics refer to plates.